Infection Control in Clinical Practice

For Baillière Tindall:

Commissioning Editor: Ninette Premdas
Project Development Manager: Karen Gilmour
Project Manager: Jane Dingwall
Design Direction: George Ajayi

Infection Control in Clinical Practice

Jennie Wilson BSc(Hons) RGN
Senior Nurse Manager and Surveillance Co-ordinator
Nosocomial Infection Surveillance Unit
Central Public Health Laboratory
London, UK

Foreword by

Elizabeth A. Jenner BSc(Hons), RGN, MEd, Nurse Tutor, Hon Dip.HIC
Principle Lecturer in Infection Control
University of Hertfordshire
Faculty of Health and Human Sciences
Department of Post-Registration Nursing
Hatfield, UK

SECOND EDITION

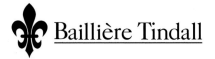

EDINBURGH LONDON NEW YORK OXFORD PHILADELPHIA ST LOUIS SYDNEY TORONTO 2001

BAILLIÈRE TINDALL
An imprint of Elsevier Limited

First edition 1995
Second edition 2001
    Reprinted 2002, 2003 (twice), 2005

ISBN 0 7020 2554 2

British Library Cataloguing in Publication Data
A catalogue record for this book is available from the British Library

Library of Congress Cataloguing in Publication Data
A catalogue record for this book is available from the Library of Congress

Note
Medical knowledge is constantly changing. As new information becomes available, changes in treatment, procedures, equipment and the use of drugs become necessary. The editors, contributor and the publishers have taken care to ensure that the information given in this text is accurate and up to date. However, readers are strongly advised to confirm that the information, especially with regard to drug usage, complies with the latest legislation and standards of practice.

The Publisher

ELSEVIER your source for books, journals and multimedia in the health sciences
www.elsevierhealth.com

Working together to grow
libraries in developing countries

www.elsevier.com | www.bookaid.org | www.sabre.org

ELSEVIER   BOOK AID International   Sabre Foundation

Printed in China
C/05

Contents

A colour plate section can be found between pages 144–145

Foreword

Those of us who teach infection control are hardly spoilt for choice when it comes to compiling reading lists of books on the subject, especially ones written by British authors. It is particularly pleasing therefore to see that Jennie Wilson's book has merited a second edition and I am delighted to have been asked to write this Foreword.

Jennie is eminently qualified to write a book about infection control in clinical practice for she not only has a degree in microbiology but has also accrued a wealth of experiential learning during her time as an infection control nurse. It would be understandable if readers inferred that this is a book written by a nurse for nurses. However, the title, clearly chosen with great foresight, points the way to multi-professional, shared learning. By not limiting the target audience to nurses, it is to be hoped that teachers of medicine and other subjects allied to medicine will realize that they too have a key role to play in teaching students about the prevention and control of infection in clinical practice.

Over the years, Jennie and I have worked together on various infection control projects and papers. During these collaborative efforts, we have enjoyed some challenging and rewarding discussions about the practice of infection control and how it should be taught. It has been argued elsewhere that infection control is an academic discipline in its own right and there are those who teach it as a discrete subject. The success of this approach is dependent on the student's prior knowledge of the supporting sciences such as microbiology, immunology and epidemiology. However, as we know to our cost, these subjects generally receive scant, if any, attention in pre-registration curricula.

An alternative approach, and the one favoured by Jennie Wilson, is to ensure that the basics of the subjects that inform the practice of infection control are taught contemporaneously. Hence, the early chapters of this book are devoted to microbiology, immunology and epidemiology. Thereafter, the principles are integrated throughout the remainder of the text that is illustrated with relevant cameos to aid the application of theory to practice. In this way, the student has easy access to the basic knowledge that underpins the practice of infection control and a solid foundation is laid. This style of writing undoubtedly aids students' understanding of these difficult subjects and is, I believe, this book's winning formula.

Since the seminal study on the efficacy of hand washing in the prevention of cross-infection, conducted by Semmelweis over 150 years ago (Newsom 1993), the evidence base for various infection control practices has been slowly accumulating. The 1960s and 1970s might be regarded as the 'Golden Era' of infection control research for during this period various major studies were conducted which have formed the foundation for many of today's practices. For example, work conducted by Williams et al. (1960) enhanced our understanding about the transmissibility of staphylococci; research on the closed urinary drainage system showed us how to reduce the incidence of urinary tract infections in the catheterised patient (Gillespie et al. 1960 and Lowbury et al. 1975) presented evidence for the efficacy of various skin antiseptics.

Of course, the last two decades have also seen the publication of important studies which have aided our understanding about the prevention and control of cross-infection. These include papers arising from doctoral theses which have been written by Infection Control Nurses on topics such as surveillance, hand washing, causes of central line infections and the psychological problems associated with being nursed in isolation. They are discussed, along with the findings of many other studies, in the relevant specialist chapters of this book. However, the evidence base for many infection control practices is yet to be determined and ritualistic practices, which are not cost-effective, can still be observed. Jennie Wilson's common sense approach to infection control does much to promote reason and dispel current myths and mysteries.

Data from both the latest survey on the prevalence of infection in hospitals in England and Wales and the study on the socio-economic impact of hospital-acquired infection are reviewed in some detail. Putting the fiscal costs aside, patient suffering should be reason enough for all healthcare workers to reappraise their role in the prevention of cross-infection. Clinical governance provides the framework for which reasons for non-adherence with infection control practices can be sought. Solutions must be found to effect behavioural change. A good place to start is by changing attitudes through education. This book has a place in this endeavour and must surely head the list of 'essential reading' for all students of health sciences.

Hertfordshire, 2001   Elizabeth A. Jenner

REFERENCES

Gillespie WA, Linton KB, Miller A, Slade N (1960) The diagnosis, epidemiology and control of urinary tract infection in urology and gynaecology. *Journal of Clinical Pathology*, **13**: 187–94.

Lowbury EJL, Ayliffe, GAJ, Geddes AM, Williams (JD 1975) *Control of Hospital Infections: A Practical Handbook*. Chapman and Hall, London.

Newsom SWB (1993) Pioneers in infection control. Ignaz Philipp Semmelweis. *Journal of Hospital Infection*, **23**: 175–187.

Williams REO, Blowers R, Garrod LP, Shooter RA (1960) *Hospital Infection. Causes and Prevention*. Lloyd Luke, London.

Preface

Infections acquired as a result of healthcare have a major impact on both the affected patient and the providers of healthcare. For the patient, the acquisition of infection causes anxiety and discomfort, delays recovery, and in some instances results in long-term morbidity or even death. It is therefore not surprising that many patients affected in this way are seeking redress in the courts and that healthcare providers are looking more closely at the management of infection prevention and control within their facilities.

Since the first edition of this book was published much has changed. The new framework for the National Health Service (NHS) in the UK that was introduced in 1997 placed considerable emphasis on the provision of a high-quality service. NHS Trusts now have a clear responsibility to ensure that quality improvement processes, such as clinical audit and risk reduction programmes, are in place, and that evidence-based practice is implemented. Infection prevention and control clearly have an important role to play in ensuring that patients receive a high quality of care. The importance of managing the health environment to minimize the risk to patients and staff has been recognized in recent 'controls assurance standards' for infection control. There is also growing concern about the emergence of antimicrobial resistance in a range of important human pathogens, and infection control forms an essential part of managing this threat to public health.

In this second edition of *Infection Control in Clinical Practice*, I have retained the accessible style and as far as possible have made the information relevant to the wide range of settings where healthcare is now practised. Each chapter has been revised, the references updated and new information incorporated.

Chapter 1 provides the basic principles of microbiology that underpin the practice of infection control. Chapter 2 examines how specimens are investigated in the microbiology laboratory, including new molecular techniques. Chapter 3 explains how micro-organisms are transmitted, factors that influence their spread in both hospital and community, and the NHS structures that are in place to manage and control them. New sections on risk management, control assurance, surveillance and the role of the infection control team have been added. Chapter 4 covers the basic principles of immunology, and a number of new figures have been incorporated to aid understanding of this complex subject. Chapter 5 describes how antimicrobial agents may be used to treat infections, and reviews the problem of antimicrobial resistance. It contains new sections on multidrug-resistant tuberculosis, glycopeptide-resistant enterococci and methicillin-resistant *Staphylococcus aureus*. Chapter 6 reviews micro-organisms commonly encountered in healthcare settings and has been revised to include emerging pathogens such as prions.

The remaining chapters focus on the practice of infection prevention and control, beginning in chapter 7 with the basic principles, which has been revised to take account of recent guidance and new products. Chapters 8 to 11 review the factors that contribute to infections in wounds, intravascular devices, urinary catheters and the respiratory tract. These have been updated to reflect the current evidence base. Chapter 12 describes the principles of food hygiene and the prevention of gastrointestinal infections, and Chapter 13 covers the decontamination of equipment; both have been revised to reflect current guidance. Chapter 14 reviews the principle of isolation and includes a revised guide to the transmission and management of common infections. Chapter 15 describes the measures required to treat ectoparasitic infections and infestation of the environment.

As in the previous edition, a comprehensive set of references and suggestions for further reading are provided at the end of each chapter. This should provide an invaluable resource for those interested in evidence-based practice. A glossary of terms is also included to facilitate reading.

I envisage that this book will be a useful reference for a wide range of nurses practising in both hospitals and the community; infection control specialists and link nurses; health educators; and other healthcare professionals. It should also be of value for nurses, healthcare assistants and other support workers in training who are undertaking higher National Vocational Qualifications, diploma or degree level courses.

I have been extremely touched by the positive feedback I received after the first edition from so many readers and hope that this second edition will be equally well appreciated.

London 2001   Jennie Wilson

Acknowledgements

I would like to thank the many people whose support has made the production of this book possible. In particular, I thank Dr Dinah Barrie, Jacqui Prieto, Peter Hoffman and Dr Tyrone Pitt for their invaluable advice, but also all those readers of the first edition whose enthusiasm about it inspired me to find the time to write a new edition.

My thanks must also go to my family: Philip, Sarah, Josie and Claire, for their support and forbearance.

Figure acknowledgements

Figs 1.11, 1.13, 2.1 were reproduced with kind permission of Dr D Barrie, Charing Cross and Westminster Medical School, London, UK.

Figs 1.2, 1.3, 1.4, 1.7, 1.12, 4.6, 4.8 were reproduced with kind permission from Ackerman and Dunk-Richards.

Figs 2.4, 2.5 were redrawn from Ayton M (1982) Microbiological investigations. *Nursing* **2**(8): 226–30 with permission of Mark Allen Publishing.

Figs 4.11 and 6.2 are Crown Copyright and were redrawn with permission from Controller of Her Majesty's Stationery Office.

Fig. 7.1 was redrawn by kind permission from Taylor LJ (1978) An evaluation of handwashing techniques. *Nursing Times* **74**: 108–10.

Figs 7.2, 12.1, 13.3, 14.4 were reprinted with kind permission of Glenys Griffiths.

Figs 7.6, 7.8 were reproduced with permission of Riverside Health Authority; original artwork by Linda Foreman.

Fig. 9.1 was reproduced with kind permission from Elliot TSJ (1988) Intravascular device infections. *J. Med. Microbiol.* **27**, 161–7.

Fig. 15.1 was reproduced with kind permission of Community Hygiene Concern.

Fig. 15.2 was reprinted with kind permission of Dr J Lane, London School of Hygiene and Tropical Medicine.

Fig. 15.3 was redrawn with permission from Kettle DS (1990) *Medical and Veterinary Entomology*, CAB International, from an original drawing by HJ Hawthorne.

Figs 15.4, 15.5, 15.6 were reproduced with kind permission of Mr L Baker.

List of colour plates

Plate 1.1 A filamentous fungus. Tubular hyphae with groups of spores.

Plate 1.2 *Candida albicans*. When incubated in serum the cells produce characteristic outgrowths called germ tubes.

Plate 1.3 *Entamoeba histolytica*. These protozoa cause amoebic dysentery. The black dots are red blood cells which have been engulfed. The nucleus can be seen in the lower right of the cell.

Plate 2.1 A clump of Gram positive staphylococci in or on a neutropil ('pus cell') and surrounded by other neutrophils.

Plate 2.2 There are four main groups of bacteria: (a) Gram-positive cocci, (b) Gram-positive bacilli (rods), (c) Gram-negative cocci, and (d) Gram-negative bacilli (rods).

Plate 2.3 Cerebrospinal fluid from two cases of meningitis. Large mononuclear cells and neutrophils can be seen with a number of small Gram-negative rods. Provisional diagnosis: *Haemophilus influenzae* meningitis.

Plate 2.4 Large colonies of *Bacillus cereus*.

Plate 2.5 *Staphylococcus aureus*.

Plate 2.6 Streptococcus group A. Haemolysins produced by streptococcus lyse the red blood cells in blood agar, producing a clear area around the colonies.

Plate 2.7 *Pseudomonas aeruginosa*. The colonies of *P. aeruginosa* appear green when grown on nutrient agar.

Plate 2.8 *Serratia marcescens*. The colonies of *S. marcescens* have a characteristic red coloration.

Plate 2.9 Mixed growth of organisms. Specimens often contain more than one type of bacterium, illustrated by the different forms of colony on this plate.

Plate 2.10 Each chamber contains a different biochemical test. Positive tests are indicated by a colour change and the set of results are used to identify the species of bacteria present.

Plate 2.11 Antibiotic sensitivity testing. Antibiotics in each disc diffuse into the agar. Bacteria cannot grow around the discs unless they are resistant to the antibiotic in the disc.

Plate 2.12 Sputum from a patient with suspected pneumonia. Gram-positive cocci, mostly in pairs, can be seen amongst the numerous, large, pus cells. Provisional diagnosis: pneumococcal pneumonia.

Plate 2.13 Tubercle bacilli appear as clumps of fine rods.

Plate 2.14 Biohazard label.

Plate 4.1 A macrophage extends a pseudopod to ingest a bacterium.

Plate 4.2 The first vaccination (Edward Jenner).

Plate 6.1 Staphylococcal infection of the eyes.

Plate 6.2 Erysipelas. An acute cellulitis caused by streptococcus.

Plate 6.3 Oral thrush infection caused by the yeast candida.

Plate 6.4 Herpetic whitlow caused by the herpes simplex virus.

Plate 6.5 Chickenpox infection.

Plate 6.6 Herpes zoster (shingles).

Plate 6.7 Measles infection.

Plate 7.1 The effect of handwashing. (a) Fingertips pressed on to blood agar before washing. (b) Fingertips pressed on to blood agar after washing with soap and water.

Plate 7.2 Chlorine-based granules can be used to soak up spills of blood.

Plate 8.1 Infection in a surgical wound.

Plate 8.2 A chronic wound. Slough and superficial pus is present on the surface of the wound but with no signs of infection.

Plate 9.1 A set of access points and a three-way tap used with intravascular devices.

Plate 15.1 The female head louse (*Pediculus humanus capitis*).

Plate 15.2 A louse egg (nit) attached to a hair.

Colour plate acknowledgements

Plates 1.1, 1.2, 1.3, 2.1, 2.3, 2.12, 2.13, 4.1, 6.6, 15.1 and 15.2 were reproduced with kind permission from Ackerman V, Dunk Richards G 1991 Microbiology: an introduction to the health sciences. WB Saunders, London.

Plates 2.2, 2.4, 2.10, 2.14, 7.2, 8.2 and 9.1 were reproduced with kind permission from Jennie Wilson.

Plates 2.5, 2.6, 2.7, 2.8, 2.9, 2.11, 6.1, 6.2, 6.3, 6.4, 6.5, 6.7, 7.1 and 8.1 were reproduced with kind permission from Dr Dinah Barrie.

Plate 4.2 was reproduced with kind permission from the Wellcome Institute Library, London.

1

Introduction to microbiology

INTRODUCTION

Microbiology is the study of living organisms so small that they cannot be seen with the naked eye. This generally includes any organism of between 0.1 and 1 mm in diameter, which although just visible requires magnification for detail to be seen. Organisms of less than 0.1 mm cannot be seen at all without a microscope.

Investigation of the world of the **microbe** began in the seventeenth century with the invention of the **microscope** by a Dutch merchant, Antony van Leeuwenhoek, who like many great scientists of his time made astounding discoveries in his spare time. Although modern microscopes bear little resemblance to those designed by van Leeuwenhoek, they are based on broadly similar principles (Fig. 1.1).

Van Leeuwenhoek was the first to appreciate the variety and profusion of the microbial world, as he indicated in one of his letters to the Royal Society of London:

I have had several gentlewomen in my house who were keen on seeing the little eels in vinegar; but some of them were so disgusted at the spectacle, that they vowed they'd never use vinegar again. But what if one should tell such people in future that there are more animals living in the scum on the teeth in a man's mouth, than there are men in a whole kingdom?

Microbes are found everywhere and can utilize almost any chemical substance as a source of energy. They are able to survive in almost every conceivable environment, even in conditions where other plants or animals cannot. Some can withstand temperatures of more than 95°C and live in hot water springs; others can grow at temperatures as low as −10°C.

They perform many essential functions in the ecological cycle: they form the first link in the aquatic food chain (e.g. plankton, algae), fix atmospheric nitrogen into the soil so that it can be used by plants, and release nutrients for use by other living things by decomposing dead plants and other animals.

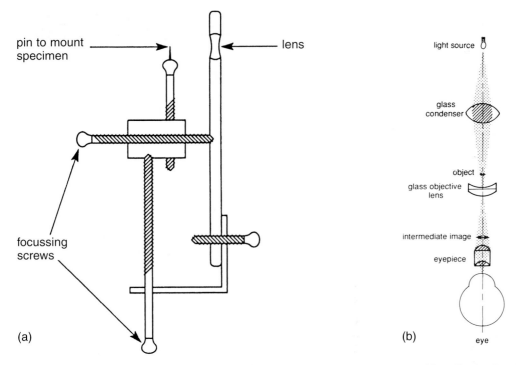

(a)

(b)

Fig. 1.1 The principles of the light microscope. (a) van Leeuwenhoek's microscope. Magnification is achieved by means of a lens with a very short focal length which is capable of high magnification. The specimen is brought into focus by moving the position of the lens relative to the specimen. (b) A modern light microscope. Visible light is directed through the specimen and magnified by the lens and eyepiece. Several lenses are used to enable images to be magnified between 100 and 1000 times.

Many foods are produced by the activities of microbes, such as cheese, yoghurt, beer, wine, bread and vinegar, and microbes are also used to manufacture drugs, such as insulin and hepatitis B **vaccine**.

CLASSIFICATION

A system of identifying individual organisms and their relationship to one another has been gradually developed since the mid-eighteenth century when Linnaeus established the first system of biological classification. Organisms are placed into groups according to similarities in their structure. Each is allocated two names; the first denotes the group or **genus** to which it belongs and the second gives it a specific name within that group, the **species**.

Bacteria of a species can often be further distinguished into different 'strains', according to slightly different characteristics. This subdivision of bacterial species usually requires complex laboratory techniques called typing, based on the analysis of cellular

characteristics or susceptibility to bacterial viruses (**bacteriophages**).

In the early days, microbial science developed independently from other biological sciences and microbial cells were considered to be very different to plant or animal cells. By the mid-twentieth century it had become apparent that there were many similarities in the biochemistry of all living organisms and the study of microbes has considerably helped our understanding of how all cells work at a molecular level.

As our knowledge and laboratory techniques have improved, organisms previously categorized together are found to be unrelated or more closely related to another genus. These **micro-organisms** sometimes change their name and are reclassified (e.g. *Streptococcus faecium* has recently been renamed as an enterococcus. Some micro-organisms are very difficult to classify as they have features of more than one genus. For example, *Pneumocystis carinii*, although currently classified as a **protozoa**, is actually very closely related to **fungi**.

THE STRUCTURE OF CELLS

A cell is the basic unit of living structures, consisting of a **nucleus** and **cytoplasm** enclosed in semipermeable membrane and, in some cases, an outer **cell wall**. The nucleus contains the genetic information unique to that cell. It is a code that, when translated, creates the specific proteins and **enzymes** necessary to build and operate the cell.

Although these basic mechanisms by which all cells function are broadly the same, two distinct types of cells can be identified (see Fig. 1.2). Plants, animals, protozoa, fungi and **algae** are all composed of **eucaryotic cells**. These have a complex structure with many distinct organelles that carry out the functions of the cell. Plants and animals are composed of many cells, extensively differentiated so that groups of cells

Table 1.1 Examples of eucaryotic and procaryotic organisms

Type of cell	Organisms
Procaryotic	
Unicellular	Bacteria
	Mycoplasma
	Rickettsia
	Chlamydia
Eucaryotic	
Multicellular (differentiated)	Vertebrates
	Invertebrates
	Seed-forming plants
	Ferns
	Mosses and liverworts
Multicellular or unicellular (undifferentiated)	Algae
	Fungi
	Protozoa

perform different tasks within the whole plant or animal. Protozoa and algae are much simpler organisms, consisting of single cells, while fungi can be unicellular or multicellular, but without any differentiation between the cells.

Procaryotic cells are far smaller and less complex; they only form single-celled organisms and include all **bacteria** (see Table 1.1).

The cell wall

There are significant differences between the cell walls of procaryotic and eucaryotic cells. Eucaryotic cells are usually enclosed by a membrane rather than a cell wall, but if a cell wall is present then it is a simple structure composed of sugars or, in the case of algae and plant cells, cellulose. Procaryotic cells have a rigid cell wall made of a network of **carbohydrates** and **amino acids** called **peptidoglycan** (see Fig. 1.3). This wall determines the shape of the cell and helps it to withstand high or low osmotic pressures outside the cell. The amount of peptidoglycan in the cell wall determines the staining properties of the bacterial cell (see Ch. 2), and provides a method for identifying and classifying bacteria.

Gram-positive bacteria have a cell wall made from a very thick mesh of peptidoglycan. Small molecules can pass into and out of the cell through this wall. The thick layer of peptidoglycan helps the cell to resist the immune system, but it is vulnerable to attack by enzymes such as lysozyme. Gram-negative bacteria have more complicated walls. They have a thin layer of peptidoglycan surrounded by an outer membrane composed of protein, phospholipid and lipopolysaccharide (LPS). The LPS is toxic to animals, especially

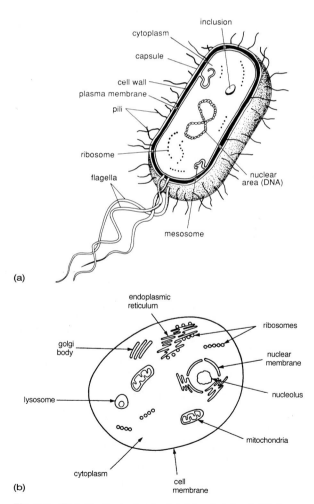

(a)

(b)

Fig. 1.2 The structure of cells. (a) A bacterial cell. (b) A eucaryotic cell.

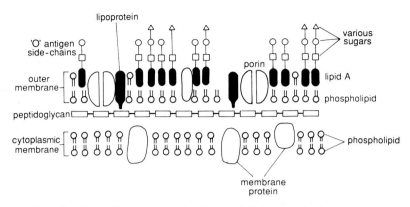

Fig. 1.3 The structure of the cell wall of a Gram-negative bacterium. Both inner and outer membranes are made of phospholipid. The porins in the outer membrane enable substances to pass into the cell. The sugars and side-chains attached to the outer membrane are antigenic. The layer of peptidoglycan between the membranes is not as thick in Gram-positive cells.

the lipid A component which causes fever and severe damage to the circulatory system. LPS is called an endotoxin because it is part of the structure of the cell rather than a secreted molecule. Although LPS is similar in all Gram-negative cells, the composition of the sugar side-chains (called O antigens) varies. Serological techniques are used to detect these differences and form an important means of identification and classification of Gram-negative bacteria. The outer membrane enables Gram-negative bacteria to resist penetration by many harmful substances (e.g. phenols), but with a much thinner layer of peptidoglycan they are more susceptible to desiccation in dry conditions. Penicillin and many other **antibiotics** destroy bacteria by interfering with the synthesis of peptidoglycan. Eucaryotic cells do not contain peptidoglycan; therefore these drugs have no effect on the cells of the animal receiving treatment.

Capsules

Many bacteria produce a layer of gelatinous material outside the cell wall that adheres strongly to the cell to form a clearly defined capsule. Capsules are an important determinant of the ability of bacteria to cause infection, protecting them from white blood cells. Some bacteria secrete a loose network of material called slime, which helps them to adhere to a range of surfaces, including teeth, plastic catheters and prosthetic devices.

Spores and cysts

These are resistant casings that form around the cell. They are made of a thick layer of peptidoglycan and a tough keratin-like protein, and are extremely difficult to destroy by heat or chemicals. Spores are made by some bacteria when they are exposed to adverse environmental conditions, e.g. no food source, or moisture (see Fig. 1.4). When conditions improve the spores germinate and the cell starts to multiply. Most spore-forming bacteria live in soil and are in the genera clostridia and bacillus. Spores can survive for very long periods; spores of *Bacillus anthrax* could still be recovered from the soil of an island off the Scottish coast used to test biological weapons many years after they had been tested there.

Some protozoa (e.g. toxoplasma and entamoeba) change into **cysts**, which enables them to survive for many months outside a host.

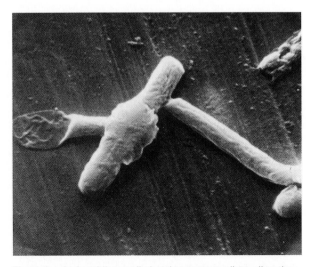

Fig. 1.4 A clostridium cell showing a spore distending the middle of the rod (electron micrograph).

The cytoplasm and cytoplasmic membrane

The biochemical reactions that maintain the cell and enable it to reproduce all take place within the cytoplasm of the cell. The cytoplasm contains a variety of nutrients that are required for the activity of the cell, and is surrounded by a cytoplasmic membrane. The cytoplasmic membrane is formed from two layers of lipid molecules interspersed with proteins. The lipids provide an impermeable barrier to most water-soluble molecules. Some of the protein molecules form pores that enable molecules to enter the cell; other proteins actively transport substances across the membrane.

In eucaryotic cells the cytoplasm contains a number of distinct structures called organelles, each containing its own set of enzymes and surrounded by a membrane. These organelles carry out the processes required by the cell (Table 1.2). Transport proteins carry substances between organelles, and a network of small tubules called the cytoskeleton is involved in cell transport, movement and chromosome separation during cell division. The cytoskeleton is also thought to enable cells making up a tissue to communicate and work together (e.g. muscle fibres).

In procaryotic cells the only structures in the cytoplasm are ribosomes, where proteins are synthesized, and inclusion bodies which are used to store lipids. Procaryotic ribosomes are smaller than those in eucaryotic cells and are only found free in the cytoplasm. In procaryotic cells nutrients can be taken up easily from the environment because of the large surface area of cytoplasmic membrane available. Small molecules, such as sugars, pass though the cytoplasmic membrane of the cell by diffusion provided their concentration is higher outside the cell. If the concentration of required nutrients is lower outside the cell, the carrier proteins are used to take them across the membrane. Large molecules cannot pass through the membrane, and bacteria often excrete enzymes into their environment to break large molecules down into smaller compounds. Procaryotic cells do not have complex transport systems and the cytoplasmic membrane also performs many of the functions of the cell, for example synthesis of cell wall components, respiration to form adenosine triphosphate (ATP) (see p. 7), secretion of enzymes and nutrient transport. Folded areas of membrane called mesosomes are thought to be involved in protein secretion and transport, in chromosome separation during cell division, and in some bacteria contain the enzymes required for respiration.

The nucleus

The structures within cells and the enzymes that regulate cellular activities are made of protein. The genetic information or genome of the cell determines what protein it can make. The genome is formed from molecules of deoxyribonucleic acid (DNA), each molecule arranged into a chromosome. The cells of higher animals have many chromosomes; for example, human cells have 46 chromosomes, procaryotic cells have very few, *Escherichia coli* for example has only one chromosome. In eucaryotic cells the chromosomes are enclosed by a nuclear membrane; in procaryotic cells they lie free in the cytoplasm.

The genetic code

DNA is made of two complementary strands of **nucleotides** held together by **hydrogen bonds** and twisted together to form a double **helix**. In bacterial cells the helix is further coiled and, although it may be 1000 times the length of the cell, it takes up only 10% of the cytoplasm. Nucleotides consist of a sugar molecule, attached to a phosphate molecule and one of four bases: **adenine, cytosine, guanine** and **thymine** (see Fig. 1.5). A **base** is a molecule that can accept a hydrogen ion and can connect with another base by forming a weak association or hydrogen bond. Adenine always bonds or pairs with thymine, whilst guanine always pairs with cytosine. Two chains or strands of nucleotides are held together by hydrogen bonds between the **pairs of bases** and are therefore mirror images of each other.

Table 1.2 The function of organelles in eucaryotic cells

Organelle	Function
Endoplasmic reticulum	Makes lipids and directs movement of lipids and proteins through the cell
Ribosome	Translates RNA sequences into proteins. Found on the endoplasmic reticulum and free in the cytoplasm
Mitochondrion	Oxidizes glucose and fatty acids to make energy in the form of ATP (respiration)
Cytoskeleton	Internal framework of the cell that enables it to move and transport substances
Golgi apparatus	Modifies and sorts proteins and lipids
Lysosome	Contains enzymes that break down unwanted large molecules

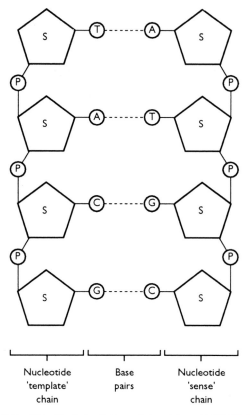

Fig. 1.5 The structure of deoxyribonucleic acid (DNA). S, sugar molecule; P, phosphate molecule; C, cytosine; G, guanine; A, adenine; T, thymine; ..., hydrogen bond.

The sequence of bases forms the code in which all the information needed to make the constituent molecules of the cell is stored. The code made by adenine, cytosine, guanine and thymine can be compared to making up three-letter 'words' with A, C, G and T. Each 'word' can be translated into one of the amino acids that are needed to make proteins (Table 1.3). Different series of amino acids can be made from the same length of DNA by changing the starting point of translation.

An average protein is composed of about 400 amino acids and corresponds to a sequence of 1200 bases

Table 1.3 The genetic code

Sequence of bases on DNA	Equivalent amino acid
GCG	Alanine
TTC	Phenylalanine
CGC	Arginine
AAA	Lysine

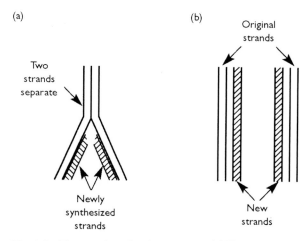

Fig. 1.6 The copying of a chromosome. (a) The two strands of DNA are separated and a copy is made of each half. (b) The two identical chromosomes.

along the nucleotide chain. Each section of DNA that codes for a protein is called a **gene**.

When cells divide, the chromosome of each new cell must contain both strands of DNA. To make an accurate copy of the DNA, the two strands are gradually separated and both then become a pattern against which a new strand is made. After replication, the two daughter chromosomes contain one strand from the parent and one new strand (see Fig. 1.6).

Plasmids

Many bacterial cells carry between one and six small circles of DNA called **plasmids** which are not incorporated into the main chromosome. Plasmid DNA can be replicated on its own and copied into each daughter cell. Plasmids do not contain any genes essential for cell viability and can be lost without damaging the cell. They often contain genes that enable the cell to resist antibiotics, adhere to surfaces (e.g. fimbriae), or synthesize **toxins**, such as **haemolysins** that destroy red blood cells and diphtheria toxin.

THE PROPERTIES OF CELLS

The activities of all cells from the smallest bacterium to the largest mammal are controlled by proteins called enzymes (see Fig. 1.7). Enzymes catalyse or speed up a whole range of chemical reactions; they control energy-making reactions, enable the cell to synthesize complex materials from nutrients, and to grow and divide into new cells.

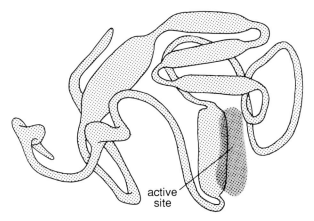

active
site

Fig. 1.7 The structure of an enzyme. The complicated folded structure of enzymes is essential for their activity. The active site is where molecules combine with the enzyme.

Cell metabolism

The chemical reactions that take place in all living cells are described as the **metabolism** of the cell. **Anabolism** is where new compounds are formed from simple molecules. **Catabolism** is where large and complicated compounds are broken down into their constituent molecules, releasing energy.

The protein structure of the cell and its enzymes are made up of amino acids and the main food reserves of the cell: carbohydrates and **fats**.

All living cells need energy to maintain the chemical and physical composition of their cytoplasm and to grow and replicate themselves. The original source of energy is solar energy from the sun. This is captured by plants and a few bacteria by a process called **photosynthesis**. Most bacteria and all animals then use plants as a source of nutrients and energy.

The biologically usable form of energy, which is present in all cells, is adenosine triphosphate (ATP). Glucose is broken down in the cell and its energy is captured in the form of ATP. There are 10 chemical reactions used to convert one molecule of glucose to carbon dioxide and water, and during these reactions 30 molecules of ATP are produced. ATP is then used by the cell to:

● make new cell components
● transport substances into the cell
● move the cell
● move the cell cytoplasm

When this energy-forming process involves the use of oxygen, it is called **respiration**. Some cells use organic compounds instead of oxygen and produce **alcohol** as the end-product instead of water. This process is called **fermentation** and is characteristic of **anaerobic** bacteria. Some bacteria can switch from respiration to fermentation in the absence of oxygen and are called facultative anaerobes. The byproducts of fermentation are used in various commercial processes such as brewing and wine-making. In eucaryotic cells, respiration occurs in the mitochondria. These have a highly folded internal membrane containing the enzymes that catalyse the energy-producing reactions.

Protein synthesis

The synthesis of a string of amino acids begins with the creation of a short length of **ribonucleic acid (RNA)** corresponding to the sequence of bases on the DNA strand. RNA has a similar structure to DNA except that it is a single chain, the sugar is ribose, not deoxyribose, and the thymine is replaced by a very similar base, **uracil**. This 'messenger RNA' (mRNA) moves to the **ribosomes** where the code is read and the appropriate amino acids are assembled into a chain. Amino acids are collected from the cytoplasm by other RNA molecules called 'transfer RNA' (tRNA). There is a specific tRNA for each type of amino acid (see Fig. 1.8).

Cell division

Procaryotic cells multiply by dividing in two in a process called **binary fission**. When the cell has grown to a certain size, the single chromosome divides into two identical copies and the cell wall and membrane grow inwards, forming a new cell wall across the cell. Eventually the cell wall splits the cytoplasm into two cells, each with a chromosome (see Fig. 1.9). Often the two cells do not completely separate from each other but remain together as clumps (e.g. staphylococci), in chains (e.g. streptococci) or in pairs (e.g. pneumococci).

Eucaryotic cells can divide by simple division, or **mitosis**, in a similar way to procaryotes. All the DNA is copied and each set enclosed in a nuclear membrane. The cytoplasm then divides to form two identical cells. This type of division will occur as the plant or animal makes new cells to grow or to repair damaged tissue.

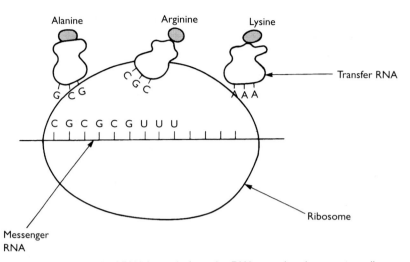

Fig. 1.8 The synthesis of protein. A length of RNA is made from the DNA strand and moves to a ribosome. The amino acids corresponding to the code on the RNA are brought from the cytoplasm by transfer RNA and assembled into a protein.

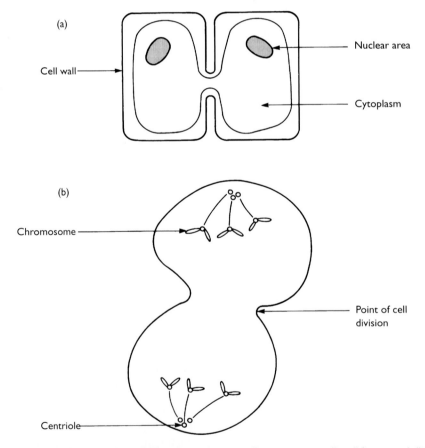

Fig. 1.9 Simple cell division. (a) A bacterial cell. The chromosome replicates, a new cell wall forms and divides the original cell into two (binary fission). (b) A eucaryotic cell. The chromosome replicates, one set is distributed to each end of the cell which then divides into two (mitosis).

Sexual reproduction

Sexual reproduction describes the process of mixing genetic information from more than one individual together and is a method of introducing variation into the population. Variation is important because it enables a species to adapt to its environment and gradually evolve.

Eucaryotes

In eucaryotic cells sexual reproduction is achieved by fusing two cells from different individuals together. As this would result in one cell with double the usual number of chromosomes, a special type of cell division called **meiosis** is required. This creates daughter cells with half the usual number of chromosomes. At **fertilization**, two cells fuse together and the new cell will contain the full number of chromosomes.

Procaryotes

Procaryotic cells do not multiply by sexual reproduction. However, transfer of genetic material between bacterial cells occurs but always in one direction, from a donor cell to a recipient cell. Transfer happens in one of three ways (see Fig. 1.10).

Transformation   Strands of DNA released from dead bacteria are absorbed through the cell wall and incorporated into the chromosome. Only DNA from closely related species will be expressed.

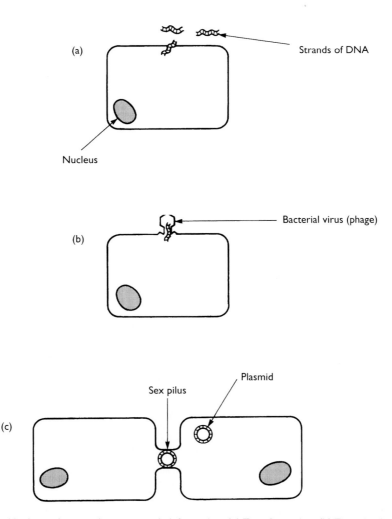

(a)   Strands of DNA

Nucleus

(b)   Bacterial virus (phage)

Plasmid

Sex pilus

(c)

Fig. 1.10   Methods used by bacteria to exchange genetic information. (a) Transformation. (b) Transduction. (c) Conjugation.

Transduction DNA from one bacterium is introduced into another cell by a bacterial virus or bacteriophage. Like other viruses, phages must incorporate into the host DNA in order to replicate. Sometimes some of the host's DNA is copied with the virus genome by mistake and is taken out of the cell with the phage. This is the method by which some bacteria acquire resistance to antibiotics.

Conjugation Plasmid DNA can transfer from one bacterial cell to another through a small tube or **sex pilus** which attaches to the sex pilus of the cell. The plasmid DNA then replicates and one copy enters the recipient cell. Plasmids commonly carry genes conferring resistance to antibiotics or toxin production, so conjugation is of major importance in the spread of these characteristics between strains of bacteria. The genetic information required to make the sex pilus and DNA transfer proteins are carried on a plasmid. Only those bacteria with this plasmid can transfer DNA by conjugation.

Recombinant DNA techniques

The study of bacterial genomes has enabled tremendous advances to be made both in our understanding of the **genetic code**, in particular the human chromosome, and in the synthesis of substances useful in medicine and industry.

Nucleases, enzymes that cut the DNA strand, can be used to break strands of DNA into small fragments. **Restriction endonucleases** are special types of nuclease that recognize specific sequences of bases in DNA strands. As each enzyme will always recognize the same sequence, the same sections of DNA are always obtained from a particular chromosome. It is therefore possible to separate a single gene known to synthesize a particular chemical. If the same endonuclease is then used to cut a DNA plasmid, the gene cut from the chromosome can be inserted into the plasmid. Plasmids can be introduced into other bacteria by conjugation, or into eucaryotic cells using specialized techniques. When the cells are cultured they then synthesize the substance coded for by the introduced gene.

This method has been used to manufacture substances used in the treatment of human disease by inserting genes from the human chromosome into bacteria. For example, the gene coding for human insulin has been inserted into a bacterium and human insulin can now be manufactured by the culture of these bacteria. Fragments of DNA from the hepatitis B virus have also been incorporated into a plasmid, which is inserted into a yeast. The viral proteins produced by the yeast as it multiplies are purified and made into a vaccine against hepatitis B virus. These recombinant DNA techniques are also used to provide rapid and specific tests for infections by detecting specific sequences of DNA.

Cell motility

Some bacteria are not capable of independent movement. Others, particularly bacilli and spirilli, have appendages called **flagella** which, by rotating like a propeller, enable them to swim (see Fig. 1.11). These motile bacteria swim towards chemicals such as nutrients to which they are attracted, and swim away from toxic substances. Many Gram-negative bacteria such as *Escherichia coli* and pseudomonas have flagella and are motile. Some species have many flagella on one cell. Flagella are rarely found on cocci. Motile bacteria thrive in moist conditions where the ability to swim is an advantage, whilst non-motile bacteria are able to survive in dry environments.

Eucaryotic cells may also have flagella or **cilia** but with a much more complex structure.

Fimbriae or pili are hair-like appendages that are thinner and shorter than flagella. They are mostly found on Gram-negative cells and their purpose is to facilitate adherence to other cells. Variation in fimbriae affects the types of cell to which the bacteria can adhere and determines their ability to cause disease. Sex pili are special types of fimbriae used in the exchange of genetic information between cells (see p. 9).

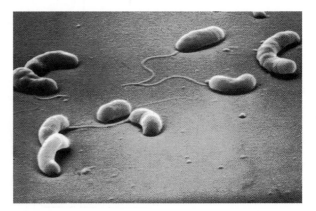

Fig. 1.11 Flagella on a bacterial cell.

THE GROWTH AND MULTIPLICATION OF BACTERIA

Since bacteria live in a wide range of environments, it is not surprising that the nutrients they need vary widely from species to species. A bacterium, such as E. coli, supplied with all the nutrients it needs will divide, on average, once every 15 min and will continue to grow at this rate until the supply of nutrients is exhausted. Some bacteria can synthesize a wide range of materials that they need to grow and multiply and can therefore survive in the presence of very few nutrients. Others need a source of specific molecules or amino acids and therefore have more exacting growth requirements. There are certain basic substances that are essential to support the growth of all bacteria.

Energy source

Energy is generally obtained from the breakdown of organic carbon-containing compounds, although some bacteria are able to capture the energy of the sun using **chlorophyll**, in the same way as plants.

Carbon source

Carbon is necessary to form the compounds that make up the structure of the cell. Most bacteria use the breakdown of organic carbon compounds such as carbohydrates to obtain energy. However, bacteria can make use of almost any form of carbon including hydrocarbons, phenol, wood and atmospheric carbon dioxide.

Nitrogen source

Nitrogen is needed to make many of the cell structures, for example proteins and nucleic acids. Nitrogen can be obtained in the form of ammonia (NH_4) or nitrates (NO_3), and some microbes can use atmospheric nitrogen. Many pathogenic bacteria need a source of organic nitrogen such as amino acids.

Inorganic ions

Sodium, potassium, magnesium, chloride and sulphate are needed both to form the structure of the cell, for example to make amino acids, and to act as cofactors for enzymes. All organisms require phosphate to make lipids and nucleic acids and to store energy as ATP.

Some bacteria will grow in very simple media containing only these substances, although usually they grow very slowly. Most of the bacteria that cause disease in humans depend on the presence of additional 'growth factors' available in the host tissue. These are usually **amino acids** or vitamins that the bacteria cannot make themselves. Other chemicals, or **trace elements** such as iron or zinc, are required to make enzymes or other proteins.

We can help to prevent the multiplication of bacteria in the clinical environment by removing potential sources of nutrients. For example, body fluid spilt on to equipment, furniture or floors will support the growth of bacteria and should be removed as soon as possible; baths or washbowls that are not properly cleaned will retain a coating of skin scales and soap on their surface which provides a plentiful supply of nutrients for the growth of bacteria (Greaves 1985).

Environmental factors

Environmental conditions also have a very important effect on the growth of bacteria. Bacteria that cause disease usually grow most rapidly under the environmental conditions found in the human body.

Water

Water is an essential requirement for the growth of bacteria and most die rapidly in the absence of water. The moisture-loving Gram-negative bacteria, in particular, thrive in damp places. They are particularly vulnerable to desiccation and will survive only for a short time on dry surfaces. The susceptibility of many bacteria to a lack of water provides us with a very useful infection control measure; we can prevent bacteria from multiplying by keeping surfaces clean and dry and by drying equipment thoroughly before it is stored. Equipment should not be immersed in liquids for prolonged periods as bacteria can grow even in **disinfectants**. Thermometers stored in disinfectant solutions or mops lingering in buckets of dirty water are commonly encountered infection hazards (Werry et al 1988). Equipment such as nebulizers or ventilator equipment that is in contact with water is particularly hazardous because bacteria can multiply rapidly in the moisture (Botman & de Krieger 1987, Cefai et al 1990).

Other bacteria are more resistant to drying out (e.g. staphylococci and mycobacteria) or are able to form spores (e.g. *Clostridium difficile*). They may be able to survive for hours or even months, recommencing multiplication if a supply of moisture is resumed. These organisms may survive in dust, and thus preventing the accumulation of dust on surfaces and floors can be an important infection control measure (Cartmill et al 1994, Casewell 1986).

Oxygen

To use respiration for energy production, bacteria must have an enzyme called catalase, which can degrade the toxic end-products of the process. Some bacteria do not have catalase and use fermentation rather than respiration to make energy. Many of these obligate anaerobes are rapidly killed when exposed to air, and special laboratory techniques are required to culture them. Some bacteria can use either respiration or fermentation to make energy, changing the method according to the prevailing environmental conditions. These are called facultative anaerobes and include enteric bacteria and the staphylococci. Obligate aerobes such as pseudomonas and mycobacteria can use only respiration and therefore cannot survive without oxygen. Anaerobes are found inside body cavities such as the intestines and vagina. Anaerobic bacteria such as *Clostridium perfringens* can cause serious infection in wounds where the tissue is extensively damaged or **necrotic** and poorly supplied with oxygen. Wounds that have a good blood supply will be well oxygenated and are unlikely to support the growth of anaerobic bacteria. *Bacteroides fragilis* is an anaerobe normally found in the intestine, which can cause intra-abdominal abscesses following surgery.

Temperature

Most bacteria grow within a wide range of temperatures but those that grow in association with humans multiply rapidly at around body temperature. Some bacteria are known for their ability to multiply even at very low temperatures. *Listeria monocytogenes*, for example, grows even at 5°C and can therefore spoil refrigerated food. Bacteria can adapt to almost any environment. Some species are even able to survive at temperatures of 100°C found in hot springs and volcanoes.

pH

The pH of a solution reflects the concentration of hydrogen ions. Most bacteria cannot maintain the neutral pH of their cytoplasm if the concentration of hydrogen ions outside the cell is too high or low, and prefer to live in approximately neutral solutions. A high pH is used to protect some body cavities from invasion by harmful bacteria; for example, the nor-

mally acidic stomach kills ingested pathogens. Lactobacilli that normally inhabit the vagina produce lactic acid, creating a local pH of 4.0 in which most pathogens are unable to survive.

Concentration of solution

Molecules that are dissolved in a solution are called **solutes**. The membrane surrounding the cell prevents the passage of solutes into the cell. If the cell is in a solution where the concentration of solutes is greater than in the cytoplasm of the cell, there is a tendency for water to diffuse out of the cell into the solution in order to equilibrate the concentrations. If the concentration of solutes in the cytoplasm is greater than outside the cell, the water will diffuse into the cell. This process is known as **osmosis**. Like all cells, bacteria have transport mechanisms operating at the membrane to make sure that the level of solutes in the cytoplasm remains at the desired concentration regardless of the concentration in their environment. In fact, the bacterial cell wall is able to withstand a wide range of very strong and dilute solutions.

The common practice of adding salt to a patient's bath to 'clean' wounds is of no actual value. The salt would need to be added in enormous quantities to achieve a final concentration in the bathwater sufficient to disrupt bacterial cells and simply adding a cupful of salt to a bath of water has no antibacterial effect at all (Austin 1988, Ayliffe et al 1975).

FUNGI

Fungi are plants. They have eucaryotic cells but lack the green pigment, **chlorophyll**, that other plants use for photosynthesis. Fungi are widely distributed in the environment and many live in soil, where they decompose organic matter. They can be grown on agar media like bacteria but, because they can survive in relatively little moisture and in high osmolarity, they are often found growing on substances that will not support the growth of bacteria (e.g. jams and other preserved foods). Some species of fungi cause disease in plants and animals. In humans, they cause superficial infection of the skin such as ringworm, oral and vaginal candidiasis, and more serious systemic infections in the immunocompromised (e.g. aspergillosis). Mycology is the term used to describe the study of fungi.

Growth

Most fungi grow as filamentous branching tubes containing cytoplasm and many nuclei. These form a mass called a mycelium. The filaments of the mycelium act like roots, penetrating into the substance on which they are growing. In some species the filaments are separated into cells by transverse walls, although these are often perforated to allow the movement of cytoplasm and nuclei. A large mass of mycelium may become visible and some species (e.g. mushrooms) produce specialized spore-bearing structures above the surface. Some species of fungi have lost the mycelial form of growth, forming small single ovoid cells instead. These are called *yeasts*, and this type of growth can be found in all the main groups of fungi. Sometimes one species can grow as either a yeast or a mycelium, depending on the temperature and availability of nutrients.

Yeast cells are between 20 and 100 times larger than a bacterial cell but can be seen only with the aid of a microscope. They can be grown on solid **agar** medium where, like bacteria, they appear as masses of cells or colonies (see Ch. 2). Most yeasts live in high concentrations of sugars such as on the surface of fruit and flowers, which they ferment. Many species are extremely useful, for example in the fermentation of sugars to produce alcohol and carbon dioxide, a process used in brewing and bread-making.

Reproduction

Fungi usually reproduce asexually by forming spores at the tips of the branched tubes. Each spore contains at least one nucleus. These are released to start a new mycelium elsewhere (Plate 1.1). Sexual reproduction occurs by fusion of cells in the mycelium to form spores, but the exact mechanism varies in each species. Yeasts multiply asexually by forming buds, where a new cell gradually grows out of the parent cell (Plate 1.2). They reproduce sexually by meiotic division of a single cell, which then forms two daughter cells or ascospores. Later two ascospores will fuse to form a new cell.

PROTOZOA

These are relatively large, but still microscopic, eucaryotic cells (Plate 1.3). They have a tough outer cell membrane instead of a cell wall, have mitochondria and can obtain nutrients by ingesting solid particles of food. These are then digested by enzymes into soluble compounds that can be transported into the cytoplasm. The cells multiply by dividing in two and some species differentiate between male and female cells. Many protozoa have complex life cycles; that is, a series of stages in their development (e.g. plasmodium species which cause malaria). They are motile in at least one of these

stages and some form thick-walled, dormant cysts which are important in transmission (e.g. *Entamoeba histolytica*). Most protozoa are aquatic and some are animal parasites.

VIRUSES

Viruses are not cells; they are simply a piece of **nucleic acid**, which may be single or double stranded and either DNA or RNA, protected by a protein coat and sometimes an envelope made of **lipids**. The protein coat is made from many identical units of polypeptide. These are often formed into symmetrical shapes such as spheres or icosahedrons. Viruses contain none of the structures necessary to synthesize the proteins or enzymes encoded by their nucleic acid. The smallest viruses contain enough nucleic acid to make three or four proteins, the largest several hundred proteins (see Fig. 1.12).

Viruses are extremely small, ranging from 27 nm in diameter to about 200 nm, compared to an average bacterial cell of about 1000 nm in diameter, and are therefore too small to be seen with an ordinary light microscope. Instead they can be seen with an **electron microscope** which uses a beam of **electrons** instead of

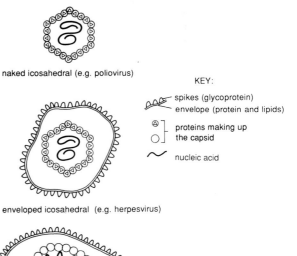

naked icosahedral (e.g. poliovirus)

KEY:

spikes (glycoprotein)
envelope (protein and lipids)

proteins making up
the capsid

nucleic acid

enveloped icosahedral (e.g. herpesvirus)

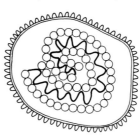

enveloped helical (e.g. influenza virus)

Fig. 1.12   The structure of viruses.

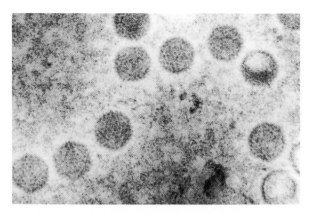

Fig. 1.13   An electron micrograph of adenovirus.

light to create an image of an object on a photographic plate. Figure 1.13 shows an electron micrograph of adenovirus.

Viral replication

Viruses can multiply only inside living cells. Receptors on the protein coat recognize and attach to specific receptors on the surface of particular cells in the host. The presence of these specific receptors determines which cells are invaded by the virus. For example, the human immunodeficiency virus (HIV) attaches to a CD4 molecule found on the surface of some lymphocytes and macrophages. The viral nucleic acid then enters the nucleus of the host cell where it instructs the cell's own mechanism to copy the nucleic acids and translate its code into viral proteins. Many copies of the viral nucleic acid and proteins are made by the host cell in this way. Some RNA viruses can be translated directly as mRNA. Retroviruses have an enzyme called reverse transcriptase, which converts the RNA to DNA to enable viral proteins to be made. The virus components are then assembled in the cytoplasm and new viruses are released from the cell either by budding out of the cell membrane or causing the cell to rupture (see Fig. 1.14). The host cells infected are usually destroyed by the virus, but because cells are rapidly replaced most viral illnesses are short and recovery is complete. Some viral infections can cause permanent damage; for example, HIV depletes the **T cells** of the immune system to such an extent that the immune system becomes defective.

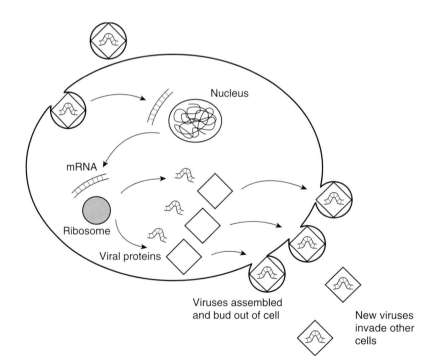

Fig. 1.14   The virus enters the host cell and its genome is released to the nucleus where it is copied and transcribed into mRNA. The mRNA is translated on the ribosomes of the host cell and many copies of the viral proteins are made. The genome and proteins are then assembled into new viruses and bud out of the cell membrane. Enveloped viruses acquire part of the membrane as they are released.

Some viruses insert all or part of their nucleic acid into the host cell's DNA, where it remains and causes the cell to become malignant by coding for unlimited cell division. This has been suggested as the mechanism by which viruses such as herpes simplex type 2 virus and human papilloma virus could cause cancer of the cervix (Mindel 1989).

Viral growth requirements

As viruses depend on living cells for their replication, it is not possible to grow them in artificial media in the same way as bacteria. Instead, viruses are grown in cultures of living cells and require an environment that will maintain the cells, including salts, amino acids and vitamins. A few viruses, for example rotavirus, cannot even be grown in these artificial cell cultures,

and thus to experiment on them live animals must be used.

Most viruses are fragile and cannot survive outside a living cell for long. However, some viruses can survive for some time on surfaces or hands and from there are transmitted to a new host (Mahl & Sadler 1975). Viruses are fairly resistant to the activity of some disinfectants such as phenol or chlorhexidine which are unable to disrupt their protein coat or lipid membrane. Outbreaks of viral gastrointestinal or respiratory infection occur frequently in hospital. Preventing outbreaks of infection caused by viruses can be extremely difficult; they are very small, can be exhaled on small respiratory droplets or be excreted in high numbers in faeces. Transmission commonly occurs on hands and may occur on inadequately decontaminated equipment such as commodes or bedpans (Ansari et al 1991).

REFERENCES

Ansari SA, Springthorpe VS, Sattar SA et al (1991) Potential role of hands in the spread of respiratory viral infections: studies with human parainfluenza virus 3 and rhinovirus 14. *J. Clin. Microbiol.*, **29**: 2115–19.

Austin L (1988) The salt bath myth. *Nursing Times*, **84**(9): 79–83.

Ayliffe G, Babb JR, Collins BJ (1975) Disinfection of baths and bathwater. *Nursing Times*, **71**(37): 22–3.

Botman MJ, de Krieger RA (1987) Contamination of small-volume medication nebulizers and its association with oropharyngeal colonisation. *J. Hosp. Infect.*, **19**: 204–8.

Cartmill TDI, Parigrahi H, Worsley MA et al (1994) Management and control of a large outbreak of diarrhoea due to *Clostridium difficile*. *J. Hosp. Infect.*, **27**: 1–16.

Casewell MW (1986) Epidemiology and control of the

'modern' methicillin resistant *Staphylococcus aureus*. *J. Hosp. Infect.*, **7** (Suppl. A): 1–11.

Cefai C, Richards J, Gould FK et al (1990) An outbreak of *Acinetobacter* respiratory tract infection resulting from incomplete disinfection of ventilatory equipment. *J. Hosp. Infect.*, **15**: 177–82.

Greaves A (1985) We'll just freshen you up, dear. *Nursing Times*, **Mar 6** (Suppl.): 3–8.

Mahl MC, Sadler C (1975) Virus survival on inanimate surfaces. *Can. J. Microbiol.*, **21**: 819–23.

Mindel A (1989) *Herpes Simplex Virus*. Springer, London.

Walzer PD (1993) *Pneumocystis carinii*: recent advances in basic biology and their clinical application. *AIDS*, **7**: 1293–305.

Werry C, Lawrence JM, Sanderson PJ (1988) Contamination of detergent cleaning solutions during hospital cleaning. *J. Hosp. Infect.*, **11**: 44–9.

FURTHER READING

Ackerman V, Dunk-Richards G (1991) *Microbiology – an Introduction for the Health Sciences*. WB Saunders/Baillière Tindall, London.

Fuerst R (1983) *Frobisher and Fuerst's Microbiology in Health and Disease*, 15th edn. WB Saunders, London.

Kedzierski M (1991) Understanding virology. *Professional Nurse*, **Nov**: 99–102.

Postgate J (1992) *Microbes and Man*, 3rd edn. Cambridge University Press, Cambridge.

Stanier RY, Ingraham JL, Wheelis ML, Painter PR (1987) *General Microbiology*, 5th edn. Macmillan Education, London.

Szekely M (1980) *From DNA to Protein*. Macmillan, London.

Watson R (ed.) (1999) *Essential Science for Nursing Students. An Introductory Text*. Baillière Tindall, London.

2

Understanding the microbiology laboratory

INTRODUCTION

In the modern age we rely extensively on antimicrobial agents to treat **infection**. It is easy to assume that at the first sign of fever we need only reach for an **antibiotic** to treat the infection and that identification and investigation of the causative organism are unnecessary. For minor infections it is reasonable to make an educated guess about the organism causing the infection; for example, skin infections such as boils or septic spots are invariably caused by *Staphylococcus aureus*, and easily treated with flucloxacillin. However, the bacteria may be resistant to the antibiotic chosen, the bacteria may continue to multiply and the patient remains ill. Confirmation of the micro-organisms causing the infection, and the most appropriate method of treatment, requires the expertise of the microbiology laboratory.

The functions of the microbiology laboratory are to:

● assist in the diagnosis of infection
● identify the causative organism
● provide advice on the best antimicrobial agent to treat the infection.

The procedures used in the microbiology laboratory aim to reproduce the environmental conditions in which **pathogenic micro-organisms** grow and to identify the causative organism by separating out the different species present in the specimen.

Micro-organisms are found on every surface of the body as part of the normal flora (see Ch. 3) and they can therefore be isolated from almost any specimen. The microbiologist must be able to find the organism that is causing infection amongst all the other micro-organisms that normally live at the site or that may have contaminated the specimen. The selection of appropriate tests and interpretation of the results rely on detailed, relevant information about the patient and the symptoms and signs. The specimen should be properly collected and stored to ensure that the results of tests reliably detect the causative micro-organisms.

The laboratory, as well as helping to interpret the results of specimens, can provide advice on how the infection should be treated, the type of antibiotic to use and for how long. This advice is provided by medical microbiologists, doctors who, in addition to their medical qualification, have a specialist knowledge of microbiology. The infection control nurse can also provide a link between the laboratory and ward staff by helping to interpret results and by advising on appropriate action.

Most acute hospitals have a microbiology laboratory on site. These laboratories may also provide a service to other local healthcare facilities such as clinics and nursing homes, as well as general practitioners. Specialist diagnostic and advisory services are provided by the Public Health Laboratories in England and Wales, and the Scottish Centre for Infection and Environmental Health (SCIEH) in Scotland. These can assist in the identification of unusual organisms, bacteria present in food, water or other environmental samples, and advise on **outbreaks of infection** in hospitals or the community.

IDENTIFICATION OF BACTERIA

Microscopy

Examination of bacterial cells on glass slides under the **microscope** can reveal some important information about their structure, shape and arrangement. The two main shapes of bacterial cells are round (cocci) or oblong (bacilli or rods), but other bacteria forms include curved rods (e.g. vibrios) or spirals (e.g. treponema). Some cocci congregate in clumps (staphylococci), whereas the cells of streptococci form into chains. Bacteria are not easy to see under a microscope as they appear colourless. In 1884 Christian Gram developed a method of colouring cells with dyes in a technique now known as the **Gram stain**. A Gram stain takes only a few minutes to carry out and is used to distinguish two main groups: Gram-positive and Gram-negative organisms. **Gram-positive** cells absorb a dark blue dye and appear blue under the microscope (Plate 2.1). **Gram-negative** cells do not absorb the blue dye, but when counterstained with a red dye, they stain pink (Plate 2.2). Other, more specialized, staining techniques are used in the identification of some bacteria, for example the Ziehl–Neelsen (ZN) stain which is used to identify mycobacteria.

Microscopy and Gram staining are often used to provide a provisional identification, particularly where the infection is life threatening. For example, when meningitis is suspected, examination of cere-brospinal fluid under the microscope may enable a provisional diagnosis to be made and appropriate antibiotic therapy to be started immediately (see Plate 2.3). **Fungi** can also have a characteristic appearance under the microscope, for example the *Candida albicans* illustrated in Plate 1.2. Whilst the conventional light microscope can establish the shape of bacteria, it cannot distinguish internal structures of the cell. For this, an electron microscope, which uses a stream of electrons instead of light to magnify an image, is required.

Culture methods

Unfortunately, bacteria cannot be reliably identified by their appearance under the microscope alone. Specimens are therefore grown in special media and a variety of tests used to identify the organism.

Solid medium is made by mixing nutrients with **agar**, a gelling agent extracted from seaweed. The most commonly used medium in a hospital laboratory is blood agar, which contains horse blood. The concentration of chemicals in the medium can be altered to reflect more closely the environment in which the pathogens are growing or to prevent the growth of the normal flora, making pathogenic species easier to identify. For example, deoxycholate agar is used to isolate shigella from stool specimens as it inhibits the growth of normal faecal flora such as *Escherichia coli*. Bacteria can also be grown in liquid media called broth. This type of culture is used to grow large numbers of micro-organisms, especially from specimens such as blood where only a few micro-organisms may be present in the sample.

Bacteria that normally live on, or cause disease in, humans grow best in media that mimic the secretions or tissues of the human body. Some bacteria will grow in very simple media containing very few nutrients; others require complex media to supply most of their growth requirements.

Incubation at around body temperature encourages most pathogenic bacteria to grow rapidly, but it can still take between 24 and 48 h before there are enough cells present to enable further testing. Some specimens will be cultured in special oxygen-free cabinets if pathogens are likely to be **anaerobes**, for example swabs taken from infected wounds.

The appearance of colonies

When bacteria are grown on solid medium, each bacterial cell will multiply many times and, after several hours, millions of bacteria will be present. The distinct group of cells appears as a **colony** and can be seen on the agar without a microscope. Their size, colour and shape vary quite markedly between different species of bacteria and an experienced microbiologist can identify some bacteria from the appearance of their colonies on different types of media. Some bacteria such as *Bacillus cereus* (Plate 2.4) produce characteristically large colonies, whilst others such as staphylococcus are smaller (Plate 2.5). **Enzymes** produced by certain bacteria lyse the red blood cells in blood agar, causing clear areas to form around the colonies (Plate 2.6). Other bacteria produce colonies of characteristic colour such as the green pigment of *Pseudomonas aeruginosa* (Plate 2.7) or red of *Serratia marcescens* (Plate 2.8).

Commonly, specimens contain a mixture of different bacteria and the skills of the microbiologist are needed to separate and identify each one (Plate 2.9). Single colonies are spread out over the surface of agar (Plates 2.5–2.8). They can then be picked off the agar and inoculated into broth to provide a pure culture. Care must be taken to ensure that micro-organisms from the air or environment do not contaminate the specimen and confuse the diagnosis.

Tests to identify the organism

Once the micro-organisms in a specimen have been **cultured**, further tests may have to be conducted to establish the exact species present. Commercially prepared kits are available that are used to distinguish bacteria by their ability to break down a range of substances. These kits enable a quick and accurate identification to be made. They are **inoculated**, incubated overnight and the subsequent colour change in each chamber is used to make the identification (see Plate 2.10).

Sensitivity to antibiotics

It is also important to establish whether different antibiotics have an effect on the organism to ensure that the right antibiotic is selected for treatment of the infection. Antibiotic sensitivity is tested by spreading the organism evenly over the surface of an agar plate, placing small circles of paper impregnated with different antibiotics on to the surface and incubating the plate overnight. The antibiotic diffuses from the paper into the agar and prevents sensitive bacteria from growing in the area around the paper. Bacteria that are not affected by an antibiotic will be able to grow right up to the impregnated paper and hence are resistant to the antibiotic (see Plate 2.11).

Detection of microbial antigens

Molecules on the surface of micro-organisms, called antigens, are recognized by the immune system. Specific antibodies will bind to a particular antigen and can be made into standard preparations, called antisera. This type of test can be applied to cerebrospinal fluid to give a rapid diagnosis for a patient with symptoms of meningitis. Laboratories use a range of these known antibody preparations that are specific to antigens on known **species** of micro-organism. The bacteria to be identified are mixed with the antisera. If they are of corresponding species, the specific antibody will bind to the bacterial cells and this reaction will be apparent as a clumping or **agglutination** of bacterial cells. Antisera can also be made to detect specific toxins, for example toxins produced by *Corynebacterium diphtheriae*.

Identification of fungi and protozoa

The identification of fungi relies mostly on the morphology of colonies and characteristics of cells viewed under the microscope. As they tend to grow slowly, identification may take up to 2 weeks. Biochemical tests are used in the identification of some yeasts.

Protozoa are identified by means of their appearance under the microscope, particularly characteristic stages in their life cycle such as cysts.

IDENTIFICATION OF VIRUSES

There are two different approaches to the identification of viral infections. The first is the culture of virus or direct detection of virus particles by electron microscopy; the second is the detection of specific antibodies in blood by **serological** testing.

Virus culture

Unlike bacteria, viruses cannot be grown on artificial media but can be cultured only in living cells (i.e. tissue cultures). Sheets of cells are grown in nutrient medium on glass or plastic. Viruses present in clinical specimens grown in the culture will alter the appearance of the cells in a characteristic manner (e.g. herpes simplex). Not all viruses will grow in tissue culture. Some are diagnosed by special staining techniques or by **electron microscopy**. Provided sufficient viral particles are present, these very powerful microscopes can be used to detect particles as small as 0.0001 μm in size (Fig. 2.1). Detection of virus in samples of body fluid can resemble the search for a needle in a haystack, and

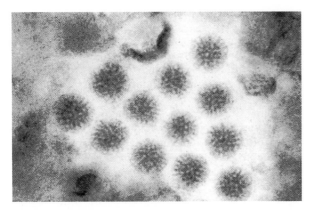

Fig. 2.1   Electron micrograph of rotavirus.

the absence of virus under the electron microscope should not be considered as conclusive evidence of the absence of infection.

Serological tests

Infection by a virus may be followed by the appearance of antibodies to the virus in the blood. The detection of these antibodies is the basis of serological testing and is used extensively to diagnose viral infections. There are several methods of diagnosing viral illnesses based on the same principle of detecting antibodies. The most widely used method is the **enzyme-linked immunosorbent assay (ELISA). Antigen** specific to the antibody to be detected is placed into small wells on special plates and incubated with **serum** from the patient. If an antibody specific to the antigen in the well is present in the blood, it will bind to it. Then an enzyme attached to an antibody that recognizes and binds to other antibodies is added and attaches to those wells containing the patient's anti-

body. This reaction is detected by a colour change caused by the enzyme.

Serum antibodies

Different types of antibody appear in the blood during the course of an infection (see Ch. 4). The type of antibody detected in the blood indicates whether the person has had the infection in the past or is recovering from the infection. This method is used to diagnose several viral infections including rubella and hepatitis. In the case of hepatitis B, identification of the types of antibody present is used to indicate whether infection has persisted and the patient is a chronic **carrier** of the virus (see Ch. 3). Relating symptoms of an infection to a particular virus is difficult if only one sample of the patient's blood is examined. Antibodies to the virus may already be present as the result of a previous infection. A second sample of blood, taken about 10 days after the first, can be examined to see whether the level of antibodies is greater than in the first sample. If a considerable increase in antibodies is found, this is evidence that the virus is causing the infection. This test is described as 'paired sera'. The different tests used to identify viral infections are summarized in Table 2.1.

Distinguishing microbial strains

Identification of different variants or strains of the same micro-organisms can be important in the investigation of outbreaks of infection. The recovery of the same strain from more than one patient or member of staff is an indication that cross-infection has occurred. The tests required to 'type' strains are complex and usually carried out in specialist reference laboratories. A variety of techniques are used, for example

Table 2.1   Some methods of identifying viral infections

Infection	Specimen	Test	Viruses
Respiratory tract infection	Throat swab, nasopharyngeal washings	Culture	Influenza, para-influenza, RSV
	Paired sera	Serology	Influenza, para-influenza, RSV adenovirus, mumps
Vesicular skin lesions	Fluid from lesion	Electron microscopy, culture, serology	Herpes simplex, varicella zoster
Erythematous skin rash	Paired sera	Serology	Measles, rubella
Hepatitis	Serum	Serology	Hepatitis B, hepatitis A
Eye infections	Conjunctival scrapings	Culture	Herpes simplex, adenovirus
Gastroenteritis	Faeces	Electron microscopy	Rotavirus, calicivirus, small round virus

Paired sera = serum from two samples of blood taken 10 days apart. RSV, respiratory syncytial virus.

susceptibility to bacterial viruses (bacteriophages), production of inhibitory substances or possession of specific antigens. More recently molecular techniques that can be used directly to compare the nucleic acids of strains have been developed and are now in wide-spread use.

Molecular techniques used in the microbiology laboratory

A range of specialized techniques is now available which identify micro-organisms by detecting specific sequences of DNA or RNA. These methods are sensitive and specific and, because they do not require culture of the micro-organisms, they are also safe.

Molecular diagnosis is most valuable for the identification of some viruses. For example, tests that detect hepatitis B virus DNA can be used to determine the stage of infection and infectivity of an affected individual. These techniques are also increasingly used to distinguish strains of bacteria in outbreaks of infection (e.g. streptococci).

Electrophoresis

In this method the DNA of the micro-organism is cut into small fragments by restriction endonucleases, enzymes that recognize specific nucleic acid sequences and cleave the DNA at points where these sequences occur. The resulting fragments are separated out on a flat gel, using an electric current which attracts the charged particles and causes small and large fragments to move at different rates. The fragments are then made visible by staining and the pattern of spread is compared to identify related and unrelated strains (Fig. 2.2).

Genetic probes

These are small sections of DNA, which are used to detect sequences from pathogens present in clinical specimens. The DNA probe is labelled with a radioactive nucleotide and then mixed with DNA from the sample under investigation. It will bind to identical sequences in the test DNA in a process called hybridization. These sequences can be detected and quantified by measuring the amount of radioactive label. If the specific DNA sequence is present only in small amounts in the specimen, the technique is used in combination with a polymerase chain reaction (PCR) method. Gene probes can be used to detect toxins produced by *Escherichia coli or Vibrio cholerae* in faeces, or *Mycoplasma pneumoniae* in sputum.

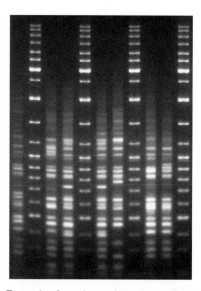

Fig. 2.2 Example of an electrophoresis gel. Each column contains DNA from a micro-organism and each band represents a differently sized fragment of DNA. Similar patterns of fragments are used to identify strains or specific micro-organisms.

Polymerase chain reaction

This method is used to detect micro-organisms that are present in very small amounts in a specimen by amplifying specific sequences of DNA. Primers for DNA replication that are known to hybridize with a specific section of DNA in the test micro-organisms are used to activate polymerase enzymes. These enzymes then repeatedly make copies of the specific segment of DNA so that after a few hours millions of copies will be present. These can then be detected by gene probes or electrophoresis. Although used mostly in research, PCR has been used to diagnose a range of infections including those caused by *Helicobacter pylori, Legionella pneumophilia* and herpes and hepatitis B viruses.

THE COLLECTION OF SPECIMENS FOR MICROBIOLOGICAL INVESTIGATION

The quality of the specimen received in the laboratory can have a major impact on the subsequent microbiological diagnosis. The correct method of collection and storage is therefore an important part of the process. False results may occur if specimens are kept for prolonged periods before examination in the laboratory, as some species may outgrow others and other delicate organisms will not survive. Samples should be taken aseptically to avoid contamination of the material with micro-organisms not causing the infection. In addition, accurate information about the patient's illness and treatment is important for interpretation of the results. Ideally, specimens should be taken before antimicrobial therapy is started, making the micro-organisms causing the infection more difficult to culture.

The following section describes the important principles to be considered when collecting clinical specimens. The laboratory will be able to advise where there is doubt about the type of specimen or investigation required.

Urine

Bladder urine should be sterile but is easily contaminated during collection by bacteria that colonize the perineum. Contamination can be reduced by discarding the first few millilitres of urine and collecting the mid-stream of urine in a sterile container. Cleaning the perineum before the specimen is collected is of questionable value in reducing the risk of contamination (Holliday et al 1991).

If the patient has a urinary catheter, the specimen must always be withdrawn from the designated sampling sleeve on the tubing with a sterile needle and syringe (Fig. 2.3). Urine obtained from the catheter bag will provide misleading results as bacteria may have multiplied in the stagnant urine (Bradley et al 1986). The bag must not be disconnected from the catheter to obtain a specimen as this is likely to introduce bacteria

into the system (Platt et al 1983). A urine sample of between 5 and 10 ml is usually sufficient for microbiological examination.

Urine specimens readily support the growth of bacteria, and the multiplication of bacteria in specimens stored at room temperature can produce misleading results. The specimen should therefore be examined in the laboratory within 2 h, but if refrigerated can be stored for up to 24 h. The microbiologist investigates the number of white blood cells present in the specimen. Large numbers of white cells suggest that the body is mounting an immune response to infection and help to confirm that an organism present in the urine is actually causing infection. The number of bacteria present in the urine is calculated by culturing a drop of urine on solid medium. If the patient has a urinary tract infection the specimen will probably contain at least 100 000 bacterial cells per millilitre and several white cells will be visible on examination under the microscope. Reagent strip tests are sometimes used to provide a rapid indication of possible infection by detecting blood protein and nitrite in the urine. However, their reliability in detecting infection is questionable (Tincello & Richmond 1998).

In the presence of a catheter, bacteria commonly **colonize** the bladder but do not necessarily invade the tissue to cause infection. In catheterized patients several species of bacteria are commonly present, although their significance is difficult to establish and

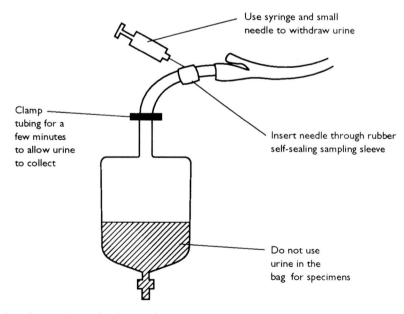

Fig. 2.3 The collection of a specimen of catheter urine.

antibiotic treatment is often unnecessary in the absence of clinical signs of infection such as pain or fever (Garibaldi 1993).

Sputum

The lower part of the respiratory tract is normally sterile but the upper respiratory tract, mouth and nose are colonized by large numbers of different bacteria, some of which are able to cause **pneumonia**. A diagnosis of respiratory tract infection is therefore made by a combination of clinical examination, history, chest radiography and microbiological examination of sputum to confirm the diagnosis and identify the causative organism.

Specimens of saliva are of no value, so it is important to ensure that the specimen is mucoid or mucopurulent. The physiotherapist may be able to help a patient who is having difficulty producing a specimen of sputum. Suctioning, using a sputum trap, may be required if the patient is unable to cough. For patients in intensive care units, bronchoscopy may be required to obtain an adequate specimen. Sputum specimens should be sent to the laboratory immediately as respiratory pathogens will not survive for prolonged periods.

The laboratory will examine the specimen for organisms likely to cause respiratory tract infection. If large numbers are present, identification can sometimes be assisted by **Gram-staining** and viewing under the microscope prior to culture (Plate 2.12).

Tuberculosis

The organism that causes tuberculosis, *Mycobacterium tuberculosis*, grows extremely slowly. Colonies of the bacteria do not appear before a minimum of 1 week of incubation and can take up to 6 weeks. Microscopic examination of sputum is therefore used to make an initial tentative diagnosis of tuberculosis. The numbers of mycobacteria in the sputum may be quite low and to increase the chance of detection three separate specimens, preferably collected in the early morning, should be examined (Plate 2.13). Gastric washings may be used to obtain these specimens in children.

Mycobacteria have particularly resistant **cell walls**; they are stained using a special dye (hot carbol fuchsin) which cannot be removed by acid or alcohol. This method is used to detect mycobacteria under the microscope, thus the term 'acid-fast bacilli' or AFB. Atypical mycobacterial infections caused by other species, for example *Mycobacterium avium intracellulare*

(MAI), cannot be distinguished from tuberculosis under the microscope and therefore several weeks of incubation are necessary before the species causing the infection can be identified.

Faeces

Faeces normally contains millions of micro-organisms. The detection of the bacteria or viruses responsible for diarrhoea or gastroenteritis is therefore not easy as pathogens need to be distinguished from **normal flora** before identification is possible. Faecal specimens can therefore take the laboratory 3–4 days to process and more than one specimen may be required to eliminate infection as a cause of symptoms.

If *Clostridium difficile* is isolated from a specimen, additional tests are necessary to establish whether it is a pathogenic, **toxin**-producing **strain**.

Viruses that cause gastrointestinal infections cannot be cultured but are detected by examination of faeces under the electron microscope. Faecal specimens are often not automatically examined for viruses; therefore, if infection is suspected as the cause of diarrhoea, two specimens should be sent to the laboratory, one requesting examination for bacteria, the second for viruses.

A walnut-sized sample of faeces, or approximately 15 ml of a liquid stool, is sufficient for microbiological investigation. It should be examined within 12 h, unless faecal **parasites** are suspected when a fresh, warm stool is required.

Wound swabs

A wound infection is recognized by the presence of clinical signs of infection rather than the isolation of bacteria from a wound swab. A wide range of bacteria able to cause infection may be grown from a wound swab, but many of these organisms may be harmless colonizers of the wound or the surrounding skin. Bacteria isolated from a wound swab should not be considered as infecting the wound unless there is also evidence of an infection process occurring in the wound, for example pus, inflammation, **erythema** or fever. A swab need be taken only when the wound exhibits these signs of infection. This is particularly the case in chronic wounds such as pressure sores or ulcers, where wounds may be colonized by several different bacteria with no adverse effect (Gilchrist & Reed 1989).

The most accurate method of identifying micro-organisms causing infection in a wound is by aspiration using a fine needle or biopsy of the underlying tissues (Gilchrist 1996). In practice, these invasive methods are rarely used and the wound swab is the most common means of sampling. To improve the accuracy of the swab, it is probably preferable to take it before the wound is cleaned and whilst the maximum number of bacteria is still present. However, some authors recommend first removing gross exudate by gentle irrigation with saline (Cooper & Lawrence 1996). The swab should be taken directly from the area of the wound suspected to be infected. Swabs taken from dry areas are unlikely to provide useful results. Samples of pus are preferable to swabs as they are likely to provide a more accurate indication of the pathogens present (Public Health Laboratory Service 1997). If **pus** is present it can be drawn up in a sterile syringe and transferred to a sterile container or, if a small amount is present, on to a swab. Most types of swab are accompanied by a tube of transport medium; this will prolong the survival of micro-organisms for several hours and should be refrigerated when immediate transport to the laboratory is not possible. In the laboratory, the swab is spread over an agar plate and the most likely cause of infection is assessed from the numbers of bacteria present.

It is extremely important to label the wound swab accurately, indicating the exact site from which it has been collected. This helps the laboratory predict the types of micro-organisms to expect in the swab and to identify the site of infection should the patient have more than one wound. However, the difficulty of distinguishing between bacteria infecting or colonizing the wound means that the results of wound swabs should be interpreted with caution.

Other swabs

Nose swabs are sometimes necessary to detect carriage of potential pathogenic bacteria such as antibiotic-resistant strains of *Staphylococcus aureus*. A standard swab can be used but should first be moistened in the transport medium or some sterile saline, and then rubbed inside the anterior nares. One swab can be used to sample both nostrils.

Pernasal swab of the nasopharynx is required when whooping cough is suspected and should be taken by a trained member of staff. The swab is fixed on to a long flexible wire and accompanied by charcoal transport medium (see Fig. 2.4).

Throat swabs should be taken by depressing the tongue and gently rubbing the swab over the pillars of the fauces, especially the inflamed area (see Fig. 2.5). Care should be taken to avoid touching other parts of the mouth which may contaminate the swab with other bacteria. The laboratory will examine the swabs for the presence of known pathogens such as streptococci and the bacilli causing diphtheria.

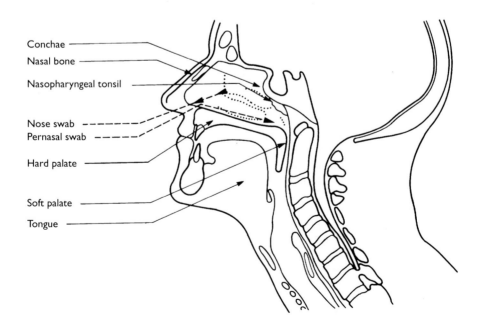

Fig. 2.4 Areas to be swabbed when sampling the nose.

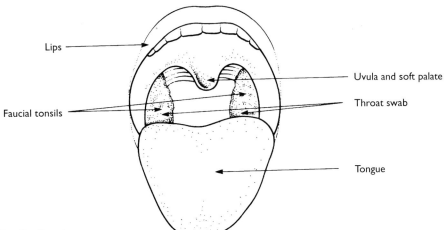

Fig. 2.5 Sampling the throat.

Swabbing exudate from the eye can be used to identify organisms responsible for 'sticky eye' in babies, but conjunctival scrapings are preferred for other infections of the eye (e.g. chlamydia) and these are usually carried out in ophthalmology departments.

Infections of the outer ear can be swabbed carefully, ensuring that the swab is introduced gradually and is not inserted very far. If infection of the inner ear is suspected, a deeper swab is required which should be taken by medical staff using a speculum.

Vaginal swabs should be taken through a vaginal speculum and always sent to the laboratory in transport medium to protect the more fragile pathogens that could be present in the specimen. Investigation for some sexually transmitted diseases requires special transport media.

Occasionally swabs of skin (e.g. groin, axilla) are requested to look for antibiotic-resistant strains of bacteria which may colonize the skin, particularly methicillin-resistant *Staphylococcus aureus* (MRSA) (Ch. 5). Swabs should first be moistened in transport medium or sterile saline solution to improve the efficiency of sampling.

Viruses do not survive well on swabs or in samples. To detect viruses in skin lesions special transport medium, obtained from the laboratory in advance, should be used. The swab should be broken off into the vial and taken to the laboratory as soon as possible.

Skin scrapings for the detection of fungal infections or scabies should be collected by a dermatologist or trained technician.

Blood cultures

A patient with a high fever may have small numbers of the bacteria responsible for the infection circulating in the bloodstream. To identify bacteria in the blood, a sample must be taken very carefully to avoid contamination by skin flora, using a clean needle to inoculate the bottles and cleansing the skin first with alcohol. Blood is inoculated into two bottles, one which supports the growth of anaerobic bacteria, the other **aerobic** bacteria. The bottles must be transported to the laboratory rapidly where they will be incubated for at least a week, but checked daily for signs of growth. Automated monitoring systems are available. As bacteria are not normally present in the blood, any growth from the bottle is usually significant. Some species (e.g. *Staphylococcus epidermidis*) are common skin contaminants, but can infect the blood via intravenous devices, particularly in the immunocompromised. A **Gram stain** will be performed immediately to provide early evidence of the cause of infection. Sometimes a third culture bottle is used containing sulfonate to neutralise antibiotics.

Cerebrospinal fluid (CSF)

In suspected meningitis, specimens should be collected by a spinal tap as aseptically as possible, preferably before antibiotics are commenced. The skin site should be disinfected with an antiseptic solution before the needle is inserted. The specimen should be transported to the laboratory immediately to increase the chance of growing meningococcus, which is extremely fragile. Viral transport medium is not necessary for CSF specimens.

Sampling the environment

Bacteria are normally present in the environment on all types of surface and in the air, and usually present no risk to the patient. The results of sampling of the environment are difficult to interpret, because the number of bacteria isolated is extremely variable and will depend on the exact area sampled. Little is known about what constitutes unacceptably high levels of contamination.

Routine sampling of equipment to demonstrate sterility is generally unnecessary; instead the efficiency of the decontamination process itself should be monitored.

Environmental sampling may be of value in outbreaks of infection where an environmental reservoir of infection may be contributing to spread of the organism (Barrie et al 1992; Ravn et al 1991).

The air quality of operating theatres may sometimes need to be assessed, for example to test the efficacy of the ventilation in newly commissioned theatres. This requires the use of a microbiological air sampler which can measure the number of bacteria per cubic metre of air. Agar 'settle plates', although often used, are not easily interpreted and do not accurately reflect levels of contamination (Holton & Ridgway 1993).

BIOHAZARD LABELS

Laboratory staff regularly handle body fluid specimens containing pathogenic organisms and are therefore at particular risk of acquiring infection.

The use of biohazard labels is recommended to indicate, both to staff who transport the specimens and to the laboratory, specimens that may contain particularly hazardous pathogens (Health Services Advisory Committee 1998) (Plate 2.14). The indication for use of biohazard labels may vary between hospitals but usually they should be applied to specimens known or suspected to contain bloodborne viruses or tuberculosis (Advisory Committee on Dangerous Pathogens 1994). If viral haemorrhagic fever is suspected, special precautions are required in the laboratory and the infection control team must be contacted before specimens are taken (Advisory Committee on Dangerous Pathogens 1996).

TRANSPORT OF SPECIMENS

Potentially infectious material presents a hazard when it is being transported and care must be taken to ensure that risk to other people is kept to a minimum. The Health Services Advisory Committee (1998) recommends procedures for the safe transport of specimens which include carriage in leak-proof boxes and a procedure for dealing with spillages. Specimens to be sent through the post must be specially packaged; advice should be sought from the microbiology laboratory.

The member of staff who collects the specimen has a responsibility to ensure the following:

- the specimen container is leak-proof and securely sealed
- all traces of body fluid have been removed from the outside of the container
- the specimen container is not overfilled
- biohazard labels are placed on the container and form where appropriate
- the specimen is accompanied by a fully completed request form in a separate pocket
- the container is sealed inside a plastic bag

INFORMATION ON REQUEST FORMS

The request form provides a very important source of information for the laboratory staff. It assists them in the identification of the causative organism and indicates factors that may influence the tests and methods to be used. The request form should therefore always be completed accurately.

Of particular importance is an accurate indication of the site of the specimen. Some bacteria may form part of the normal flora in one site of the body and yet be pathogenic if isolated elsewhere. Anaerobes may be a likely cause of infection at some sites (e.g. pressure sores) and require special culture techniques. If the patient is receiving antibiotic therapy, antibiotic present in the specimen may inhibit the growth of bacteria in laboratory cultures and produce misleading results. Ampicillin-resistant klebsiella, an unlikely cause of respiratory tract infection, is commonly isolated from the sputum of patients receiving ampicillin for a chest infection because ampicillin present in the specimen inhibits the growth of the causative organism. The date and time of specimen collection indicates whether prolonged storage has occurred which may change the number of micro-organisms present. A relevant history, including symptoms of infection, suspected site of infection or recent travel abroad can assist in the interpretation of the results and will direct the laboratory to perform a relevant range of tests. For example, information on the nature and frequency of vomiting and diarrhoea should accompany a specimen of faeces.

INTERPRETATION OF LABORATORY REPORTS

The results of a microbiological examination must always be interpreted in combination with a clinical evaluation; without this the microbiological data are often meaningless. Some bacteria isolated from a specimen may be there as part of the normal flora and not capable of causing infection (e.g. diphtheroids in a wound swab). Sometimes bacteria may be present in a specimen as a result of contamination during its collection but, in the absence of clinical signs of infection, antibiotic treatment is not indicated. For example, *Staphylococcus epidermidis* in a blood culture is often significant but in about 25% of cases organisms from the skin contaminate the blood culture bottle, and if the patient is not pyrexial treatment would not be indicated. Where treatment is indicated, the laboratory report provides information on suitable antibiotics to prescribe. Some examples of laboratory report forms are shown in Fig. 2.6.

Advice and information about the interpretation of microbiology laboratory forms can be obtained from the consultant microbiologist.

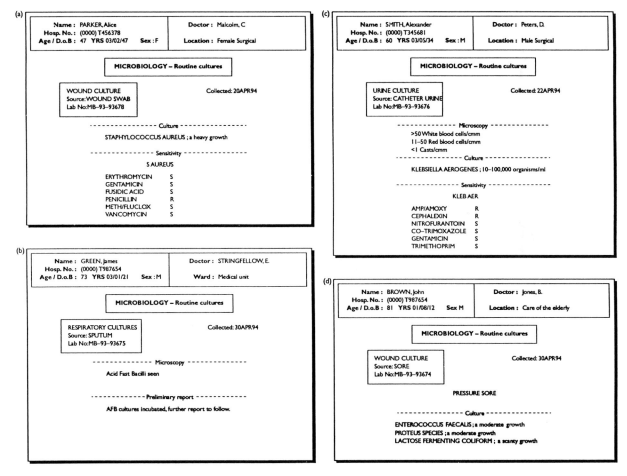

Fig. 2.6 Interpretation of a laboratory request form. (a) The heavy growth of *S. aureus* in this wound indicates that this is the most likely cause of infection. In common with most hospital isolates of this organism it is resistant to penicillin. The exact site of the wound has not been indicated on the request form and this may cause some confusion if the patient has more than one wound. (b) This patient has pulmonary tuberculosis and requires isolation to minimize the risk of cross-infection. Isolation can be discontinued after 2 weeks of treatment; repeat specimens of sputum are not usually necessary. The specimen will now be cultured to determine the species of mycobacterium and antibiotic sensitivities. (c) The presence of klebsiella and a large number of white cells in a specimen of catheter urine is not necessarily unusual. Treatment would be indicated if the patient had signs of infection, for example a pyrexia. The organism is resistant to ampicillin and cephalexin and these antibiotics should not be used to treat the infection. (d) It is not unusual to isolate several different species of bacteria from a chronic wound. Treatment for infection would be indicated only if clinical signs such as pus or inflammation were present.

REFERENCES

Advisory Committee on Dangerous Pathogens (1994) *Categorisation of Biological Agents According to Hazard and Categories of Containment*, 4th edn. HSE Books, Sudbury.

Advisory Committee on Dangerous Pathogens (1996) *The Management and Control of Viral Haemorrhagic Fevers*. The Stationery Office, London.

Ayton M (1982) Microbiological investigations. *Nursing*, **2**(8): 226–30.

Barrie D, Wilson JA, Hoffman PN et al (1992) *Bacillus cereus*, meningitis in two neurosurgical patients: an investigation into the source of the organism. *J. Infect.*, **25**: 291–7.

Bradley C, Babb J, Davies J et al (1986) Taking precautions. *Nursing Times*, **5 March**: 70–3.

Cooper R, Lawrence JC (1996) The isolation and identification of bacteria from wounds. *J. Wound Care*, **5**(7): 335–40.

Garibaldi RA (1993) Hospital-acquired urinary tract infections. In *Prevention and Control of Nosocomial Infections*, 2nd edn (RP Wenzel, ed.), pp. 600–13. Williams and Wilkins, Baltimore, MD.

Gilchrist B (1996) Wound infection. *J. Wound Care*, **5**(8): 386–92.

Gilchrist B, Reed C (1989) The bacteriology of leg ulcers under hydrocolloid dressings. *Br. J. Dermatol.*, **121**: 337–44.

Health Services Advisory Committee (1998) *Safe Working and Prevention of Infection in Clinical Laboratories*. The Stationery Office, London.

Holliday G, Strike PW, Masterton RG (1991) Perineal cleansing and midstream urine specimens in ambulatory women. *J. Hosp. Infect.*, **18**: 71–6.

Holton J, Ridgway GL (1993) Commissioning operating theatres. *J. Hosp Infect.*, **23**: 153–60.

Platt R, Polk BF, Murdock B, Rosner B (1983) Reduction of mortality associated with nosocomial urinary tract infection. *Lancet*, **i**: 893–7.

Public Health Laboratory Service (1997) *Standard Operating Procedure – Investigation of Skin and Superficial Wound Swabs*. B.SOP 11. Issue 1. Technical Services, PHLS, London.

Ravn P, Lundgren JD, Kjaeldgaard et al (1991) Nosocomial outbreak of cryptosporidiosis in AIDS patients. *BMJ*, **302**: 277–80.

Tincello DG, Richmond DH (1998) Evaluation of reagent strips in detecting asymptomatic bacteriuria in early pregnancy: prospective case series. *BMJ*, **316**: 435–7.

FURTHER READING

Glenister H (1983) Diagnosis of the patient and specimen collection. *Nursing*, **2**: 6–7.

McFarlane A (1989) Using the laboratory in infection control. *Prof. Nurse*, **4**(8): 393–7.

McKune I (1989) Catch or bag your specimen? A comparative study of the contamination rates between clean-catch and bag specimens of urine in children aged two years and under. *Nursing Times*, **85**(37): 80–2.

Mims CA, Playfair JHL, Roitt IM et al (1998) *Medical Microbiology*, 2nd edn. Mosby-Year Book, London.

Zaaijer HL, Borg F, Cuypers HTM et al (1994) Comparison of methods for detection of hepatitis B virus DNA. *J. Clin. Microbiol.*, **32**(9): 2088–91.

3

The epidemiology of infection

INTRODUCTION

The term **epidemiology**, derived from the Greek, means the study of things that happen to people. It is used to describe the study of disease and ill-health in human populations, and is particularly concerned with the frequency with which they occur and the factors that influence their distribution.

The interaction between humans and microbes has changed considerably through history. The microbes responsible for the great **epidemics** of the past have largely been controlled through improvements in living conditions, **immunization** and chemotherapy. However, many parts of the world have yet to benefit from our ability to understand and control **infectious** disease, whilst the re-emergence of old diseases such as tuberculosis and the appearance of new diseases, such as acquired immune deficiency syndrome (AIDS) and new variant Creutzfeldt–Jakob disease, present new challenges.

A knowledge of potential sources of micro-organisms and an understanding of how they spread and who may be susceptible to them enables appropriate measures to be taken to prevent transmission of infection. This chapter reviews the epidemiology of infection; it outlines how micro-organisms are spread from person to person and how epidemiology has informed the development of public health services in the UK. Finally it reviews the epidemiology of infection associated with healthcare, and the strategies in place for their prevention and control.

THE INTERACTION BETWEEN MICROBES AND THEIR HOSTS

The surface of the body is densely populated by a wide variety of micro-organisms which use it as their habitat. These micro-organisms are commensals; they live on the host without causing harm and are referred to as the 'normal flora' of the body. The species present at different sites on the body vary according to the local conditions, in particular the availability of nutrients and oxygen and the temperature and humidity (Table 3.1). In many circumstances, the relationship between micro-organisms and their human host is symbiotic; that is, they both gain advantage from it. The key benefit to the host is that the presence of the normal flora prevents other harmful micro-organisms from occupying the surface. This is particularly important in the intestine. In ruminants, bacteria and protozoa living in the stomach are also actively involved in the digestion of cellulose.

Some micro-organisms have a parasitic relationship with their host; they not only use their host as a habitat but actively cause it harm. These harmful effects are recognized as a disease, and micro-organisms able to cause disease are known as pathogens. Pathogens account for only a small proportion of the microbial population, but are often difficult to define because many species are neither always harmful nor always harmless. Bacteroides, which helps to digest cellulose in ruminants, acts as a harmless commensal in the human gut, but can cause infection if it enters damaged tissues following surgery on the bowel. The commensals that make up the normal flora of the body are harmless in their usual habitat but may cause disease if transferred to a different part of the body; for example, *Escherichia coli* from the intestines causes urinary tract infection if it enters the bladder. Disruption of the hosts' normal barriers against infection, for example the insertion of an invasive device through the skin or a urinary catheter into the bladder, can facilitate this process. The ability of a pathogen to cause disease is also affected by the susceptibility of the host. Commensal micro-organisms may cause infection in

people with an impaired immune response. These are known as opportunistic pathogens; an example is *Pneumocystis carinii*, a fungus that is a common commensal of the respiratory tract but which causes a severe pneumonia in an immunocompromised host.

Pathogens may not be a normal commensal of the host, but still inhabit part of the body without causing adverse effects or symptoms of infection. This is described as colonization, and the colonized individual is called a carrier. The carriage may be short lived or may continue indefinitely. In some situations the carrier spreads infection to others. Patients in hospital who are colonized with antibiotic-resistant bacteria provide a source from which the organisms may spread easily to other patients. In extreme examples a carrier can spread infection to many other people; in the late nineteenth century 'Typhoid Mary', a carrier of *Salmonella typhi*, infected 54 people over a period of 10 years through her employment as a cook. Viruses are the ultimate example of a parasite as they are totally dependent on the host for their replication, but can also exist in a latent colonizing form. For example, varicella zoster virus remains dormant in the nerve ganglion following chickenpox infection.

Some pathogens invariably cause disease when they enter a host, although the severity of the infection may vary depending on the susceptibility of the host. Some cause a specific and characteristic disease, for example shigella, which causes an acute diarrhoeal illness called dysentery. Other pathogens can cause a wide variety of infections; for example, *Staphylococcus aureus* can infect the skin, causing abscesses, impetigo and wound infection, but also causes osteomyelitis, pneumonia and gastroenteritis.

The process of infection

The adverse effects caused by pathogens invading and multiplying in tissues are recognized as signs and symptoms of infection. These will vary according to the affected site (Table 3.2). If the invading micro-organisms overcome the local immune defences, systemic symptoms such as fever and malaise may develop. To establish infection the micro-organisms must first be able to resist the defences of the host, such as the gastric acid in the stomach. The susceptibility of the host to infection varies; some individuals may acquire infection through exposure to a smaller dose of the same organisms than others, and people with impaired immune defences are particularly vulnerable to infection (see Ch. 4). Once the defences have been bypassed, several stages in the infection process follow.

Table 3.1 The normal flora of body surfaces

Site of body	Common commensal micro-organisms
Skin	*Staphylococcus epidermidis*, streptococci, corynebacterium (diphtheroids), candida
Throat	*Streptococcus viridans*, diphtheroids
Mouth	*Streptococcus viridans*, *Moraxella catarrhalis*, actinomyces, spirochaetes
Respiratory tract	*Streptococcus viridans*, moraxella, diphtheroids, micrococci
Vagina	Lactobacilli, diphtheroids, streptococci, yeasts
Intestines	Bacteroides, anaerobic streptococci, *Clostridium perfringens*, escherichia, klebsiella, proteus, enterococci

Table 3.2   Symptoms of some common infections

System of the body	Symptoms of infection
Skin	Inflammation Pain Swelling Heat
Respiratory tract	Increased respiratory secretions Cough
Urinary tract	Pain (cystitis) Frequency Urgency
Central nervous system	Confusion Drowsiness Stiff neck Headache
Gastrointestinal tract	Abdominal pain Vomiting Diarrhoea

Box 3.1   Bacterial toxins

Exotoxins
These are proteins secreted by bacteria at the site of infection that may cause adverse effects at other sites if transported in the bloodstream. Some intestinal pathogens release exotoxins called enterotoxins which irritate the mucosal cells causing profuse diarrhoea. *Clostridium botulinum* produces a powerful neurotoxin which, if ingested even in minute amounts, causes paralysis within hours.

Endotoxins
These are lipopolysaccharides (LPS) which form part of the structure of the outer membrane of Gram-negative bacteria. They are released when the cell is destroyed and can cause serious systemic effects such as high fever, hypotension and coagulation defects. These effects, called septic or endotoxic shock, are associated with bloodstream infections caused by Gram-negative bacteria and often result in the death of the patient.

Penetration of tissues   For this to occur, the micro-organisms must first adhere to cells. Bacteria have several mechanisms to facilitate this, for example special hairs on their surface (fimbriae) or extracellular secretions such as slime or dextran. Viruses are able to penetrate cells by recognizing and binding to specific molecules on their surface.

Multiplication   The ability of the invading micro-organisms to multiply will depend on the availability of nutrients and required environmental conditions. The number of micro-organisms introduced can have an important effect on the outcome of the invasion. A few micro-organisms may be easily overpowered by the host defences or by other harmless commensals, and therefore unable to establish infection. Some micro-organisms are able to produce disease even when the infective dose is very low. For example, the ingestion of only a few hundred campylobacter can cause disease as this micro-organism multiplies readily in the gastrointestinal tract. Other gastrointestinal pathogens must be present in high concentration (more than 10^5 per g) in the ingested food to cause infection (e.g. *Clostridium perfringens*).

Spread to other tissues   Some pathogens cause a local infection only at the site of invasion, others may spread to more tissues or invade the bloodstream and be carried to other parts of the body. For example, infection by *Salmonella typhi* begins with symptoms of gastrointestinal infection but may progress to a systemic illness, associated with high fever, when the bacteria invade the bloodstream. Polio virus enters via the gastrointestinal tract but causes paralysis by infecting and destroying motor neuron cells.

Damage to tissues   The invading micro-organisms may damage cells through the release of enzymes (e.g. proteases or collagenases) or toxins, substances that have specific adverse effects on tissues (Box 3.1). The toxin may damage tissue at a site remote from the infection. For example, in diphtheria, the infection remains localized in the upper respiratory tract, but the toxin released by the organisms circulates in the bloodstream and causes serious damage to the heart, nerves and kidneys. Viruses often destroy the host cell as the new viruses are released. The immune response mounted against the infection can also result in damage to the hosts' own cells, with the affected area becoming inflamed and swollen, and invaded cells being destroyed by phagocytes (see p. 66).

Microbial virulence and transmissibility

The ability of an organism to cause disease is described as virulence. Virulence may depend on a number of factors that assist micro-organisms to invade, multiply and cause damage to tissues. These include fimbriae or slime production, which assist adhesion; extracellular enzymes, which facilitate invasion; capsules that confer protection against the immune system; and toxins that cause tissue damage. The genetic information determining these traits may not be carried by all members of a particular species; some strains will therefore be more virulent than others. For example, only strains of *Corynebacterium diphtheriae* able to produce the diphtheria toxin can cause the neurological and cardiac effects associated with the disease.

Some micro-organisms are transmitted readily from person to person and the infections they cause are termed infectious or contagious diseases. The capacity to spread easily may relate to the whole species; for example, varicella zoster virus causes an extremely contagious infection, or may be strain specific. For example, some strains of methicillin-resistant *Staphylococcus aureus* (MRSA) have a greater capacity to spread than others, although the reasons for these differences are unclear (CDR 1997).

SOURCES AND RESERVOIRS OF MICRO-ORGANISMS

Micro-organisms have a **reservoir** where they live, grow and multiply; this may be in the environment, animals or people (Table 3.3). Viruses, which cannot replicate outside living cells, rely on human or animal reservoirs, and survive by passing from one to another. The human body is also the reservoir for many bacteria and fungi that colonize the bowel, skin and respiratory tract. Other micro-organisms, for example clostridium and legionella, normally inhabit the environment in soil, dust or water.

A microbial reservoir can become a source of infection when the micro-organisms have a means of transferring into a susceptible host (see Box 3.2). In clinical settings, environmental reservoirs of micro-organisms are most likely to occur where moisture is present. However, a reservoir does not necessarily become a source of infection. For example, vases of flowers probably contain a variety of potentially **pathogenic Gram-negative** bacteria but since these bacteria are unlikely to find a way out of the vase and into the patient, the vase is an improbable source of infection. Similarly, the outlet pipes and overflows of washbasins are a reservoir of many micro-organisms, particularly Gram-negative bacilli, but these are usually of low pathogenicity, not readily transferred to

Box 3.2   How a reservoir may become a source

Legionella pneumophila normally lives and multiplies in water but if inhaled by a susceptible person may cause a severe pneumonia known as Legionnaires' disease. An ornamental pond may be a reservoir of this micro-organism, but to act as a source of infection aerosols of water droplets that can be inhaled must be generated, for example by a fountain.

susceptible sites on patients, and therefore an unlikely source of infection (Levin et al 1984, Orsi et al 1994).

The most common reservoir and source of micro-organisms in clinical areas are patients themselves, particularly their excretions, secretions and skin lesions. A patient does not need to have an overt infection to act as a source. Transmission may occur during the incubation period before symptoms develop. Even once symptoms have resolved, micro-organisms may continue to be excreted or secreted. Sometimes a person becomes a long-term carrier of the disease. Approximately 10% of people infected by the hepatitis B virus do not completely clear the infection and continue to carry the virus in their blood asymptomatically. *Salmonella typhi* may remain in the gallbladder or kidneys following a gastrointestinal infection and be excreted intermittently in the faeces or urine for months.

Sometimes a person who acquires a micro-organism does not develop infection themselves, but acts as a source of infection to other susceptible individuals. This is a common feature of meningococcal disease. Many people carry *Neisseria meningitidis* asymptomatically in their respiratory tract, but if it is transferred to a susceptible person it can invade the tissues and cause meningococcal meningitis or septicaemia. Reservoirs of colonized patients are also an important factor in the spread of infection caused by antibiotic-resistant micro-organisms such as MRSA and glycopeptide-resistant enterococci.

If the micro-organisms causing an infection are acquired from another person or the environment, this is described as an **exogenous** source and the transmission is referred to as **cross-infection**. For example, streptococcus infecting a leg ulcer may be transferred by the hands of staff to the wound of another patient. **Endogenous** or **self-infection** occurs when a micro-organism **colonizing** a site on the host enters another site and establishes infection. For example, the Gram-negative bacilli of the intestine are a common cause of wound infection following abdominal surgery or of urinary tract infections in catheterized patients. In practice, it can often be very difficult to determine whether an infection has been acquired endogenously or exogenously.

Table 3.3   Examples of reservoirs of human pathogens

Reservoir	Micro-organism	Disease
Environment		
Soil	*Clostridium tetani*	Tetanus
Water	*Legionella pneumophila*	Legionnaires' disease
Animals		
Cow	*Escherichia coli* (toxigenic strains)	Gastroenteritis
Poultry	Salmonella spp.	Gastroenteritis
Humans		
Respiratory tract	Rhinovirus	Common cold
Gut	Rotavirus	Gastroenteritis

Identification of the source of a micro-organism can be important during the investigation and control of outbreaks of infection. Once a source has been found, action can be taken to prevent further transmission (see Box 3.3).

ROUTES OF MICROBIAL TRANSMISSION

To cause disease a **pathogen** must have a way to enter the body – a portal of entry. Once a micro-organism has gained access to the body, it may spread to other tissues and then be expelled by the same or different route – a portal of exit. To transmit to another host it must be able to leave the body via a portal of exit. For example, enteric infections enter via the mouth and leave in the faeces, while micro-organisms that cause respiratory tract infection both enter and are expelled via the mouth and nose (Fig. 3.1). As pathogens leave the body in excretions and secretions, these are important sources of infection.

Micro-organisms use a range of different routes to find new hosts, and a particular microbe may be able to spread by using more than one method. For example, chickenpox may be acquired through inhalation of respiratory droplets or contact with fluid from

Box 3.3   How routinely used equipment became an infection hazard

The problem was first noticed when three patients on the same ward developed wound infections caused by an antibiotic-resistant strain of klebsiella. Despite strict isolation, new cases of the same infection occurred in other wards. A wide range of ward equipment, including ventilators, humidifiers and suction equipment, was investigated to identify the source of the organism. The resistant klebsiella was found on a portable electric suction pump and immediately all other portable pumps were removed and examined in the laboratory. The organism was found in the collection bottles, internal tubing, filters, oil reservoirs and exhaust outlet of six of the seven pumps.

The suction pumps had been used for draining wound cavities and had been shared between several wards. Of the 66 patients affected by this organism, 80% had been nursed in areas where the portable suction had been used. The suction pumps became contaminated because drainage fluids were allowed to overfill the collection bottles and because filters designed to prevent contamination were not replaced regularly.

The equipment was sterilized, improved air filters and overflow prevention devices were introduced and no further cases of infection were reported (Davies & Blenkharn 1987).

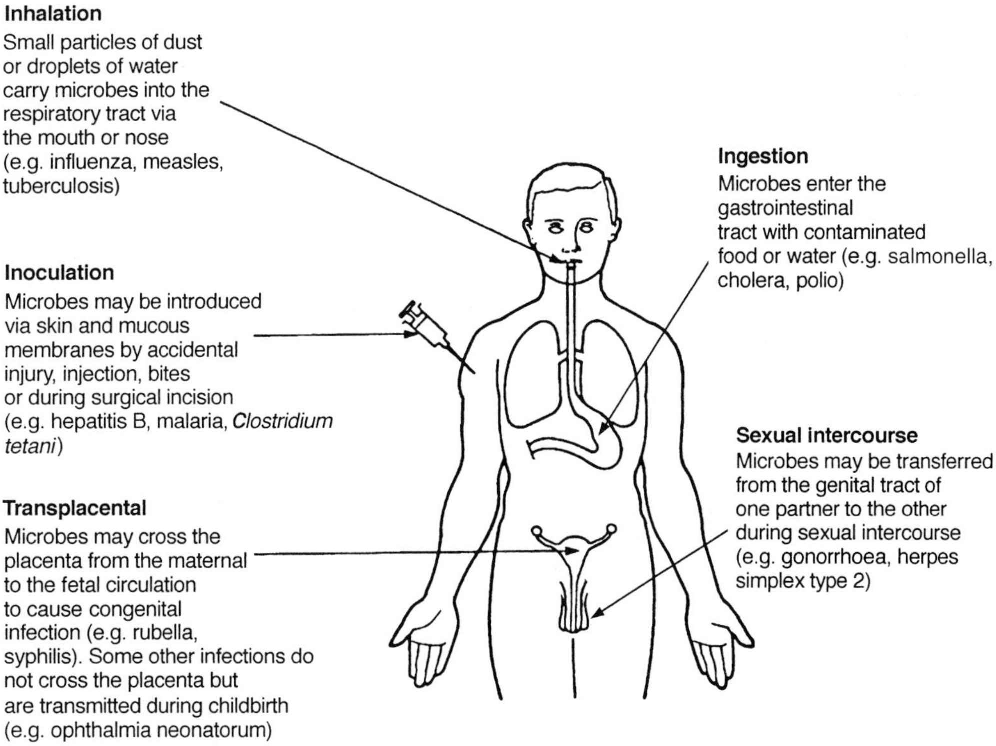

Inhalation
Small particles of dust or droplets of water carry microbes into the respiratory tract via the mouth or nose (e.g. influenza, measles, tuberculosis)

Inoculation
Microbes may be introduced via skin and mucous membranes by accidental injury, injection, bites or during surgical incision (e.g. hepatitis B, malaria, *Clostridium tetani*)

Transplacental
Microbes may cross the placenta from the maternal to the fetal circulation to cause congenital infection (e.g. rubella, syphilis). Some other infections do not cross the placenta but are transmitted during childbirth (e.g. ophthalmia neonatorum)

Ingestion
Microbes enter the gastrointestinal tract with contaminated food or water (e.g. salmonella, cholera, polio)

Sexual intercourse
Microbes may be transferred from the genital tract of one partner to the other during sexual intercourse (e.g. gonorrhoea, herpes simplex type 2)

Fig. 3.1   Routes of microbial invasion.

the lesions. However, micro-organisms cannot move themselves from one host to another. They cannot fly or jump, but transmit either as a result of direct physical contact or indirectly using another person, animal or inanimate object (fomite). Establishing the source and route of transmission of a particular micro-organism is clearly important if the appropriate control measures are to be instituted. For example, pulmonary tuberculosis is known to be transmitted from an infected person through the inhalation of airborne droplet nuclei expelled from the respiratory tract. Effective control therefore depends on ventilation to ensure dilution of airborne droplet nuclei and prompt treatment of the infected person to reduce the number of droplet nuclei expelled from the respiratory tract. Fomites play no part in the transmission of this micro-organism and therefore do not require special control measures.

Transmission by direct contact

Micro-organisms may spread to a susceptible host as a result of direct contact with body surfaces or fluids of an infected individual. There are several examples of this type of transmission. They include infections transmitted from mother to baby in utero (e.g. rubella), sexually transmitted diseases such as *Neisseria gonorrhoeae*, and infections transmitted by direct contact with respiratory secretions, for example by sneezing respiratory droplets on to the mucous membranes of others or kissing (e.g. glandular fever and respiratory viruses). Some infections, such as *Clostridium tetani*, may be acquired directly from the environment as a result of injury.

Transmission by indirect contact

Many micro-organisms are transferred from their reservoirs to a new host indirectly on people, animals or inanimate objects. In clinical settings, indirect transmission may involve vehicles such as hands, equipment, food and water, or airborne particles. Common-source transmission is where infection is acquired by several people following exposure to the same contaminated item, such as food, water or equipment. Indirect transmission by vectors (insects or animals) also occurs but is an unusual mode of transmission in hospitals.

Hands

The first clear indication of the important role that hands play in the transmission of infection emanated from the work of Semmelweis in the 1850s. Semmelweis noticed that puerperal fever was more common on the maternity ward where the medical students worked than on the ward where midwives provided care. He thought that the medical students might be transferring the disease on their hands from cadavers they were dissecting, and ordered that they must wash their hands in chlorinated lime after dissection and before examining patients. This simple measure resulted in a dramatic reduction in the rates of infection and mortality. Later, he ordered that hands should be washed between examinations of all patients to prevent cross-infection within wards (Jarvis 1994, Newsom 1993).

Unfortunately, until the late 1960s, the significance of hands as vectors of hospital-acquired infection was not fully appreciated and airborne transmission was considered more important. This view was changed by a study published in 1966 (Mortimer et al 1966) in which babies in the same nursery were divided into two groups attended by different staff. Although both groups occupied the same room, transmission of staphylococci occurred mostly between babies in the same group. When hands were not washed after handling the babies, the rate of transmission was even greater. The results strongly implicated hands as the main vector of infection whilst illustrating that air was not a significant route of transmission.

Microbes acquired on hands through contact with excretions, secretions or infected lesions are readily transferred to another host by touch (Mackintosh & Hoffman 1984) (see p. 135). This type of contact is probably responsible for the transmission of a large number of infections, particularly among hospital patients where healthcare workers have frequent and intimate contact with secretions and excretions of patients (Conly et al 1989, Larson 1988, Reybrouck 1983, Sanderson & Weissler 1992). Most micro-organisms acquired on the hands are not able to survive for long and are usually transferred rapidly to the next object or patient that is touched. Some species, including antibiotic-resistant strains of klebsiella and acinetobacter, have been found to survive for several hours (Casewell & Desai 1983, Musa et al 1990), providing plenty of opportunity for them to be transferred to another patient.

Food or water

Some bacteria, viruses and protozoa may be transmitted by food or water. Many foods are contaminated by pathogens in their raw state and, if these are not destroyed by thorough cooking, will cause infection when the food is eaten. Food may also be indirectly contaminated by hands in what is described as a faecal–oral route of transmission (Fig. 3.2). The microbe is ingested, causes gastrointestinal infection and is excreted in faeces. Transmission to another host occurs when the infected person contaminates his or her hands with micro-organisms in their faeces, and the hands transfer the organism to food which is then ingested by someone else. Food that is cooked, handled prior to ingestion and then eaten cold, such as cold meats, desserts, sandwiches, salads, etc., may easily be contaminated by an errant food-handler with poor hand hygiene and could easily transmit infection as the organism will not be destroyed by further cooking. Food that is cooked after handling is less likely to transmit infection because the organisms will be destroyed unless the **inoculum** is extremely large and the food not cooked thoroughly.

Water may be readily contaminated by faecal pathogens and must be filtered and treated with chemicals to ensure that it does not transmit infection. Common waterborne infections include *Vibrio cholerae* (the bacterium that causes cholera), giardia and cryptosporidium. Gastrointestinal viruses such as Norwalk virus can contaminate shellfish grown near to sewage outlets.

In hospitals, hydrotherapy pools or other treatment baths may transmit infection if water filtration or chlori-nation is inadequate. The presence of agitation channels that are difficult to disinfect are a particular hazard (Hollyoak et al 1995). The risk is particularly great where patients using the pool are faecally incontinent or have infected wounds, as the warm water will encourage the growth of micro-organisms contaminating the water.

Airborne particles

Contrary to popular belief, microbes cannot travel through the air on their own but may be carried on airborne particles, such as dust, water or respiratory droplets.

Dust Dust is largely composed of skin squames and lint fibres released from clothing and other fabrics. Skin squames are flat flakes of dead skin about 10–20 µm in diameter, which are shed from the surface of the skin into the air at a rate of about 300 million per day. The rate of release is particularly high during movement, when 10^4 skin squames may be shed from one person in a minute (Hambraeus 1988). About 10% of these squames carry micro-organisms. The larger particles of dust settle within a few minutes on to exposed horizontal surfaces such as the floor, furniture and equipment. Small particles may remain airborne for several hours and microbes carried on them may be inhaled into the respiratory tract or settle into wounds. Most

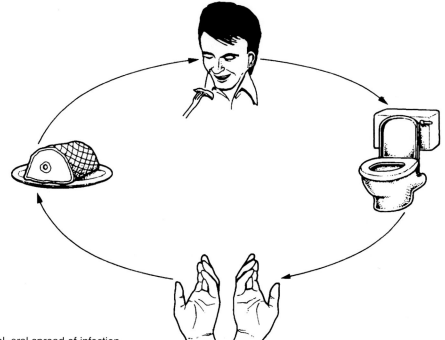

Fig. 3.2 Faecal–oral spread of infection.

micro-organisms cannot survive for long on dust particles. However, bacteria that form spores may survive for many months. The spores of *Clostridium difficile* are released from the faeces of infected patients who have diarrhoea. If allowed to accumulate in dust, the environment may act as a source of infection (Hoffman 1993), although there is little evidence that spread occurs in relation to geographical location of patients (Johnson et al 1990). Some species of fungus release spores into the air, which can remain airborne for prolonged periods and gain access to buildings from the outside. Whilst most of these fungal spores are not harmful to humans, aspergillus can cause serious infection if inhaled by immunocompromised patients (Rhame 1998).

The main significance of airborne dust particles is in the operating department where there is a strong correlation between the numbers of airborne particles and the number of personnel in the operating room. **Pathogens** carried on these particles may settle into the wound or on to surgical instruments and subsequently cause wound infection (Howarth 1985, Whyte et al 1982). Barrie et al (1992) reported an outbreak of surgical wound infection caused by *Bacillus cereus*, where this spore-forming bacterium probably entered surgical wounds on airborne lint particles released from contaminated scrub-suits. In wards, activities such as bedmaking can increase the number of bacteria carried in the air, although they will settle rapidly on to surfaces (Overton 1988).

Respiratory droplets Droplets of saliva are expelled from the respiratory tract by coughing, sneezing and talking. These droplets may contain a small number of pathogenic organisms from the respiratory tract. The large droplets (more than 0.1 mm in diameter) fall to the ground within a few seconds and are not inhaled. Small droplets (less than 0.1 mm in diameter) evaporate rapidly to a size of between 1 and 10 µm in diameter. These very small particles, called droplet nuclei, can remain airborne for hours and be inhaled in the same way as small dust particles, and carried deep into the alveoli of the lungs.

Although some infections are transmitted by respiratory particles in the air, most notably *Mycobacterium tuberculosis* (Riley et al 1959), the probability of inhaling particles carrying pathogenic organisms is quite low. Many respiratory infections are more commonly transmitted through contact with respiratory secretions, for example on tissues, handkerchiefs and hands (Ansari et al 1991). Pathogens in droplets expelled on to the hand that covers the sneezer's mouth will be readily passed on to others unless they are removed by handwashing.

Water droplets The inhalation of aerosols of contaminated water may also transmit infection. The bacterium *Legionella pneumophila* commonly colonizes static water and is responsible for the respiratory infection, Legionnaires' disease (see pp. 112, 207). Infection is acquired through inhalation of aerosols generated from contaminated water sources by fountains, whirlpools, showers or air-conditioning systems (Bartlett et al 1986).

Inanimate objects and equipment

Inanimate objects that become contaminated with pathogenic bacteria and then spread infection to others are often referred to as **fomites**. These objects include beds, curtains, bedclothes, toys, bedpans and sphygmomanometers. Most micro-organisms are not able to survive in the absence of moisture, warmth and nutrients. The presence of pathogenic micro-organisms on a range of fomites is frequently reported during outbreaks of infection. However, it is usually difficult to establish whether these micro-organisms have a role in transmission or are there as a result of contamination of the environment by the patient. Unless the micro-organisms are able to multiply on the fomite, the numbers present are unlikely to be sufficient to transmit infection in most situations (Rhame 1986). An important exception are some respiratory and gastrointestinal viruses, where contamination of the environment has been implicated in transmission and may occur as a result of touching the mouth or nose after handling contaminated objects (Green et al 1998, Hall and Douglas 1981, Patterson et al 1997). Provided that equipment is kept clean and dry bacteria will not be able to multiply and their presence on surfaces will be transitory. Occasionally, outbreaks of infection associated with inadequate decontamination of fomites have been reported (Barrie et al 1994). Hands may acquire micro-organisms when handling heavily contaminated fomites, for example during bedmaking or through handling used linen or equipment in the sluice (Ansari et al 1991, Sanderson & Weissler 1992).

Wet environments present a particular hazard. Some bacteria, particularly pseudomonas, acinetobacter and other Gram-negative bacilli, are able to survive and multiply easily in moisture, which may become a source of infection. Equipment that is filled with fluid, for example humidifiers, bowls of disinfectant or wash bowls, is particularly prone to contamination (Gormon et al 1993, Greaves 1985). Again it is important to distinguish between sources and reservoirs. Many bacteria may be found in a washbasin but are unlikely to be transferred to a patient, whereas bacteria contaminating a nebulizer chamber are highly likely to be inhaled into the respiratory tract of the patient (see Box 3.4).

Most outbreaks of infection associated with inanimate objects are caused by items that should be sterile but have been inadequately decontaminated. Instruments that enter sterile parts of the body or are in close contact with mucous membranes present particular cross-infection hazards. Infection can also be transmitted by accidental injury with a sharp contamined instrument such as the transmission of bloodborne viruses following a needlestick injury (see p. 119).

Animal and insect vectors

Some micro-organisms are spread by animal or insect vectors. Cockroaches, ants, rats or mice are often blamed for transmission of infection by carrying pathogens on the surface of their bodies, but there is little evidence to substantiate such claims. The main significance of these pests is in food preparation areas where severe infestation may result in the contamination of food with enteric pathogens.

Other animals and insects act as a reservoir for human pathogens and transmit disease by bites. For example, rickettsia, which causes typhus, is carried by lice (human and rat lice) and transmitted by their bites. Malaria (a protozoon) and yellow fever (a virus) are transmitted by the bite of mosquitoes. In some cases

humans act as a host for part of the life cycle of an animal (e.g. parasitic worms).

EPIDEMIC AND ENDEMIC INFECTION

Within a population a disease can be *endemic* (i.e. it is always present at a static level) or *epidemic* (i.e. a definite increase in the incidence of the disease above its normal or **endemic** level).

A typical epidemic curve shows a gradual increase in the number of infections until all the susceptible individuals have become infected, followed by a fairly rapid decline in new cases of infection (Fig. 3.3a). Some epidemics occur every few years, for example whooping cough and measles. Children who are not **immune** through previous exposure or **vaccination** may acquire the infection. When all susceptible children have been infected, the number of new cases falls. Three to five years later there will be another increase in infections among the new population of non-immune children.

Other infections are associated with seasonal epidemics, for example influenza, rotavirus and chickenpox (Fig. 3.3b). Infections that induce long-term **immunity** usually cause epidemics amongst the very young or elderly who have either not been previously exposed or have a diminished immunity.

Epidemics of infection associated with a single exposure to infection (e.g. food poisoning) present with a sudden rise in the number of infections followed by a rapid fall. If the infection can be transmitted to others from infected individuals during the incubation period, then a second epidemic due to cross-infection may follow shortly after the first (Fig. 3.3c).

Two measures are commonly used to represent the occurrence of a disease within a population. A **prevalence** rate measures the number of infections present in a particular population at a particular time, for example 'the number of patients who have an infection on a particular ward on a specific day expressed as a percentage of the total number of patients on the ward on that day'. An **incidence** rate measures the number of new infections that occur in a particular population over a specified period of time, for example 'the number of patients who develop surgical wound infections during the year expressed as a percentage of the total number of operations performed during the same time'. Sometimes it is necessary to take account of the period of exposure to a particular risk. For example, the rate of bloodstream infection associated with intravenous devices may be

---

Box 3.4   The problem with mattresses...

Despite strict isolation precautions, infections caused by an antibiotic-resistant strain of acinetobacter continued to colonize and infect patients on the burns and intensive care units. Whilst investigating the source of this organism, it was noticed that one patient's bedlinen was wet, yet she was not incontinent or perspiring and there was no leakage from her burns. When the linen was removed, a badly stained mattress cover was revealed and inside it the mattress was found to be wet. Further investigation found 23 mattresses with stained covers and all stained parts were no longer impermeable to fluid. Bacteria were isolated from inside 15 mattresses and the resistant strain of acinetobacter was found in nine. The damage to the mattress covers may have been related to the use of phenolic disinfectants to clean the mattress cover and silver nitrate applied to burns. No further cases of the resistant acinetobacter occurred once the stained mattresses had been replaced, a regular system of mattress inspection implemented, and the use of phenolic agents to clean mattresses discontinued (Loomes 1988).

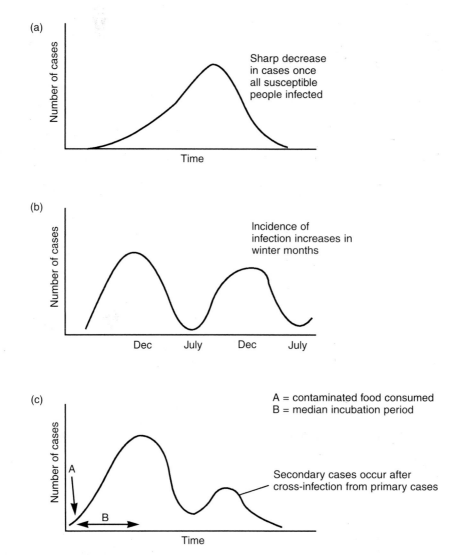

Fig. 3.3 Epidemic curves. (a) Classical epidemic curve. (b) Seasonal epidemic. (c) Single point epidemic of food poisoning with secondary spread by cross-infection.

expressed as the number of infections per 100 days of device use (see Box 3.5).

INFECTION ACQUIRED IN THE COMMUNITY

The principles of epidemiology were first recognized in the time of Hippocrates, 300 years BC. In Britain, the first form of record-keeping began in the early sixteenth century with the introduction of 'Bills of Mortality' which provided information on deaths and disease. Epidemics of disease such as plague, typhus, smallpox and syphilis were commonplace in the Middle Ages

and, although some attempts to control spread through quarantine were employed, the widespread belief that diseases were punishment from God prevailed for hundreds of years.

Giralano Fracastoro, who published *De Contagione* in 1546, realized that disease could be transmitted by contact with sick people, their bedding and excreta, or through the air. The connection between **contagious** disease and the bacteria first seen under van Leeuwenhoek's microscope was not universally accepted until Louis Pasteur and Robert Koch began the study of micro-organisms in the late nineteenth century. These two scientists had to overturn the widespread

---

Box 3.5 Prevalence and incidence of infection

Prevalence rate
This measures the number of people in a population who have the disease or infection at a given time.

Incidence rate
This measures the number of new cases of a disease or infection that occur in a population over a specified period of time. It can be expressed as a risk (the proportion of people who develop one or more infections) or a ratio (the number of infections that occur within the given population). The ratio takes into account the fact that the same person may develop the infection more than once.

Relationship between prevalence and incidence
The prevalence rate depends on the incidence of the disease and duration of illness. Chronic diseases are more likely to be detected at a given point in time, and their prevalence will therefore be relatively larger than the incidence within a given population.

---

and strongly held belief in evil humours released by decomposing matter and dirt as the cause of disease.

Pasteur was able to prove that **fermentation** was initiated by microbes and that cultures of anthrax bacillus would cause the disease in sheep. Koch demonstrated that microbes were responsible for anthrax and tuberculosis. He isolated the microbes from infected tissue, cultured them outside the body, reinfected another animal with the culture and finally recovered the same microbes from the animal. Once the link between micro-organisms and human disease was established, other workers studied immunization as a method of protection against infection and the use of antimicrobial drugs to kill microbes without harming the host.

The public health reform acts

The progress made in the understanding of microbiology had an enormous effect on the control of infectious disease, but of parallel importance was the revolution in public health that took place in the second half of the nineteenth century. The Industrial Revolution of the 1800s brought with it rapid development of towns, which were built with no provision for water supply or sewage drainage. These newly industrialized towns, with overcrowded, squalid conditions, and sewage and rotting carcasses filling the streets, were associated with frequent epidemics of disease, particularly typhus, typhoid fever, cholera, smallpox, scarlet fever and measles. Infant mortality of 200 deaths per 1000 births was recorded in some places.

The cholera epidemic of 1831, which killed 60 000 people in Britain, mostly those living in poor and densely populated areas, resulted in demands for action to improve the living conditions of the poor. The Poor Law Commission was established in 1832 to consider how the Poor Laws should be amended. Edwin Chadwick, a barrister, was appointed Secretary to the Poor Law Commissioners. His report in 1842 on 'The sanitary condition of the labouring population of Great Britain' highlighted the problems of inadequate sewage disposal, pointed to contaminated water as a cause of disease, and suggested that a network of earthenware pipes, flushed with running water, should be used to drain sewage away. It also recommended the removal of refuse, improvement of water supplies and street cleansing. This report had an immense impact, although it was some years before the Act for Promoting Public Health was passed in 1848, in response. This Act established the role of district medical officers responsible for initiating sanitary improvements and inspectors to monitor their implementation.

Unfortunately, the provisions in this first Public Health Act were not obligatory and it was not until Gladstone became Prime Minister in 1868 that a national Public Health Service was created by parliamentary acts in 1872 and 1875. These acts resulted in the appointment of Medical Officers for Health (MOH) in each local authority. The MOH was responsible for all aspects of public health including sewage disposal, water supply, food hygiene, infectious disease control, child welfare, maternity and venereal disease clinics, the school medical service and, until the formation of the National Health Service (NHS) in 1948, the municipal hospitals.

The compulsory registration of births and deaths, enacted in 1836, enabled accurate data to be produced on which decisions about public health issues could be made. Between 1840 and 1900, the death rate in Britain fell from 25 to 15 per 1000 and life expectancy increased from 40 to 50 years. By the end of the nineteenth century the combined effects of improved standards of hygiene, nutrition, drinking water supply and sewage control virtually eliminated the threat of epidemic disease in developed countries. Today, vaccination is widely used to control the spread of many infectious diseases, but different challenges in disease control develop as a result of changes in lifestyles. For example, the increase in sexual freedom has been associated with a rise in sexually transmitted diseases and the emergence of human immunodeficiency virus.

The public health service of today

In the 1970s, the NHS was restructured and many of the community health services previously under the control of the local authority moved to the newly formed District Health Authorities (DHAs). Monitoring of environmental services such as water and sewage supply, food hygiene and housing remained with the local authorities within Environmental Health Departments. The old Public Health Inspectors became Environmental Health Officers (EHOs). The EHOs also retained responsibility for the control of communicable disease and food poisoning within the community. The office of MOH was abolished and replaced by a Medical Officer for Environmental Health (MOEH) employed by the health authorities. The medical specialty of community medicine was established to train doctors in all aspects of public health and the planning of health services.

Since 1988, the monitoring of disease and the investigation of outbreaks of infection have been the responsibility of the health authorities (Health Boards in Scotland). Each health authority appoints a Director of Public Health (DPH) to advise it, the local authority and the general public on issues related to public health. The DPH is also closely involved in drawing up health improvement programmes for local communities and in the planning and development of local services. The Consultant in Communicable Disease Control (CCDC) (Consultant in Public Health Medicine, Communicable Disease and Environmental Health in Scotland) works with the DPH and has responsibility for monitoring, preventing and controlling outbreaks of infection. The CCDC will liaise between the Environmental Health Officers of the local authority, who have responsibility for food hygiene and pollution control within the local area, and the health authority. They are also designated as 'proper officer' to whom cases of infectious disease must be notified (NHS Management Executive 1993).

The regional offices of the NHS Executive, together with the regional DPHs, have an important role in overseeing the work of the NHS locally and in monitoring the progress of local health improvement programmes (Department of Health 1998a). Regional epidemiologists are based in the regional offices of the NHS Executive and have a role in monitoring the occurrence of disease within the local community and in providing expert advice on prevention and control.

Notification of infectious disease

A system of recording cases of infectious disease was recognized as an essential part of the control of epidemics in the early 1900s. Local authorities have a statutory responsibility to control infectious diseases within their boundaries, and to facilitate this some diseases must be notified to the Proper Officer, usually by the doctor who makes the diagnosis. Box 3.6 shows the infectious diseases that are notifiable in England and Wales, and in Scotland.

There are several reasons why notifications of infectious disease are necessary. First, close family or other contacts may have been exposed to the infection and require treatment or monitoring for signs of infection (e.g. tuberculosis, meningococcal meningitis). Second, the infection may have been acquired from contaminated food or water and require investigation to identify the source of infection (e.g. food poisoning).

Box 3.6 Notifiable diseases

Public Health (Control of Diseases) Act 1984
Cholera
Food poisoning
Plague
Relapsing fever
Smallpox
Typhus

Public Health (Infectious Diseases) Regulations 1988

Acute encephalitis	Ophthalmia neonatorum
Acute poliomyelitis	Paratyphoid fever
Anthrax	Rabies
Diphtheria	Rubella
Dysentery	Scarlet fever
Leprosy	Tetanus
Leptospirosis	Tuberculosis
Malaria	Typhoid fever
Measles	Viral haemorrhagic fever
Meningitis	Viral hepatitis
Meningococcal	Whooping cough
septicaemia	Yellow fever
Mumps	

Local authorities have the power to add to, or subtract from, this list in order to prevent the spread of infectious diseases. Acquired immune deficiency syndrome is not a notifiable disease but doctors are asked to report cases to a voluntary, confidential scheme at the Communicable Disease Surveillance Centre. Sexually transmitted diseases are reported anonymously by genitourinary clinics to the Department of Health.

Additional diseases notifiable in Scotland

Chickenpox	*Foodborne infections*
Erysipelas	Botulism
Legionellosis	Brucellosis
Lyme disease	Campylobacter
Membranous croup	Cryptosporidiosis
Puerperal fever	*Escherichia coli* 0157
Toxoplasmosis	Giardiasis
	Listeriosis
	Q fever
	Rotavirus
	Salmonellosis
	Yersiniosis

Finally, the information is analysed and used at both a local and national level to monitor fluctuations in the levels of infection and the effect of vaccination programmes, to detect epidemics at an early stage and to inform the planning of preventive programmes.

Public Health Laboratory Service (PHLS)

A network of laboratories providing microbiological services to local public health departments was established during the Second World War. These laboratories are distributed throughout England and Wales, many on the site of NHS hospitals.

PHLS laboratories provide comprehensive clinical, public health and microbiological services. They can provide advice in the investigation and control of outbreaks of infection and use specialized techniques to culture food, water and environmental specimens. Reference laboratories specialize in the identification and typing of a range of micro-organisms. Many of these reference laboratories are sited at the Central Public Health Laboratory in Colindale, London.

The Communicable Disease Surveillance Centre (CDSC)

The CDSC is based at the headquarters of the PHLS in Colindale, London. It receives data on a voluntary basis from laboratories and CCDCs throughout England and Wales. Its main role is to analyse and disseminate data on communicable diseases. It provides epidemiological expertise and assistance in the investigation and management of major outbreaks of infection. Data on the incidence of infectious diseases are published weekly in the *Communicable Disease Report*. The CDSC also provides advice and information about infectious diseases to public health departments and local authorities.

In Scotland, the Scottish Centre for Infection and Environmental Health (SCIEH) is responsible for monitoring infection, publishing data (in the *SCIEH Weekly Report*), and providing expert advice on the investigation and control of outbreaks.

INFECTION ASSOCIATED WITH HEALTHCARE

A **nosocomial** or **hospital-acquired infection** (HAI) is any infection that develops as a result of hospital treatment from which the patient was not suffering or incubating at the time of admission to hospital. The types of infection acquired by patients in hospital are usually quite different from those acquired at home.

The risks of infection associated with hospitalization have been recognized for thousands of years. Before the development of effective antimicrobial agents, the mortality rate due to infection following surgical intervention was extremely high. Advances in technology have enabled many patients with previously fatal conditions to be treated, and an increasing proportion of healthcare is now provided in the community rather than in hospitals. However, the use of invasive devices and immunosuppressive therapy increases patients' vulnerability to infection.

Occasionally epidemics of HAI occur as a result of a breakdown of infection control procedures or spread from a patient with an infectious disease. In recent years, strains of bacteria resistant to antimicrobial agents have emerged. The infections they cause can be extremely difficult to treat and preventing their transmission is of paramount importance.

Historical perspective of HAI

Hospitals for the sick existed in the civilized world as early as 500 BC, in particular in Asia, Egypt, Palestine and Greece. The standards of hygiene in these early hospitals were based on religious rituals and were far superior to those found in the hospitals of later centuries. Patients were generally housed in separate beds or rooms, good ventilation was considered essential, and many of the rudiments of infection control were practised, such as not touching wounds, isolation of infected patients and use of cleaning and hot ovens to 'sterilize' instruments (Selwyn 1991).

Unfortunately, after the fall of the Roman Empire, standards deteriorated because of the influence of Christianity, which was associated with an aversion to washing and an absence of laws on hygiene. Severe overcrowding, with several patients sharing one bed, and poor ventilation were features of hospitals until the late nineteenth century, and it is therefore not surprising that the mortality rate due to infection was extremely high and death rates from postoperative infection of more than 50% were frequently reported.

John Simpson, Professor of Medicine and Midwifery at Edinburgh University and an early advocate of infection control measures, made a detailed study of the epidemiology and prevention of 'surgical fever'. He observed a significantly higher rate of infection amongst patients operated on in hospital than in those operated on by a country surgeon (Simpson 1869).

Various attempts over the centuries to implement simple infection control measures met with considerable opposition. Many doctors recommended cleanliness of clothes, hands and dressings, but surgeons preferred to blame 'intrinsic defects' in the patient or the 'atmosphere'. An increasing understanding of bacteria, asepsis and transmission of disease, combined with improvements in hospital conditions introduced by Florence Nightingale, finally brought HAI under some control by the end of the nineteenth century (Nightingale 1863). In the 1940s, further reductions in the incidence of HAI were associated with the emergence of antimicrobial drugs as effective treatments for infection.

In the early twentieth century, streptococcus was the main problem of cross-infection. Later, in the 1950s, this was replaced by staphylococci, already resistant to a number of antibiotics. The HAI problems of today reflect the nature of the hospital population: highly susceptible patients who in the past would have died from their illness and extensive use of invasive procedures – each with an attendant risk of infection.

The development of an organized structure within hospitals to prevent and control infection began in the 1940s with the appointment of part-time Control of Infection Officers and the formation of Infection Control Committees. In 1959 the first Infection Control Nurse was appointed to provide a full-time infection control service. The increasing complexity of medical care, the cost of HAI and the effects of adverse outbreaks of HAI (Fig. 3.4) have established infection control as an essential hospital service (Department of Health 1995).

Factors that affect the risk of acquiring infection in hospital

Healthcare exposes patients to an increased risk of infection. This risk is particularly high when care is provided in a hospital setting, where contact with healthcare staff and equipment occurs frequently and other patients may act as a source of infection. However, although patients in hospital are likely to be exposed to more factors that increase their risk of infection, the boundaries between hospital and community care are no longer clearcut. Day-case procedures now account for a significant proportion of surgery and, even where an inpatient stay is required, the length of time spent in hospital after operation has reduced markedly (Goodman 1997). In 1974 the average postoperative stay was 9 days, compared with 4.5 days in 1997. Similarly, patients in elderly care now spend an average of 19 days in hospital, compared with 100 days in 1974

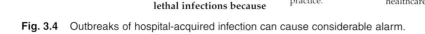

Fig. 3.4   Outbreaks of hospital-acquired infection can cause considerable alarm.

(Appleby 1997). Distinguishing infections acquired in hospital from those acquired in the community may not be possible. Patients with invasive devices such as urinary catheters or central vascular catheters may be cared for in their own homes, and others receive treatment at home for chronic illnesses such as renal disease or cystic fibrosis. The principles of infection prevention and control are therefore applicable in both hospital and community settings, although adaptation for local circumstances may be necessary.

There are several factors associated with healthcare that increase vulnerability to infection and these are described below.

Underlying disease

The ability of the immune system to respond to infection may be affected by severe underlying diseases such as carcinoma or leukaemia, and immunosuppressive therapy. Some conditions (e.g. diabetes or vascular disease) affect the perfusion of the skin, leading to poor wound healing or tissue necrosis and increased susceptibility to infection. Symptoms of the disease process may also increase the risk of infection; for example, faecal incontinence increases vulnerability to urinary tract infection.

Extremes of age

The immature immune system of neonates and young children increases their susceptibility to infection. Immunity may also gradually be lost with increasing age, so that the elderly are likely to be susceptible to infections such as rotavirus, first encountered in childhood, and reactivation of chronic infection such as varicella zoster or tuberculosis.

Breach of defence mechanisms

The natural defences of the body, which protect us against invasion by micro-organisms, are frequently damaged or breached as a result of hospital treatment. The integrity of the skin may be interrupted by surgery, intravascular or other invasive devices, or debicutous ulceration. Intubation or respiratory ventilation may bypass the activity of cilia in the upper respiratory tract, and normally sterile organs may be exposed to contamination by invasive procedures such as urinary catheterization and endoscopy. Antibiotic therapy may destroy bacteria that normally colonize and protect mucosal surfaces, enabling harmful micro-organisms to establish infection.

Exposure to infection

Places where many people are in close proximity with one another encourage the spread of disease. However, the problem is exacerbated in hospitals because of the regular and intimate contact that occurs between patients and healthcare workers, and which enables micro-organisms to transfer from person to person. A patient may have contact with many different healthcare workers, for example nurses, doctors, physiotherapists, occupational therapists, social workers and porters.

Hospital pathogens

Antimicrobial therapy is a common feature of hospital care, both for treatment and for prevention of infection. Types of micro-organisms intrinsically resistant to commonly used antimicrobial agents (e.g. enterococci, pseudomonads and strains that have acquired genetic determinants of resistance (e.g. MRSA) are favoured in this environment. Patients admitted to hospital, particularly those who are critically ill, rapidly change their normal bacterial flora for these more resistant organisms (Noone et al 1983). A patient previously treated with antimicrobial therapy may be more likely to develop infection with resistant micro-organisms, such as glycopeptide-resistant enterococci, *Clostridium difficile*. Once infection or colonization has established, the organisms may be transferred to other patients in close proximity (Casewell & Desai 1983, Wade et al 1991).

Patients who are critically ill are also more vulnerable to a range of pathogens that are unlikely to cause infection in the healthy. *Staphylococcus epidermidis* causes 20% of bacteraemia in hospital patients, normally in association with intravenous devices (PHLS 2000b). Candida takes advantage of a normal flora altered by antimicrobial therapy and is an increasingly common cause of systemic infection in the immunocompromised (Lipman & Saadia 1997). Many Gram-negative bacteria such as pseudomonas, klebsiella and acinetobacter are able to establish infection in damaged skin sites or invasive devices.

Assessing a patient's susceptibility to infection

Some patients are at greater risk of acquiring infection than others. Bowell (1992) developed a scoring system to enable the risk in individual patients to be assessed. It takes into account underlying disease, invasive procedures and treatments (Box 3.7). By identifying patients at risk of infection, actions required to manage or prevent infection can be incorporated into the planning of care (Kingsley 1992), for example the safe management of an intravenous infusion or urinary catheter, measures to improve nutrition or hydration.

The size of the problem

It is difficult to make precise estimates of the number of infections acquired as a result of healthcare. The presence of infection is often not accurately recorded in medical or nursing records and few hospitals have systems in place to routinely collect and analyse information about infections. Endemic infections commonly associated with invasive devices or procedures account for most hospital or healthcare-associated

infections. A national prevalence study undertaken in 157 hospitals in the UK and Ireland found that, on average, nine of every 100 patients had a HAI at the time of the survey. However, there were marked differences between hospitals, with the prevalence ranging from 2 to 29% and a higher rate of HAI in teaching hospitals (11.2%) than in non-teaching hospitals (8.4%) (Emmerson et al 1996). Infections of the urinary tract, lower respiratory tract, surgical wounds and bloodstream accounted for about 60% of all HAI identified in the survey (Fig. 3.5). Factors that predispose to these infections are summarized in Box 3.8 and described in more detail in subsequent chapters.

Prevalence surveys tend to overestimate the true level of infection because patients who develop an

---

Box 3.7   Identifying patients at risk of infection. From Bowell (1992) with permission

General factors	Local factors	Invasive procedures	Drugs	Diseases
Age	*Oedema*	*Cannulation*	Cytotoxics	Carcinoma
Very young	Pulmonary	Peripheral	Antibiotics	Leukaemia
Very old	Ascites	Central	Steroids	Aplastic anaemia
		Parenteral nutrition		Diabetes mellitus
Nutrition	*Ischaemia*			Liver disease
Emaciated	Thrombus	*Surgery*		Renal disease
Thin	Embolus	Anaesthesia		AIDS
Obese	Necrosis	Wound		
Dehydrated		Wound drainage		
	Skin lesions	Wound/colostomy		
Mobility	Trauma	Implant		
Limited	Burns			
Immobile	Ulceration	*Intubation*		
Temporary		Endobronchial suction		
Permanent	*Foreign body*	Humidification		
	Accidental	Ventilation		
Mental state	Planned			
Confused		*Catheterization*		
Depressed		Intermittent		
Senile		Closed drainage		
		Irrigation		
Incontinence				
Urine				
Faeces				
Temporary				
Permanent				
General health				
Weak				
Debilitated				
General hygiene				
Dependence				
Mouth/teeth				
Skin				

Each factor listed increases the risk of a patient acquiring infection. An infection risk assessment can be made by counting the risk factors for an individual patient. The higher the number counted, the greater the risk that the patient will develop an infection.

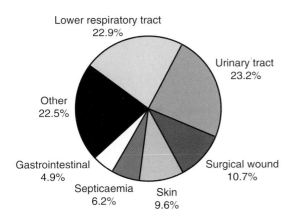

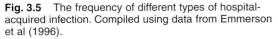

Fig. 3.5 The frequency of different types of hospital-acquired infection. Compiled using data from Emmerson et al (1996).

infection are more likely to stay in hospital for longer and will therefore account for a disproportionate number of hospital inpatients at a single point in time. A more accurate estimate is provided by incidence studies which measure how many patients acquire infection during hospitalization or after exposure to a specific event. These suggest that around 8% of patients admitted to hospital acquire an infection during their stay (Glenister et al 1992, Plowman et al 1999).

The risk of acquiring a HAI has probably increased over recent decades as a result of more complex medical care and more acutely ill patients. However, such changes are difficult to measure, as the trend towards early discharge or treatment outside hospital means that many infections are not likely to be detected while the patient is in hospital. The study by Plowman et al (1999) estimated that at least a further 19% of patients developed a HAI after discharge.

Some patients in hospital may be infected or colonized with micro-organisms that have a particular propensity to spread to others and may do so easily in hospital or other healthcare environments. These include infectious diseases such as chickenpox or tuberculosis, or hospital pathogens such as MRSA. Isolation procedures are used to prevent the spread of these pathogens, but occasionally transmission does occur. The main causes of outbreaks of infection in hospitals are listed in Box 3.9. Whilst outbreaks of infection are uncommon, probably accounting for less than 4% of all HAI (Haley et al 1985a, Wenzel et al 1983), considerable resources may be required to control them. Barnass et al (1989) calculated the costs of an outbreak of salmonella, in which 17 patients and

Box 3.8 Epidemiology of common hospital-acquired infections

Urinary tract infections
These are some of the most common infections associated with healthcare, accounting for 23% of HAI. Most are related to urethral catheterization as this device facilitates the entry of bacteria into the bladder, either along the outside of the tube or through its lumen. Once in the bladder, micro-organisms may spread to the kidneys or invade the bloodstream. Urinary tract infection occurs most commonly in patients likely to be catheterized, such as those treated in urology, gynaecology and orthopaedic units (Glynn et al 1997).

Lower respiratory tract infections
These infections account for 23% of HAI. Infection is acquired through aspiration of micro-organisms from the oropharynx or inhalation of airborne particles. The risk is increased by devices that bypass the normal defences (e.g. endotracheal and nasogastric tubes), and by reduced levels of consciousness (e.g. sedation). Opportunistic pathogens such as aspergillus may cause pneumonia in the immunocompromised.

Surgical wound infections
These account for nearly 11% of HAI, although the risk of infection is highest for procedures more likely to encounter microbial contamination (e.g. operation on the bowel). Prolonged procedures, damaged tissue and the skills of the surgeon are important risk factors in the development of surgical wound infection.

Bloodstream infections
These account for approximately 6% of HAI, but are responsible for considerable morbidity and mortality. Some 38% are directly related to intravenous therapy, particularly central vascular devices, and are commonly caused by skin commensals such as *Staphylococcus epidermidis* (PHLS 2000b). Other bloodstream infections develop from another focus of infection (e.g. urinary or respiratory tract). Those caused by Gram-negative bacteria are particularly difficult to treat because these organisms produce a range of toxins that have severe systemic effects.

two staff were affected, to be over £21 000. Preventing the spread of MRSA can be particularly expensive as it may require staff and patients to be swabbed to detect carriage, treatment of those affected with topical creams or expensive antibiotics, ward or bed closures, and additional staff to manage isolation precautions (Cox et al 1995).

Costs of healthcare-associated infections

Infections acquired as a result of healthcare cause considerable morbidity and mortality. Plowman et al (1999)

Box 3.9 Detecting epidemiologically significant infections amongst hospital patients

Early detection of infections likely to transmit readily in a hospital setting is achieved by monitoring laboratory specimens and identifying patients with signs or symptoms suggestive of infection. Examples of these 'alert organisms' and 'alert conditions' are given below.

'Alert organisms'

Infection control precautions should be initiated when these micro-organisms are identified, either from a laboratory specimen or as a result of a clinical diagnosis, to prevent their spread to other patients.

Clostridium difficile

Antibiotic-resistant organisms, e.g. MRSA, vancomycin-resistant enterococci (VRE), penicillin-resistant pneumococci

Salmonella, shigella or other gastrointestinal pathogens

Group A streptococci

Mycobacterium tuberculosis

Gastrointestinal viruses, e.g. rotavirus, small round structured virus, Norwalk agent

Respiratory viruses, e.g. influenza, respiratory syncytial virus

Chickenpox

'Alert conditions'

Infection control precautions should be taken when a patient develops any of the following signs or symptoms until an infectious cause has been excluded.

Diarrhoea

Vomiting

Symptoms of respiratory tract infection, e.g. cough, sputum

Fever of unknown origin

Skin rash

---

assessed the general health of patients following hospitalization using a Health Status Questionnaire that measured aspects of physical, social, emotional and mental health. They found that patients who acquired a HAI had significantly lower health status scores, particularly if they had symptoms of infection after discharge from hospital. Return to employment and normal activities was delayed in patients who developed a HAI in hospital, by 6 and 12 days respectively.

Some infections may be serious enough to cause the death of the patient. It has been estimated that approxi-mately 10% of patients who acquire an infection in hospital die (Haley 1986, Plowman et al 1999). Many of these patients would have died despite the infection; however, in one third of cases the infection is likely to be a major contributory factor to death, and in an estimated 10% of cases infection is the main cause of death (Haley 1986).

In addition to the effect that a HAI may have on the patient and the outcome of care, HAIs have important resource implications for hospitals, community health-care services and society as a whole. In hospital, patients who acquire an infection incur nearly three times more costs than those who do not. These additional costs include specialist care, antimicrobial and other drug therapy, tests and treatments, and the costs

associated with extra days spent in hospital (Plowman et al 1999). Overall, patients who acquire a HAI spend nearly three times longer in hospital (Table 3.4). These extra costs vary according to the specific site of infection. Multiple infections (where a patient acquires more than one HAI affecting different sites) are the most expensive to treat but occur infrequently, affecting only 1.4% of patients. Urinary tract infections incur greater costs because, although they are inexpensive to treat, they occur more commonly, affecting 2.7% of patients.

Many infections acquired as a result of care in hospital are not detected until after the patient has been discharged. The costs of consultation, drug therapy and treatment fall to the general practitioner and community nursing services, although these costs are much lower than those incurred by hospitals (Elliston et al 1994, Plowman et al 1999). There are also costs to society in terms of loss of earnings, productivity and social security payments, which may impinge on both the patients and their carers (Plowman et al 1997, 1999).

The effect that HAIs have on the resources of the NHS are considerable. In 1993 Coello et al estimated that the costs of HAI in surgical patients in England was over £170 million. Plowman et al (1999) extrapolated the data on the costs of HAI at a single district general hospital

Table 3.4 Additional costs and days spent in hospital by patients who develop a hospital-acquired infection

Site of infection	Additional costs (£ per patient)	Ratio of costs (compared to non-infected)	Additional days in hospital (per patient)	Incidence of HAI (%)
Urinary tract	1122	1.7	5	2.7
Lower respiratory tract	2080	2.3	8	1.2
Surgical wound	1594	2.0	7	1.0
Bloodstream	6209	4.3	4*	0.1
Skin	1615	2.0	11	0.6
Other	2465	2.5	12	0.8
Multiple	8631	6.3	29	1.4
Any infection	3154	2.8	11	7.8

* Two patients died. Estimates derived by regression modelling to control for confounding variables (e.g. age, sex, diagnosis, number of co-morbidities) that could have contributed to the increased costs. Data from Plowman et al (1999).

and estimated that these infections cost the NHS in England £986 million annually, £930 million incurred during hospitalization and £55 million postdischarge. The hospital costs represent 9% of the national budget for acute, elderly care and obstetric services.

These figures point to the value of measures to prevent HAI. In an average hospital £300 000 of additional resources would be released by preventing 10% of HAIs. A considerable proportion of these resources would be the release of additional bed-days for the treatment of other patients. The costs of establishing an infection control programme and employing sufficient specialist staff to maintain it are likely to be outweighed by the savings made through the prevention of HAI, the elimination of costly and ineffective practices, and reduction in unnecessary pollution of the environment (Currie & Maynard 1989, Daschner 1991, Haley 1986, Plowman et al 1999).

Implications for service quality

The acquisition of infection as a result of hospital or other healthcare treatment has important implications both for the patients affected and the organizations concerned. HAIs are seen as important quality indicators, and as such their prevention is key to ensuring that services provided by the NHS are of a high quality (Box 3.10) (Quality Indicator Study Group 1995, Thomson et al 1997).

> **Box 3.10** What is a quality indicator?
>
> 'a quantitative measure that can be used to monitor and evaluate the quality of important governance, management, clinical and support functions that affect patient outcomes' (Joint Commission on the Accreditation of Healthcare Organisations 1989).

Clinical governance

In 1998, a new framework for the NHS was introduced with particular emphasis on quality (Department of Health 1998a). The framework requires accountability for quality at a corporate level, with clear lines of responsibility for the overall quality of care within the organization and a range of mechanisms in place to establish and monitor the quality of services (Box 3.11). In addition, there is a requirement for healthcare professionals to be responsible for maintaining their standard of practice at a high level with the support of professional development programmes and codes of professional practice. The Commission for Health Improvement (CHIMP) is responsible for policing the

> **Box 3.11** Clinical governance framework
>
> **Corporate accountability**
> - Chief Executive accountable
> - clear lines of responsibility
>
> **Internal mechanisms**
> - individual accountability
> - professional regulation
> - professional development
>
> **External support structures**
> - Commission for Health Improvement (CHIMP)
> - National Institute of Clinical Excellence (NICE)
>
> **Core principles**
> - clinical audit
> - evidence-based practice
> - clinical effectiveness
> - risk management
> - risk reduction programmes
> - monitoring outcomes of care
> - learning lessons from complaints
> - dissemination of good practice
>
> Source: Wilson (1998), with permission

systems introduced by Trusts to establish and monitor service quality. The National Institute of Clinical Excellence (NICE) has been established to facilitate the development of evidence-based clinical guidelines and to promote their use (Wilson 1998).

Infection prevention and control has a key role to play in the clinical governance framework, both in terms of identifying areas where quality of care may be improved (e.g. by measuring the incidence of infection), and in ensuring that appropriate procedures to prevent and control infection are in place, are evidence based and regularly audited.

Control assurance

The success of clinical governance depends on an organizational structure that provides a foundation for clinical excellence and quality care. In the past, NHS Trusts were required to demonstrate that internal financial controls were in place. This principle has now been extended to other aspects of the organization to ensure that patients, staff and the public are, as far as possible, protected from risks. This framework of organizational controls underpinning clinical governance is called controls assurance. Controls standards and assessment criteria have been defined for a range of operational activities, for example catering and food hygiene, contract control, environment management, medicines management, security (NHS Executive 1999a). The importance of the infection control programme and the structures required to support it have been recognized in a controls assurance standard for infection control (NHS Executive 1999b). This standard requires acute hospital Trusts to provide 'a managed environment, which minimises the risk of infection to patients, staff and visitors'. The criteria contained within the standard define good practice and provide a measure against which Trust boards can assess their performance.

Risk management

Risk management is an important part of the clinical governance and controls assurance framework. It involves a systematic approach to identifying events that could have adverse consequences for either patients or staff, implementing measures to control them, and ensuring that appropriate structures and policies are in place. It also requires the investigation of adverse events to ensure that lessons are learnt from them and that these are incorporated into practice (Dickson 1995). For example, needlestick injuries to staff are known to carry a significant risk of transmission of bloodborne viruses. Effective management of this risk requires a clearly stated policy on the safe disposal of used needles, training of staff who handle them, the provision of sufficient disposal containers, and a system for reporting and monitoring injuries.

There are financial benefits associated with risk reduction systems as they will minimize the exposure of NHS organizations to litigation (Moss 1995). This has taken on increasing importance since the removal of Crown Immunity in the late 1980s and early 1990s, which in the past exempted hospitals from prosecution and prevented enforcement of some legislation, for example food safety.

Infection control has an important part to play in risk management, with the safe care of patients, equipment and body fluids being fundamental to preventing patients or staff from acquiring infection in hospital.

Programmes for the prevention and control of infection

It may not be possible to prevent all HAIs as many patients in hospital have compromised immune systems and are highly vulnerable to infection. However, the value of an effective programme to prevent HAI was demonstrated by a major American study carried out in the 1980s, called the Study of the Efficacy of Nosocomial Infection Control (SENIC). It evaluated the infection control activity in 338 hospitals and, through the review of clinical records, measured how the rate of HAI changed in the 5-year period after infection control programmes were established. Those hospitals with the most comprehensive infection control programmes, featuring all the components described in Box 3.12, were able to reduce the

---

Box 3.12 Components of an infection control programme (SENIC)

Infection control personnel coordinating the programme
- trained infection control doctor
- one infection control nurse to every 250 beds

Control activities
- detect, investigate and control outbreaks of infection
- produce, implement and monitor policies
- educate staff

Surveillance activities
- identify infections
- analyse data
- disseminate results

Source: Haley et al (1985b), by permission of Oxford University Press

rate of HAI by 32% during this period. In hospitals with a poor or non-existent infection control programme, the rate of HAI increased by 18% over the same period.

The results of this study have important implications for clinical practice. They suggest that a significant proportion of HAI can be prevented and that the quality of the infection control programme makes a difference. The study also highlighted the combination of activities that were important for an effective infection control programme, identifying surveillance of HAI as a key component and the important role of specialist staff – the infection control nurse and infection control doctor. Although 15 years have elapsed since the SENIC study, and there have been considerable changes in the provision of healthcare, a recent study in England reported that the majority of acute NHS Trusts considered there was scope to reduce HAI by at least 15% (National Audit Office 2000). Data collected on the incidence of HAI in several hospitals indicated significant differences between them. For example, the incidence of urinary tract infection in gynaecological patients varied from 1.4 to 3.3 infections per 1000 catheter-days (Glynn et al 1997).

The Chief Executive of each NHS Trust is responsible for ensuring that effective arrangements for infection control are in place and a planned programme has been defined and is regularly reviewed. This programme should be specified in the service level agreement between the NHS Trust and the health authority (NHS Executive 2000). The infection control programme should define the focus of infection control activity, identify policies for development or review, and include targets and objectives for surveillance, audit and education. Planning and implementing an infection control programme requires the expertise of specialist staff, and all hospitals are recommended to employ a trained infection control nurse and infection control doctor to take on this role (Department of Health 1995, Scottish Office 1998). These staff work as a team, liaising with each other regularly, to ensure that measures required by the programme are implemented. The infection control team (ICT) is supported by an infection control committee (Fig. 3.6).

Infection control nurse (ICN) The ICN is usually the only full-time member of the ICT and carries the main responsibility for ensuring that the infection control programme is carried out, liaising with a wide range of departments and groups of staff within the Trust (Fig. 3.7). Every NHS Trust should employ an ICN; many employ more than one, but few have the ratio of one ICN for every 250 beds found in those SENIC hospitals with the most effective infection

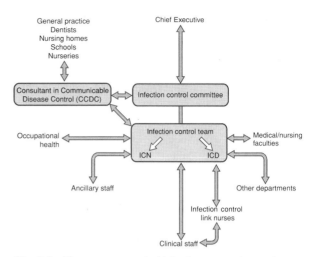

Fig. 3.6 The management of infection prevention and control in hospitals.

control programmes (Haley et al 1985b, National Audit Office 2000).

The ICN is usually a registered nurse with specialist training, who operates at the level of a Clinical Nurse Specialist, the characteristics of which have been defined by Hamric (1989) (Box 3.13). The ICN is required to act as an expert practitioner, interpreting laboratory and other relevant data, and providing advice to clinical staff, patients and their families (Prieto 1994). A range of courses is available for training nurses in the role (Box 3.14).

Box 3.13 Defining characteristics of the Clinical Nurse Specialist role

Primary criteria
- graduate study in specialty
- certification
- focus of practice on patient/client and family

Skills and competencies
- change agent
- collaborator
- clinical leader
- role
- model
- patient advocate

Subroles
- expert practice
- education
- consultation
- research

Source: Hamric (1989)

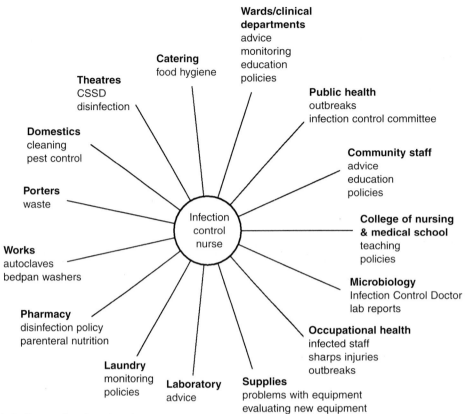

CSSD, central sterile supplies department.

Fig. 3.7 The role of the infection control nurse. The ICN liaises with many departments and personnel within a hospital.

Box 3.14 Training for infection control nurses
Professional certificates ENB 329 Foundation course in infection control ENB 910 Principles of infection control N26 Developments in infection control nursing **Academic courses** Diploma in infection control BSc (Hons) in infection control Postgraduate diploma in infection control MSc in infection control

Many ICNs are now being appointed to positions in Community Healthcare Trusts or public health, where they provide an advisory service and contribute to the infection control programme for community healthcare staff, nursing homes, general practitioners and practice nurses.

Infection control doctor (ICD)   The ICD is usually a consultant microbiologist based in an acute hospital with access to microbiology laboratory facilities. The ICD does not usually work full time in the role and is often unable to devote the recommended amount of time to the role (National Audit Office 2000). ICDs should have specialist training in infection control and play a key part in developing the infection control programme, influencing the prescribing of antimicrobial agents, the treatment of HAI, and the training of medical students and qualified doctors.

Infection control committee (ICC)   Every hospital should have an infection control committee (Department of Health 1995). In addition to the ICT, the committee will draw its membership from the Chief Executive (or a senior member of the management team), Director of Nursing, Consultant in Communicable Disease Control (CCDC), occupational health physician or nurse, senior clinical medical staff, pharmacy and sterile services supplies. The role of the committee is to endorse infection control policies, advise the ICT, and act as a forum through which key groups can be consulted. The ICC will also approve the infection control programme and monitor progress in its implementation.

Other key personnel

Consultant in communicable disease control The CCDC is a doctor appointed in the Department of Public Health Medicine of each health authority (in Scotland, Consultants in Public Health Medicine are appointed by Health Boards) to coordinate the surveillance, prevention and control of all communicable diseases in a health district (see p. 40). The CCDC is a member of the ICC and liaises with the hospital's ICT to coordinate the infection prevention and control activities between hospital and community. CCDCs have an important role in ensuring the effective management of outbreaks of infection and advising health authorities on contractual arrangements for infection control. Many CCDCs now work directly with ICNs to provide a service in community health-care Trusts.

Infection control link nurses (ICLNs) Many hospitals use ICLNs to improve awareness of infection control in clinical areas. These staff receive some basic training in the principles of infection control and then help to pro-vide information to other staff, undertake surveillance and audit, and report on infection control problems in their own area of practice (Teare & Peacock 1996).

Occupational health department (OHD) Close liaison between the ICT and OHD is essential to ensure the health and safety of staff and the protection of patients from healthcare workers with infection. The OHD will undertake health surveillance for infectious diseases that may affect fitness to work (e.g. tuberculosis), health surveillance in relation to hazards (e.g. glutaraldehyde) and the ergonomic design of workplaces. They will also play an important role in formulating and implementing infection control policies (e.g. management of sharps injuries) and in monitoring their effectiveness (e.g. analysing sharps injury statistics). The OHD will be closely involved in outbreaks of infection, monitoring staff and ensuring that they remain off work whilst suffering from an illness that may affect patients. OHD staff should also be available to provide advice and support to staff who have been exposed to infection, such as those concerned about acquiring a bloodborne virus following a needlestick injury, and those who may be particularly susceptible to infection themselves, such as staff infected with HIV (Health Service Advisory Committee 1993, Royal College of Nursing 1991).

Key components of an infection control programme

The ICT will be responsible for establishing and maintaining a comprehensive programme of activities to ensure that high standards of infection prevention and control are maintained in all clinical areas. The programme will be reviewed annually to define the focus of activity, identify policies that require development or revision, and plan audit, surveillance and educational targets. There are several key areas of activity, as described below.

Advisory service

The ICT provides advice on a wide range of issues related to infection control such as the management of patients with infection, purchase and decontamination of equipment, cleaning, catering and waste management. They will also be required to attend various committees (e.g. Health and Safety, Waste Management, Supplies and Laundry Users).

Surveillance of hospital-acquired infection

Surveillance is the systematic monitoring of the occurrence of disease in a population. The importance of surveillance in the control of infectious diseases was recognized at the beginning of the twentieth century, and there is now a statutory requirement for doctors to notify cases of infectious disease. Surveillance in a hospital setting has, until recently, been focused on detecting cases of infectious disease that have the potential to cause outbreaks of infection (see Box 3.9). Now, many more hospitals are recognizing HAI as an important quality indicator and are using surveillance to assess the quality of care as part of the clinical audit process (Fig. 3.8) (Gaynes & Solomon 1996). If the data are disseminated to clinical staff whose practice is key in preventing infection, it can help to reinforce good practice and identify areas where improvements could be made (Glynn et al 1997). However, surveillance data need to be interpreted with care because differences in methods of data collection, criteria for defining infections and the mix of patients can all affect the results and need to be considered when comparing data from different hospitals (Public Health Laboratory Service 2000a,b, Wilson 1995).

The Nosocomial Infection Surveillance Unit (NISU), based at the Central Public Health Laboratory in London, coordinates a programme to help hospitals in England to collect data on specific HAIs using standard methodology and definitions, and to make national data on their incidence available for comparison. The

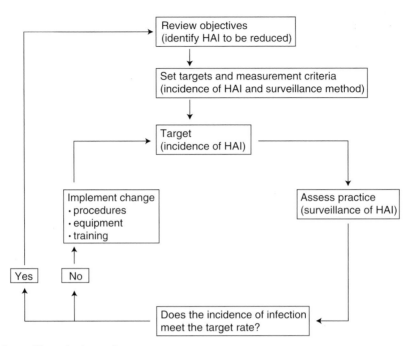

Fig. 3.8 The role of surveillance in the audit process.

scheme currently coordinates surveillance on blood-stream infections and surgical site infections associated with several different categories of surgical procedure. Hospitals participating in this scheme can compare their incidence of infections with other participating hospitals and, if their rates are found to be high, initiate an investigation of underlying causes and identify any changes of practice that may be indicated (Public Health Laboratory Service 2000 a, b).

Detection, investigation and control of outbreaks of infection

Outbreaks or epidemics of infection can occur in any community, but are a particular problem in institutions where many people live in close proximity (e.g. schools, universities, residential homes and military barracks). The risks are even greater in hospital settings, where many patients have underlying illnesses that increase their susceptibility to infection. An outbreak may develop rapidly and be related to an event that exposed many people to the pathogen (e.g. food poisoning), or may develop gradually over many days or weeks as the pathogen is spread from person to person (e.g. viral gastroenteritis). The deaths of several patients during an outbreak of salmonella at Stanley Royd Hospital in Wakefield in 1985 (Box 3.15) high-lighted deficiencies in the management of outbreaks of

Box 3.15 Outbreak of salmonella at Stanley Royd Hospital

In 1984, a large number of patients and staff at Stanley Royd Hospital for mentally ill patients in Wakefield acquired salmonella poisoning after eating beef served by the hospital kitchens. Of a total of 788 residents, 355 had been ill with suspected salmonella poisoning and a further 81 were symptom-free but had positive specimens. Of the 980 staff, 109 had been ill with suspected salmonella and a further 29 had positive specimens but no symptoms. Many of the affected patients were elderly and there were 19 deaths due to, or partly contributed to, the infection. The inquiry that followed identified many deficiencies in the way that food was handled, stored and prepared, and in the way the outbreak of infection was managed.

At the time of this incident, hospitals were protected from prosecution by Crown Immunity so that, while Environmental Health Officers could inspect hospital kitchens, they had no means of enforcing their recommendations or preventing the continuation of unsafe practices. In 1987, following the Stanley Royd Inquiry, Crown Immunity was removed from health service catering facilities and formal requirements for infection control advice and the management of outbreak of infection were established (Department of Health and Social Security 1988).

infection and led to advice to introduce more careful controls and clearer lines of responsibility in the future (Department of Health 1995).

When an outbreak of infection occurs within a hospital, the ICT will investigate the source of infection, identify people who have been in contact with the infection, advise on the control measures that are required and monitor their implementation. The ICT may establish an Outbreak Control Group, involving clinicians and senior nurses from affected departments, the CCDC, occupational health physician and other staff whose help may be required to ensure that the outbreak is controlled effectively (Department of Health 1995). Clinical staff may be crucial in the early detection of outbreaks of infection. They should be aware of symptoms indicative of infection amongst patients or staff, and report to the ICT when two or more cases with similar symptoms occur. Relevant clinical specimens can also help to determine the cause of infection and whether cases are related to the outbreak (Box 3.16).

Policies and procedures to prevent and control infection

Written information in the form of policies, guidelines or procedures is required to define routine practices and standards of care expected by the organization and to provide guidance when members of the ICT are not available. These policies and procedures are a key component of effective risk management. Infection control policies may refer to specific areas of practice, for example isolation of infectious patients, management of equipment, the environment and waste materials, use of protective clothing. Others may contain aspects of infection control practice within a broader practice guideline, for example recommended practices for the insertion and management of invasive devices such as nasogastric tubes, intravenous cannulae or urinary catheters. The ICT, in conjunction with other staff, is responsible for developing many of these policies. The ICC will decide on the priorities for policy development and revision, and approve them when completed. In some situations staff will develop their own policies but seek the advice of the ICT on recommended practice.

There are often conflicting views about what constitutes best practice in terms of infection control. A recent analysis demonstrated considerable variation in practices recommended for the prevention of infection in a range of policies from 19 hospitals across England and Wales (Glynn et al 1997). The publication of some simple clinical guidelines for preventing infection associated with a range of commonly used invasive devices may help to focus on those practices that have been most clearly demonstrated to reduce the risk of infection (Pratt et al 2001, Ward et al 1997).

A range of strategies, in addition to manuals or protocols, may be necessary if evidence-based practice is to be adopted. These include local opinion leaders such as ward sisters, senior medical staff or link nurses, the audit of practice and surveillance of infection with feedback of results to relevant clinical staff (Richardson 1999).

Epic project The Department of Health in England has commissioned the development of national evidence-based guidelines on some key aspects of infection control practice, for example indwelling urethral catheters, intravenous catheters and general principles of infection control. These guidelines contain the broad principles of good practice, derived from research evidence and expert review, and are intended to inform the development of more detailed operational policies at a local level. Evidence has been gathered by systematically reviewing the literature and then critically appraising the study design, methodology, analysis and relevance to practice. Relevant evidence has then been graded into three categories:

Category 1 generally consistent findings in a range of evidence derived from well-designed experimental studies

---

Box 3.16 Key steps in the control of suspected outbreaks of gastrointestinal infection

Where more than one patient or member of staff is affected by unexplained diarrhoea or vomiting, the following actions should be taken.

In a hospital
- inform the doctor in charge of the patients
- inform the infection control doctor or nurse
- ensure sufficient supplies of gloves and aprons
- collect stool specimens from affected patients for viral and bacterial culture
- wash hands after contact with affected patients
- use protective clothing for handling body fluids
- change gloves and wash hands between patients
- transfer affected patients to single rooms and follow isolation precautions
- ensure that affected staff attend the occupational health department

In a nursing home
- inform the general practitioner responsible for affected patients
- inform the CCDC
- ensure sufficient supplies of gloves and aprons
- collect stool specimens from affected patients for viral and bacterial culture
- wash hands after contact with affected patients
- use protective clothing for handling body fluids
- change gloves and wash hands between patients
- ensure affected staff consult their general practitioner

Category 2 evidence based on a single acceptable study, or a weak or inconsistent finding in some multiple acceptable studies

Category 3 limited scientific evidence that does not meet all the criteria of 'acceptable studies' or an absence of directly applicable studies of good quality. This includes published or unpublished expert opinion. (Pratt et al 2001)

Dissemination and implementation of policies

National guidelines can help to ensure consistent evidence-based practice, but more detailed policies and guidelines should be developed that take into account local practices and attitudes. Written policies alone may not be sufficient to ensure effective practice if staff are not aware of them or do not understand their content. There must, therefore, also be a system for implementation and dissemination, to ensure that the relevant staff know about the policy and understand its contents and the rationale for recommended practice (Cheater & Closs 1997, Seto et al 1991).

Education and training

ICNs spend a considerable proportion of their time in the education of a wide range of the staff who work in clinical settings (Griffith-Jones 1991). This can take place informally, for example discussing the management of a particular patient whilst visiting a ward or clinic, during feedback sessions following audits, or more formally as lectures and study days. Infection control should also form part of the basic training and continuous professional development of all groups of healthcare professionals and support staff such as domestics and porters (NHS Executive 1999b).

There is a close relationship between health and safety and many aspects of infection control. The health and safety legislation recognizes the importance of training as a means of ensuring that staff understand procedures and know what is expected of them. Staff who join a healthcare organization should be made aware of local infection control policies, and the ICT should be involved in their orientation programmes.

A basic knowledge of microbiology underpins the practice of infection control, and several workers have pointed to the lack of this knowledge amongst nurses and doctors (Courtenay 1991, Emmerson & Ridgway 1980). The fears and misunderstandings that surrounded the first patients diagnosed with AIDS demonstrates how important education is if such problems are to be avoided (Välimäki et al 1998). Staff who have received education are more able to educate others, both patients and other staff, and, as in the case of infection control link nurses, can provide a valuable adjunct to the ICT (Teare & Peacock 1996). Ching & Seto (1990) have used ICLNs to support the teaching activity of the ICN and were able to demonstrate significant improvements in adherence to an infection control policy when ICLNs were providing tutorials on the ward.

Monitoring clinical practice

Routine visits to clinical areas provide the ICN with the opportunity to monitor aspects of clinical practice and detect potential problems. However, in some situations a formal audit can be used to provide a systematic measurement of the quality of care and to identify where improvements could be made (Milward et al 1993). This involves marking observed practice against predefined criteria and feeding back the score generated from the process to the clinical staff in the department concerned (Fig. 3.9). Such a process can identify where information about infection control policies, additional equipment or in-service education may be required; any problems identified should be discussed during the feedback session and solutions agreed (Friedman et al 1984).

Standard : Sharps will be handled safely to negate the risk of sharps injury

- A container as specified by the infection control committee is in use ☐
- The container is less than two-thirds full ☐
- The box is free from protruding sharps ☐
- Sharps box is available on the arrest trolley ☐
- Sharps box available on the medicine trolley ☐
- Sharps box is correctly assembled ☐
- Sharps box is labelled according to hospital policy ☐
- Sharps are disposed of directly into a sharps box ☐
- What action would you take following a needlestick injury? (question to a member of staff at random) ☐

Comments:

Fig. 3.9 Infection control audit tool. Source: Milward et al (1993).

REFERENCES

Ansari SA, Springthorpe S, Sattar SA et al (1991) Potential role of hands in the spread of respiratory infections: studies with human parainfluenza virus 3 and rhinovirus 14. *J. Clin. Microbiol.*, **29**: 2115–19.

Appleby J (1997) The English patient. *Health Services Journal*, **10 April**: 36–40.

Barrie D, Wilson J, Hoffman PN et al (1992) *Bacillus cereus* meningitis in two neurosurgical patients: an investigation into the source of the organism. *J. Infect.*, **25**: 291–7.

Barrie D, Hoffman PN, Wilson JA, Kramer JM (1994) Contamination of hospital linen by *Bacillus cereus*. *Epidemiol. Infect.*, **113**: 297–306.

Barnass S, O'Mahony M, Socket PN et al (1989) The tangible cost implications of multiply-resistant salmonella. *Epidemiol. Infect.*, **103**: 227–34.

Bartlett CLR, Macrae AD, Macfarlane JD (1986) *Legionella Infections*. Edward Arnold, London.

Bowell B (1992) Protecting the patient at risk. *Nursing Times*, **88**(3): 32–5.

Casewell MW, Desai N (1983) Survival of multiply-resistant *Klebsiella aerogenes* and other Gram-negative bacilli on fingertips. *J. Hosp. Infect.*, **4**: 350–60.

Cheater FM, Closs SJ (1997) The effectiveness of methods of dissemination and implementation of clinical guidelines for nursing practice: a selective review. *Clin. Effect. Nurs.*, **1**: 4–15.

Ching TY, Seto WH (1990) Evaluating the efficacy of the infection control liaison nurse in the hospital. *J. Adv. Nurs.*, **15**: 1128–31.

Coello R, Glenister H, Fereres J et al (1993) The cost of infection in surgical patients: a case control study. *J. Hosp. Infect.*, **25**: 239–50.

Communicable Disease Report (1997) Epidemic methicillin resistant *Staphylococcus aureus*. *CDR*, **7**(22): 191.

Conly JM, Hill S, Ross J et al (1989) Handwashing practices in an intensive care unit: the effect of an educational program and its relationship to infection rates. *Am. J. Infect. Control*, **17**: 333–9.

Courtenay M (1991) A study of the teaching and learning of biological sciences in nurse education. *J. Adv. Nurs.*, **16**: 1110–16.

Cox RA, Conquest C, Mallghan C et al (1995) A major outbreak of methicillin-resistant *Staphylococcus aureus* caused by a new phage type (EMRSA 16). *J. Hosp. Infect.*, **29**: 87–106.

Currie E, Maynard A (1989) *Economic Aspects of Hospital Acquired Infection*. Discussion paper 56. Centre for Health Economics, University of York, York.

Daschner FD (1991) Unnecessary and ecological costs of hospital infection. *J. Hosp. Infect.*, **18** (Suppl. A): 73–8.

Davies B, Blenkharn I (1987) On the right track. *Nursing Times*, **83**(22): 64–8.

Department of Health (1995) *Hospital Infection Control – Guidance on the Control of Infection in Hospitals*. DH/PHLS/ Hospital Infection Working Group. HMSO, London.

Department of Health (1998a) *A First Class Service in the New NHS*. The Stationery Office, London.

Department of Health (1998b) *Our Healthier Nation. A Contract for Health*. The Stationery Office, London.

Department of Health and Social Security (1988) *Hospital Infection Control*, HC (88)33. HMSO, London.

Dickson G (1995) Principles of risk management. *Qual. Health Care*, **4**: 75–9.

Elliston PRA, Slack RCB, Humphreys H et al (1994) The cost of postoperative wound infections. *J. Hosp. Infect.*, **28**(3): 241–2.

Emmerson AM, Ridgway GL (1980) Teaching asepsis to medical students. *J. Hosp. Infect.*, **1**: 289–92.

Emmerson AM, Enstone JE, Griffin M et al (1996) The second national prevalence survey of infection in hospitals – overview of the results. *J. Hosp. Infect.*, **32**: 175–90.

Friedman C, Richter D, Skylis T et al (1984) Process surveillance: auditing infection control policies and procedures. *Am. J. Infect. Control*, **12**: 228–32.

Gaynes RP, Solomon S (1996) Improving hospital-acquired infection rates: the CDC experience. *Joint Comm. J. Qual. Impr.*, **22**(7): 457–67.

Glenister HM, Taylor LJ, Cooke EM et al (1992) *A Study of Surveillance Methods for Detecting Hospital Infection*. PHLS, London.

Glynn A, Ward V, Wilson J et al (1997) *Hospital Acquired Infection: Surveillance Policies and Practice*. PHLS, London.

Goodman H (1997) Home is where the heart is. *Nursing Times*, **93**(18): 56–7.

Gormon LJ, Sanai L, Notman W et al (1993) Cross-infection in an intensive care unit by *Klebsiella pneumoniae* from ventilator condensate. *J. Hosp. Infect.*, **23**: 17–26.

Greaves A (1985) We'll just freshen you up, dear. *Nursing Times*, **Mar 6** (Suppl.): 3–8.

Green J, Wright PA, Gallimore CI et al (1998) The role of environmental contamination with small round structured viruses in a hospital outbreak investigated by reverse-transcriptase polymerase chain reaction assay. *J. Hosp. Infect.*, **39**: 39–46.

Griffith-Jones A (1991) Are we giving value for money. *Nursing Times*, **87**(11): 64–8.

Haley RW (1985) Surveillance-by-objectives: a new priority-directed approach to the control of nosocomial infections. *Am. J. Infect. Control*, **13**: 78–89.

Haley RW (1986) *Managing Hospital Infection Control for Cost Effectiveness*. A Strategy for Reducing Infectious Complications. American Hospital Publishing, Chicago.

Haley RW, Tenney JH, Lindsay JO et al (1985a) How frequent are outbreaks of nosocomial infection in community hospitals? *Infect. Control*, **6**: 233–6.

Haley RW, Culver DH, White JW et al (1985b) The efficacy of infection surveillance and control programs in preventing nosocomial infections in US hospitals (SENIC Study). *Am. J. Epidemiol.*, **121**: 182–205.

Hall CB, Douglas RG Jr (1981) Modes of transmission of respiratory syncytial virus. *J. Pediatr.*, **99**: 100.

Hambraeus A (1988) Aerobiology in the operating room – a review. *J. Hosp. Infect.*, **11** (Suppl. A): 68–76.

Hamric AB (1989) History and overview of the CNS role. In: Hamric AB, Spross JA (eds) *The Clinical Nurse Specialist in Theory and Practice*, 2nd edn. WB Saunders, Philadelphia.

Health Services Advisory Committee (1993) *The Management of Occupational Health Services for Healthcare Staff*. HMSO, London.

Hoffman PN (1993) *Clostridium difficile* and the hospital environment. *PHLS Micro. Digest*, **10**(3): 91–2.

Hollyoak V, Allison D, Summers J (1995) *Pseudomonas aeruginosa*, wound infection associated with a nursing home's whirlpool bath. *CDR*, **5**(7): R100–2.

Howarth FH (1985) Prevention of airborne infection during surgery. *Lancet*, **i**: 386–8.

Jarvis WR (1994) Handwashing – the Semmelweis lesson forgotten? *Lancet*, **344**: 1311.

Johnson S, Clabots CR, Linn FV et al (1990) Nosocomial *Clostridium difficile* colonisation and disease. *Lancet*, **336**: 97–100.

Joint Commission on the Accreditation of Healthcare Organisations (1989) Characteristics of clinical indicators. *Qual. Rev Bull.*, **15**: 330–9.

Kingsley A (1992) First step towards a desired outcome. Preventing infection by risk recognition. *Prof. Nurse*, **7**(11): 725–9.

Larson E (1988) A causal link between handwashing and risk of infection? Examination of the evidence. *Infect. Control Hosp. Epidemiol.*, **9**: 28–36.

Levin MH, Olsen B, Nathan C et al (1984) *Pseudomonas* in the sinks of an intensive care unit: relation to patients. *J. Clin. Pathol.*, **37**: 424–7.

Lipman J, Saadia R (1997) Fungal infections in critically ill patients. *BMJ*, **315**: 266–7.

Loomes S (1988) Is it safe to lie down in hospital? *Nursing Times*, **84**(49): 63–5.

Mackintosh CA, Hoffman PN (1984) An extended model for the transfer of micro-organisms via the hands: differences between organisms and the effect of alcohol disinfection. *J. Hyg.*, **92**: 345–55.

Milward S, Barnett J, Thomlinson D (1993) A clinical infection control audit programme: evaluation of an audit tool used by infection control nurses to monitor standard and assess effective staff training. *J. Hosp. Infect.*, **24**: 219–32.

Mortimer EA, Wolinsky E, Gonzaga AJ et al (1966) Role of hands in the transmission of staphylococcal infections. *BMJ*, **1**: 319–22.

Moss F (1995) Risk management and the quality of care. *Qual. Health Care*, **4**: 102–7.

Musa FK, Desai N, Casewell MW et al (1990) The survival of *Acinetobacter calcoaceticus* inoculated on fingertips and formica. *J. Hosp. Infect.*, **15**: 219–228.

National Audit Office (2000) *The Management and Control of Hospital Acquired Infection in Acute NHS Trusts in England*. Report by the Comptroller and Auditor General. The Stationery Office, London.

Newsom SWB (1993) Ignaz Philip P Semmelweis. *J. Hosp. Infect.*, **23**: 175–88.

NHS Executive (1999a) *Governance in the New NHS: Controls Assurance Statements 1999/2000: Risk Management and Organisational Controls*. HSC 1999/123. Department of Health, London.

NHS Executive (1999b) Controls assurance standard. Infection Control. Available: http://www.doh.gov.uk

NHS Executive (2000) *The Management and Control of Hospital Infection*. HSC 2000/002. Department of Health, London.

NHS Management Executive (1993) *Public Health: Responsibilities of the NHS and Roles of Others*. HSG (93)56. Health Publications Unit, Heywood.

Nightingale F (1863) *Notes on Nursing*. Longman, London.

Noone MR, Pitt TL, Bedder M et al (1983) *Pseudomonas aeruginosa* in an intensive therapy unit: role of cross infection and host factors. *BMJ*, **286**: 341–4.

Orsi GB, Mansi A, Tomao P et al (1994) Lack of association between clinical and environmental isolates of *Pseudomonas aeruginosa* in hospital wards. *J. Hosp. Infect.*, **27**(1): 49–60.

Overton E (1988) Bed making and bacteria. *Nursing Times*, **84**(9): 69–71.

Patterson W, Haswell P, Fryers PT et al (1997) Outbreak of a small round structured virus gastroenteritis arose after a kitchen assistant vomited. *CDR Rev.*, **7**(7): R101–3.

Plowman RM, Graves N, Roberts JA (1997) *Hospital-acquired Infection*. Office of Health Economics, London.

Plowman R, Graves N, Griffin M et al (1999) *The Socio-economic Burden of Hospital-acquired Infection*. PHLS, London.

Pratt RA, Pellowe CM, Loveday HP et al (2001) The Epic project: developing national evidence-based guidelines for preventing healthcare associated infections. *J. Hosp. Infect.*, **47**: Suppl. A.

Prieto J (1994) The specialist role of the ICN. *Nursing Times*, **90**(38): 63–66.

Public Health Laboratory Service (2000a) *Surgical Site Infection: Analysis of Two Years' Surveillance in English Hospitals, 1997–1999*. Nosocomial Infection Surveillance Unit, PHLS, London.

Public Health Laboratory Service (2000b) *Hospital Acquired Bacteraemia: Analysis of Two Years' Surveillance in English Hospitals, 1997–1999*. Nosocomial Infection Surveillance Unit, PHLS, London.

Quality Indicator Study Group (1995) An approach to the evaluation of quality indicators of the outcome of care in hospitalised patients, with a focus on nosocomial infection indicators. *Inf. Control Hosp. Epidemiol.*, **16**: 308–16.

Reybrouck G (1983) Role of hands in the spread of nosocomial infections 1. *J. Hosp. Infect.*, **4**: 103–10.

Rhame F (1986) The inanimate environment. In *Hospital Infections* (JV Bennett, PS Brackman, eds), pp. 299–324. Little Brown, Boston.

Rhame FS (1998) The inanimate environment. In *Hospital Infections* (JV Bennett, PS Brachman, eds) 4th edn., pp. 223–50. Lippincott-Raven, Philidelphia.

Richardson R (1999) Implementing evidence-based practice. *Prof. Nurse*, **15**(2): 101–4.

Riley RL, Mills CC, Nyka W et al (1959) Aerial dissemination of pulmonary tuberculosis: a two year study of contagion in a tuberculosis ward. *Am. J. Hyg.*, **70**: 185.

Royal College of Nursing (1991) A Guide to an Occupational Health Nursing Service. A Handbook for Employers and Nurses. Scutari, London.

Sanderson PJ, Weissler S (1992) Recovery of coliforms from the hands of nurses and patients: activities leading to contamination. *J. Hosp. Infect.*, **21**: 85–93.

Scottish Office (1998) Scottish Infection Manual. *Guidance on Core Standards for the Control of Infection in Hospitals, Healthcare Premises and at the Community Interface*. Advisory Group on Infection, Scottish Office, Edinburgh.

Selwyn S (1991) Hospital infection: the first 2500 years. *J. Hosp. Infect.*, **18** (Suppl A): 5–65.

Seto WH, Ching RN, Yuen KY et al (1991) The enhancement of infection control in-service education by ward opinion leaders. *Am. J. Infect. Control*, **19**: 86–91.

Simpson JY (1869) Some propositions on hospitalism. *Lancet*, **Oct 16**: 535–8.

Teare EL, Peacock A (1996) The development of an infection control link-nurse programme in a district general hospital. *J. Hosp. Infect.*, **34**: 267–78.

Thomson RG, McElroy H, Kazandjian VA (1997) Maryland hospital quality indicator project in the United Kingdom: an approach for promoting continuous quality improvement. *Qual. Health Care*, **6**: 49–55.

Välimäki M, Suominen T, Peate I (1998) Attitudes of professionals, students and the general public to HIV/AIDS and people with HIV/AIDS: a review of the research. *J. Adv. Nurs.*, **27**: 752–9.

Wade JJ, Desai N, Casewell MW et al (1991) Hygienic hand disinfection for the removal of epidemic vancomycin-resistant *Enterococcus faecium* and gentamicin-resistant *Enterobacter cloacae*. *J. Hosp. Infect.*, **18**: 211–18.

Ward V, Wilson J, Taylor L et al (1997) *Preventing Hospital-acquired Infection. Clinical Guidelines*. PHLS, London.

Wenzel RP, Thompson RL, Landry SM et al (1983) Hospital-acquired infections in intensive care unit patients: an overview with emphasis on epidemics. *Infect. Control*, **4**: 371.

Whyte W, Hodgson R, Tinkler J (1982) The importance of airborne bacterial contamination of wounds. *J. Hosp. Infect.*, **3**: 123–35.

Wilson J (1995) Infection control: surveying the risks. *Nursing Standard*, **9** (15 Suppl. NU): 3–8.

Wilson J (1998) Clinical governance. *Br. J. Nurs.*, **7**(16): 987–8.

FURTHER READING

Essex-Cater A (1979) *A Manual of Public Health and Community Medicine*, 3rd edn. John Wright, London.

Fine P (1993) Herd immunity: history, theory, practice. *Epidemid. Rev.*, **15**(2): 265–302.

Haley RW (1998) A cost benefit analysis of infection control programs. In *Hospital Infections* (JV Bennett, PS Brachman, eds) 4th edn. pp. 249–68. Little Brown, Boston.

Infection Control Standards Working Party (1993) *Standards in Infection Control in Hospitals*. Laboratory of Hospital Infection, CPHL, London.

Jenner EA, Wilson JA (2000) Educating the infection control team – past, present and future. A British perspective *J. Hosp. Infect.*, **46**: 96–105.

Kretzer EK, Larson EL (1998) Behavioural interventions to improve infection control practices. *Am. J. Infect. Control*, **26**: 245–53.

McCormick A (1993) The notification of infectious diseases in England and Wales. *CDR*, **3**(2): R19–24.

McCulloch J (1999) Risk management in infection control. *Nursing Standard*, **13**(34): 44–6.

Morgan D (ed.) (1989) *Infection Control. The British Medical Association Guide*. Edward Arnold, London.

Mulhall A (1997) Epidemiology in infection control. *Nursing Times*, **93**(45): 68–70.

Wilson J (1997) Formulating a risk management strategy. *Br. J. Nurs.*, **6**(16): 924–5.

4

The immune system and the immunocompromised patient

INTRODUCTION

Molecules recognized by the immune system as 'non-self' are called antigens. Single molecules, complex proteins and carbohydrates, and whole micro-organisms can all be antigenic. The body possesses several different mechanisms that protect it against foreign material or invasion by micro-organisms.

Some of these mechanisms are non-specific and act as general barriers to all types of micro-organisms. These include physical barriers such as the skin and acid in the stomach, which protect points of the body vulnerable to invasion, and internal cellular responses provided by phagocytic cells and the complement proteins. The immune system can also target an attack against specific antigens. This specific response is made by two types of white blood cell: the B lymphocytes, which produce antibodies, and the T lymphocytes, which attack cells that have been invaded by micro-organisms and coordinate the activity of different components of the response. The lymphocytes retain a 'memory' of micro-organisms or other antigens that have previously invaded so that when the same antigen enters the body again the correct antibodies can be produced very rapidly and the micro-organism will be prevented from causing infection. The first line of defence against micro-organisms and other antigens are a series of physical barriers which protect potential points of entry into the body (Fig. 4.1).

NON-SPECIFIC IMMUNE RESPONSE
External defences

Skin

Intact skin provides the body with a tough outer layer that cannot be penetrated by microbes. Lactic acid and fatty acids secreted by sebaceous glands create a low

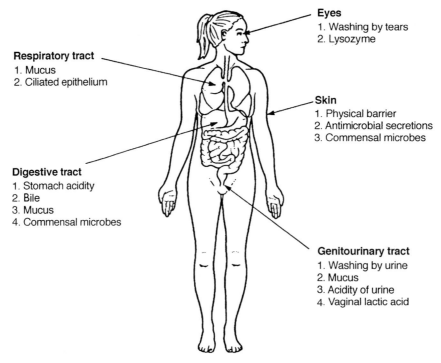

Fig. 4.1 External defences against infection.

pH which, together with an arid environment, prevents the growth of most micro-organisms. Some bacteria, for example diphtheroids and staphylococi, thrive on the surface of the skin and their presence discourages colonization by other species. Whilst this normal flora is usually harmless, some species (e.g. *Staphylococcus epidermidis*) may invade the bloodstream via invasive devices such as intravenous catheters (see Ch. 9). In hospital, the normal skin flora of patients may be replaced by strains of hospital bacteria that are more resistant to **antibiotics** and which can cause serious infections if they enter the body, for example methicillin-resistant *Staphylococcus aureus* (MRSA), klebsiella and acinetobacter species.

Skin that is damaged (e.g. burns, abrasions) or penetrated by invasive devices can be invaded by pathogens. Tetanus **spores** present in contaminated soil may be accidentally introduced through injured skin, human immunodeficiency virus (HIV) and hepatitis B virus by contact with infected blood or body fluids. Infection may also be introduced when skin is incised during surgical procedures or injured (e.g. stab wounds). Some micro-organisms are injected through the skin by the bites of insects (e.g. malaria, typhus and yellow fever).

Respiratory tract

Most micro-organisms are prevented from entering the bronchial tree by hairs in the nose, which filter particles, and the cough reflex, which prevents their aspiration. The membrane that lines the tract secretes mucus. This both traps particles that enter the airway and prevents micro-organisms from adhering to the tissues. Mucus is constantly moved by small hairs called cilia, which propel it upwards towards the mouth, where it is swallowed. This mechanism is called the ciliary escalator.

Lysozyme

This is an enzyme present in tears, nasal secretions and saliva, which breaks down bacterial cell walls and is especially active against **Gram-positive** bacteria.

Gastrointestinal tract

Gastric juices are highly acidic and a pH of between 2 and 3 destroys most ingested bacteria. Bile in the small intestine also inhibits bacterial growth. The large intestine contains many bacteria that discourage the growth of pathogens by competing for nutrients and producing inhibitory substances. Antimicrobial therapy may destroy some of the normal flora and enable other pathogenic species to establish, for example *Clostridium difficile* (see p. 105).

Genitourinary tract

These surfaces are protected by a mucous lining which prevents micro-organisms from adhering to the surface. In the urinary tract, the constant flow of urine flushes out bacteria. In the vagina, commensal lactobacilli produce lactic acid as a byproduct of their metabolism, and the consequently low pH (between 4 and 5) prevents other species from establishing.

Internal defences

When micro-organisms or other antigens penetrate the external defences of the body, the immune system starts to take action. A range of non-specific mechanisms effective against any antigen work in concert with the specific response discussed in the next section. The non-specific defences are:

- inflammatory response
- phagocytic cells
- eosinophils
- complement proteins
- interferon
- natural killer cells.

Inflammatory response

When the body is injured or invaded by micro-organisms or other antigens, a process called the inflammatory response is triggered. Cells that have been damaged by injury or infection release chemical signals called prostaglandins. These cause an increase in the permeability of blood vessels in the area and allow white blood cells and plasma proteins to pass into the tissue. In addition, if immunoglobulin (Ig) E bound to mast cells in tissues encounters an antigen it triggers the release of vasoactive amines (e.g. histamine) and chemotactic factors for phagocytic cells. These stimulate dilation of local arterioles and result in an increased flow of blood to the area. These vascular changes enable the important components of the immune response – the lymphocytes, phagocytes and complement proteins – to be concentrated in the affected area (Table 4.1).

Table 4.1 Stages in the inflammatory response

Response	Mediator	Effect	Visible sign
Dilation of blood vessels	Histamine released from mast cells	Increases blood flow to area	Redness and heat
Blood vessels become more permeable	Prostaglandins	Plasma and white blood cells migrate into tissue	Swelling
Pressure on nerve endings	Swollen tissue	Discourages movement of affected part	Pain

Fever The temperature of the body is maintained by a centre in the hypothalamus of the brain. Increased body temperature is a systemic effect of the inflammatory response. Fever is induced by pyrogens, proteins released by **white blood cells** and hormones such as **prostaglandins**. These substances stimulate the hypothalamus and produce a rise in body temperature. Aspirin inhibits prostaglandins and is used to reduce fever in adults.

Pyrexia is assumed to confer some advantage on the host, although the exact benefit is uncertain. High temperature increases the metabolic rate of the body and this may speed tissue repair and potentiate the immune response (Mackowiak 1994). Most pathogenic microbes prefer a temperature of around 37°C and therefore an increase in body temperature may help the body to destroy them.

The effect of fever on the patient can be exhausting; the heart and respiratory rates increase and violent shivering or rigors may occur in severe fever. This increased activity may cause depletion of the glycogen energy reserves in the body and so protein may need to be broken down as a source of energy, the patient becomes debilitated and tissue repair is delayed. Children have immature temperature control and may experience febrile convulsions if the pyrexia develops rapidly. Although the convulsions are usually transient with no long-term effects, they may lead to aspiration of secretions and asphyxia.

Evidence for the value of fever reduction is conflicting. The febrile patient is already responding as if to a cold environment and further cooling can increase discomfort. The use of antipyrexial drugs can disguise symptoms that may indicate a change in treatment is necessary, for example antibiotics (Styrt & Sugarman 1990).

Guidelines for practice: the care of pyrexial patients

The nursing care should aim to reduce the discomfort associated with a raised body temperature, whilst replacing body fluids lost through sweating. Cooling the skin by sponging with warm water or with a fan may be of some benefit, but frequently causes greater discomfort and stress to the patient (Kinmouth et al 1992).

- Cover with one sheet, remove nightclothes if necessary
- Administer cool drinks frequently
- Offer frequent mouth care to counter the effects of dehydration
- Administer antipyrexial drugs if prescribed

Phagocytic cells

These are white blood cells that engulf foreign substances and destroy them with enzymes by a process known as phagocytosis (Fig. 4.2). For phagocytosis to occur, the microbe (or other foreign substance) must first attach to a surface of the phagocytic cell. Recognition of foreign substances by phagocytes is not specific, but greatly enhanced by complement proteins that coat the surface of the microbe. Phagocytes are attracted to the site of infection by damaged tissues, the products from bacterial cells, antibody complexes and complement proteins.

There are two types of phagocytic cell: polymorphonuclear neutrophil leucocytes (neutrophils) and mononuclear macrophages (Plate 4.1).

Neutrophils are formed in the bone marrow (see Fig. 4.4) and are the main white cell circulating in the blood. They are short-lived, circulating for only 6–8 h, and have receptors on their surface for complement proteins and antibodies. Large granules inside the cell contain enzymes used to destroy ingested antigens.

Macrophages are also formed in the bone marrow (see Fig. 4.4) but are long-lived and mostly concentrated in the tissues. In the spleen and lymph nodes they filter out foreign material circulating through the lymph system. They pass into tissues by secreting enzymes that increase the permeability of blood vessels. Ingested micro-organisms are processed by enzymes, and antigenic components of the micro-organism are then displayed on the surface of the macrophage for recognition by T and B lymphocytes (see p. 66).

Macrophages play an important role in attacking micro-organisms living inside host cells and in fighting chronic infections. *Mycobacterium tuberculosis* is ingested by macrophages but, by preventing the release of enzymes, is able to live and multiply in the white cell. Infected macrophages congregate and become surrounded by connective tissue to form a tubercle.

Eosinophils

These are polymorphonuclear cells, similar to neutrophils, that attack large invaders such as parasitic protozoa. Protozoa are too big to be phagocytosed and instead are destroyed by enzymes released on to them by eosinophils.

Complement proteins

These are a series of proteins that, when activated, have several important effects, essential for phagocytosis to take place:

- increase blood vessel permeability
- attract phagocytes (chemotaxis)

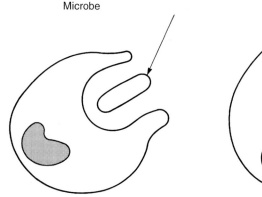
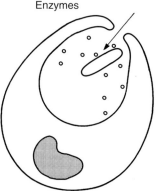

Microbe   Enzymes

Fig. 4.2   Phagocytosis.

- increase efficiency of phagocytosis (opsonization)
- destroy foreign cells by puncturing their membrane.

The complement system is similar to blood clotting in that, once the first protein in the series is triggered, the product of each reaction is an enzyme that catalyses the next stage (see Fig. 4.3). The series of reactions can be triggered in two ways. The classical pathway is initiated by the presence of antibody–antigen complexes; the alternative pathway is triggered by the attachment of the C3 convertase protein to molecules on the surface of micro-organisms. The subsequent reaction produces C3b, which acts as an 'opsonin', that is it coats the surface of a particle, making it more susceptible to phagocytosis. Other complement proteins, such as C5a and C3a, trigger the release of mediators from mast cells (see p. 61). These include chemotactic factors, which attract more phagocytes, and capillary permeability factors, which increase the flow of blood to the area. Another component, C5b, binds to the bacterial membrane and with several other proteins causes a C9 protein to be inserted into the membrane. This allows water and electrolytes to flood in, causing lysis of the cell.

Interferons

Interferons are proteins produced by all cells when infected by a virus and are also produced by T lymphocytes. There are three main types of interferon: natural killer (NK) cells and T lymphocytes produce interferon γ, epithelial cells produce interferon β, and interferon α is produced by most other cells. Interferons inhibit viral infections by binding to receptors on neighbouring cells, causing them to reduce messenger RNA (mRNA) translation and produce enzymes that degrade viral mRNA. Interferons also play an important role in coordinating the immune response. They are part of a family of cytokinins, soluble factors that act as a means of communicating between cells, mobilizing the T lymphocytes when intracellular pathogens are encountered and switching off antibody production by B lymphocytes. They also promote the activity of macrophages, causing them to degrade ingested micro-organisms and display their antigens on their surface for recognition by T lymphocytes.

Interferons are also known to be involved in mobilization of the immune response against tumour cells, and are used to treat some cancers. Their value in

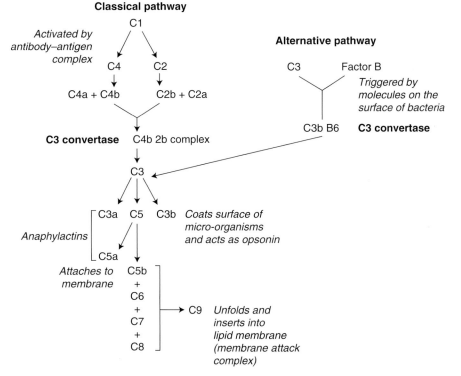

Fig. 4.3   The complement system.

therapy is limited by severe side-effects such as 'flu-like symptoms and bone marrow suppression, but these problems may be overcome by using them in combination with other drugs.

Natural killer cells

These cells resemble T lymphocytes but do not recognize specific antigens. Their main role is to attack intracellular pathogens such as viruses, parasites and malignant cells. It is not known how NK cells recognize infected cells but, once targeted, they bind to the cell and destroy it by releasing enzymes and a protein called perforin, which punches holes in the cell membrane.

THE SPECIFIC IMMUNE RESPONSE

Some microbes are not readily ingested by phagocytic cells or attacked by complement and therefore other cells in the immune system, the lymphocytes, are required to destroy them. Unlike phagocytes, lymphocytes interact with specific antigens; they are able to remember a previous encounter with an antigen and provide a very rapid response the next time the same antigen enters the body.

There are two types of lymphocytes, B and T, both of which recognize and bind to receptors on specific anti-

gens. **B lymphocytes** produce antibodies against the specific antigen, and are referred to as the **humoral immune system**. Humoral means 'of the body fluids' and is used to describe antibodies because they operate outside the cells in the blood and tissue fluids. **T lymphocytes** destroy abnormal or tumour cells and cells infected with viruses or other microbes. T lymphocytes are referred to as the cellular or **cell-mediated immune system**. The T lymphocytes also produce protein molecules (e.g. interferon) that activate other lymphocytes and **macrophages**.

The lymphocytes do not operate independently, but act collectively to destroy the invading antigen. They interact with one another, with phagocytic cells and the complement system. The differentiation of blood cells into red cells, lymphocytes, leucocytes and macrophages is illustrated in Fig. 4.4. The interaction between the different parts of the immune response is illustrated in Fig. 4.7.

B lymphocytes

B lymphocytes originate from stem cells in the bone marrow. They are referred to as B cells because in birds they mature in a structure called the 'bursa of Fabricius'. B lymphocytes are responsible for the production of antibodies.

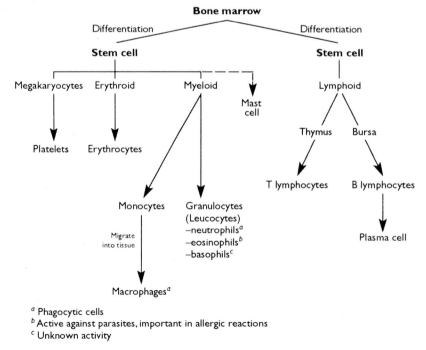

a Phagocytic cells
b Active against parasites, important in allergic reactions
c Unknown activity

Fig. 4.4 Differentiation of blood cells.

Structure of antibodies

Antibodies are Y-shaped proteins called globulins, or **immunoglobulins**. The two arms of the Y vary in structure and are the parts of the molecule that enable the antibody to recognize or fit around different molecules on the surface of an antigen (Fig. 4.5). The stem of the Y activates complement and attaches to phagocytes, triggering them to engulf the invader. There are five different types of immunoglobulin, distinguishable by their structure and number of amino acid chains (see Table 4.2). The same B lymphocytes produce all five types of immunoglobulin and each recognizes the same antigen.

Synthesis of antibodies

Thousands of B lymphocytes are produced and circulate around the body. Each B lymphocyte displays a different antibody on its surface. These attach to a specific antigen that has a complementary shape, like a lock and key. When a lymphocyte encounters an antigen that fits the antibody it is carrying, it binds to the antigen and is

Table 4.2   Different classes of immunoglobulin (antibody)

Immunoglobulin	Activity
IgG	The most abundant; diffuses from blood vessels into tissue fluids. Coats bacteria to facilitate phagocytosis and neutralize bacterial toxins. Crosses the placenta in the last three months of pregnancy
IgM	A large molecule made up of five short and five long chains of amino acids. Is the first to appear in an attack against an antigen, but is confined to blood. Assists phagocytosis by coating the antigen, and binds efficiently with complement
IgA	Acts as the early defence against microbial invasion of mucous membranes. Found in the secretions of reproductive, respiratory and gastrointestinal tract, where it coats micro-organisms and prevents them from adhering to epithelial cells
IgE	Mainly attached to mast cells where it causes the release of histamine if it encounters an antigen. Associated with allergic response (e.g. hay fever), but also thought to be involved in the destruction of parasites
IgD	Maximum levels are detected during childhood but function is unknown

triggered to convert into a plasma cell. This cell synthesizes large quantities of the particular antibody carried by the lymphocyte. The plasma cells then divide rapidly to produce a large number of identical cells or clones, all of which carry the same antibody. This mechanism enables a large amount of specific antibody to be produced when required. T lymphocytes influence the division and maturation of the plasma cells with messenger proteins (interferons) which bind to receptors on the surface of the B lymphocyte.

The first type of immunoglobulin to be synthesized by the plasma cell is IgM. After a few days T lymphocytes trigger a switch in production to IgG (Table 4.2). Production of IgG can continue for up to 1 year. As IgG is the only class of immunoglobulin that can cross the placenta, newborn infants acquire only IgG from their mother. This disappears after approximately 6 months and the child begins to synthesize its own IgM. Levels of IgG and IgA remain below those of an adult until the child is 7 and 12 years old, respectively.

One micro-organism may have several receptor sites recognized by different antibodies. Once antibodies have bound to its surface, the complement system and

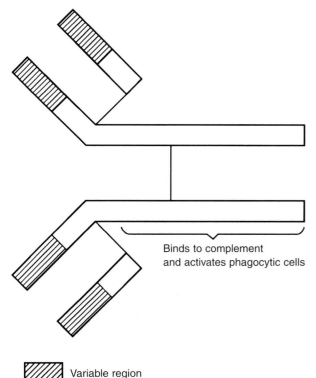

Binds to complement and activates phagocytic cells

▨ Variable region

Fig. 4.5   The structure of immunoglobulin G. IgG is made of two long and two short peptide chains. The variable regions determine the specificity of the antibody.

phagocytes are activated and the micro-organism is destroyed.

T lymphocytes

These lymphocytes are formed in the bone marrow but mature in a gland called the thymus that is situated behind the sternum. The thymus is prominent in children, continuing to grow until puberty. It then gradually diminishes in size, although it is still active in old age.

There are two types of T lymphocyte: cytotoxic T cells, which destroy infected cells and tumour cells, and T helper cells, which regulate the activity of other cells, coordinating the attack by the immune system.

Recognition of infected cells

T lymphocytes are particularly important for the control of intracellular parasites such as mycobacteria, fungi, viruses and protozoa. Antibodies can attack these microbes while they are in the blood or tissue fluid, but not if they are inside a host cell. Many micro-organisms can multiply inside phagocytes that engulf them. To attack these pathogens, the T lymphocyte must be able to identify infected cells. They do this by recognizing 'non-self' antigens on the surface of an infected cell. All cells constantly degrade proteins into small fragments which bind to a molecule called the major histocompatibility complex (MHC) and are carried to the surface of the cell. Fragments from the host cell proteins are ignored by circulating T lymphocytes, but when a 'non-self' fragment from a micro-organism infecting the cell is displayed, a T lymphocyte with the appropriately shaped receptor locks on to the combination of MHC and microbial fragment (Fig. 4.6). Like B lymphocytes, T lymphocytes are programmed at the time they are made with a unique surface receptor. Each T lymphocyte will therefore recognize a specific antigen which best fits the shape of this receptor.

Destruction of intracellular pathogens

Once the T lymphocyte has bound on to the MHC and microbial fragment, it is triggered to divide rapidly, producing a large number of T lymphocytes all carrying the same surface receptor. Cytotoxic T cells recognize viral fragments combined with the MHC and attack the infected cell with enzymes before new virus can be released (Fig. 4.7). T helper lymphocytes recognize microbial fragments on an infected macrophage and release interferon γ, which activates the suppressed macrophage to destroy the micro-organism.

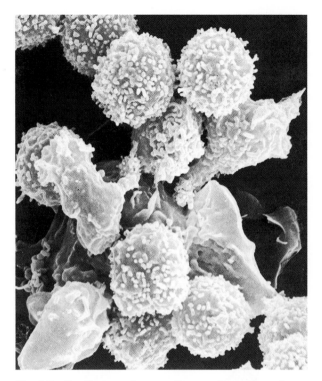

Fig. 4.6 T cells recognize an antigen on the surface of a macrophage. The T cells are the small spherical objects, the macrophage the larger, flat object.

T helper cells also produce a range of interleukins (Fig. 4.7). These are cytokines, soluble factors that act on other cells in the immune system and coordinate the response to the invasion. They play a key role in the activity of B lymphocytes, promoting antibody production in response to bacterial invasion and suppressing it in favour of T lymphocyte activity in response to intracellular pathogens.

Memory cells

Following exposure to a particular antigen both B and T lymphocytes produce memory cells to protect against subsequent infections (Fig. 4.7). These are primed to respond if the same antigen is encountered again, enabling the production of a large number of specific lymphocytes. A second exposure to a previously encountered antigen therefore results in the appearance of specific antibody at 10 to 15 times the concentration of the first response within 3 days. These memory cells enable immunity to specific infections to develop, and form the basis of active immunization to prevent the acquisition of infection (see Fig. 4.10).

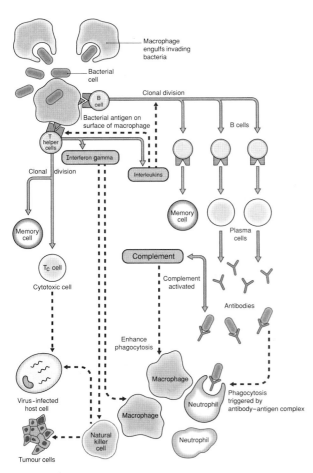

Fig. 4.7 The specific immune response. The B cells, T cells and macrophages all interact to fend off the attack from invading micro-organisms.

Monoclonal antibodies

A large amount of a single antibody can be manufactured artificially by fusing a cell producing specific antibodies with a cell from a B lymphocyte tumour. The fused cells survive and multiply indefinitely in tissue culture and produce many copies of the single specific antibody. These monoclonal antibodies are used in research on infectious diseases and the immune system and for the identification of some micro-organisms (e.g. legionella, chlamydia, viruses). They can provide very specific and sensitive tests enabling particular proteins to be isolated from complex mixtures.

The recognition of self and non-self

Defence against an invader is possible only if the immune system is able to distinguish between the cells of the host (self) and those of the invader (non-self). At birth the immune system is immature and does not respond to self and non-self antigens that it encounters, possibly because neonatal macrophages are unable to present antigens or because all the self-reacting B and T lymphocytes are inactivated. T lymphocytes are particularly important in the recognition and destruction of 'non-self' cells. They undergo a process of differentiation in the thymus that results in the elimination of any lymphocytes that might recognize self markers. The final set of T lymphocytes therefore recognizes only 'non-self' markers.

Each cell of the body also carries on its surface a distinct marker of selfness called the major histocompatibility complex (MHC), which not only differs between species but between individuals of the same species. The segment of **chromosome** that codes for these 'self-marking' molecules is called the **human leucocyte antigen (HLA) system**.

The MHC markers enable the immune system to recognize and destroy tissue grafted into the body from another person. Grafted material is less likely to be attacked by the immune system if the MHC proteins of the donated material are similar to those of the host. Tissue typing is used to find donors whose MHC proteins are very similar to those of the intended recipient of the tissue.

Organs of the immune system

The immune response is mounted from lymphoid tissue found throughout the body at points vulnerable to invasion (Fig. 4.8). These are connected by a network of small channels called the lymphatic system. There is lymphoid tissue in the liver, spleen, gut (Peyer's patches and appendix), tonsils and adenoids. It is also found in the lymph nodes – small glands distributed throughout the body at junctions between lymph and blood vessels. The cells of the immune system are made in the bone marrow. They differentiate from a single stem cell into several different lines which produce lymphocytes, macrophages and granulocytes (e.g. neutrophils). Once they have matured, the cells migrate to the lymphoid tissue.

Response to invasion by micro-organisms

When a micro-organism reaches a lymph node or other lymphoid tissue it is trapped and ingested by macrophages. These process the micro-organism and display its antigens on their surface for recognition by T lymphocytes. The T lymphocytes then bind to the antigen and trigger the specific immune response

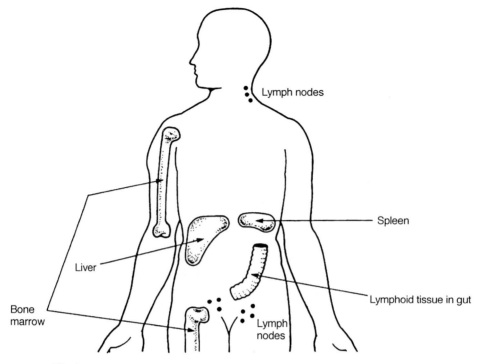

Fig. 4.8 The organs of the immune response.

against the invading micro-organism. The lymph nodes closest to the site of infection will mount the immune response and this is apparent when they become swollen and painful; for example, an infection of the leg may cause lymph nodes in the groin to swell, whilst an infection of the upper respiratory tract causes nodes in the neck to swell. Once the micro-organisms have been destroyed, B and T lymphocyte memory cells remain and are distributed throughout the lymphoid tissue, enabling a rapid response to be made should the pathogen invade again.

IMMUNITY TO INFECTION

The B and T lymphocyte memory cells enable a very rapid response to be mounted against micro-organisms encountered previously. This enables the host to develop **immunity** to infections. Immunity can be acquired naturally following an infection or artificially by the inoculation of an organism or its products into the body. Immunity can also be conferred by injecting antibody (lgG) against a specific micro-organism. This is called **passive immunity** because it does not cause the production of memory cells and the protection lasts only for the lifetime of the IgG. IgG crosses the placenta from mother to fetus so that the baby has

some protection against infection for the first few months of life (Fig. 4.9).

Immunization

In the developed world, the ravages of **infectious** disease have declined dramatically in the last 100 years and immunization is one of several factors that have played a part in this decline (Box 4.1). The principles of immunization were developed in the early 1800s. They were pioneered by Edward Jenner, who in 1796 demonstrated that humans could be protected against smallpox by inoculation with a similar virus which caused cowpox in cows; this was the first use of a **vaccine** (Plate 4.2).

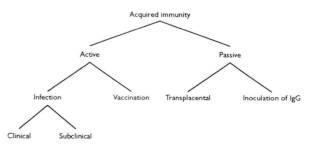

Fig. 4.9 Acquired immunity to infection.

Vaccines

The aim of vaccination is to induce a specific immune response against a particular micro-organism without causing the actual disease. Most vaccines produce their protective effect by stimulating the production of antibodies, although Bacillus Calmette–Guérin (BCG) vaccine for tuberculosis promotes cell-mediated immunity.

There are a number of different types of vaccine available (Table 4.3). Some are made from dead micro-organisms, others from live micro-organisms that have been altered (attenuated) to prevent them causing infection. A few are made from bacterial products such as altered toxins.

Killed micro-organisms These can be made from whole cells that have been killed, for example by heat, or from purified components of the cell such as capsule proteins.

Live-attenuated These use live micro-organisms that have been altered to prevent them causing infection. They induce a good immune response because the organism multiplies in the body resulting in a high level of antigen production. Some live-attenuated vaccines can induce a long-lasting immunity after just a single dose (e.g. measles, mumps, rubella (MMR) vaccine). Attenuated strains occasionally revert to their disease-causing form and the vaccines can therefore be associated with complications (e.g. encephalitis in association with measles vaccination). The BCG

vaccine against tuberculosis is a live-attenuated vaccine of a related organism *Mycobacterium bovis*.

Inactivated toxin Toxins produced by a micro-organism are inactivated by treatment with formaldehyde. Although the resulting toxoid induces an immune response, its toxic activity is destroyed. Adsorption of the toxoid on to aluminium hydroxide reduces the rate at which it diffuses from the site of inoculation and stimulates macrophage activity.

Genetically engineered Gene manipulation techniques have now been applied to vaccine production. The genes that code for specific microbial antigens (the part of the bacterium or virus recognized by the immune system) are isolated and inserted into a piece of DNA which is transferred into a yeast and cultured in a very large fermenter. The yeast makes the antigen, which is then recovered, purified and made into a vaccine. This method is used to make a vaccine for hepatitis B.

Some organisms present particular problems for vaccine production. The orthomyxoviruses, which cause influenza, undergo minor changes to the proteins on their surface (antigenic drift) and occasionally major changes (antigenic shift). The latter occurs when large sections of chromosome are exchanged with viruses from other animal hosts. Antibody made to the antigens on one strain of influenza may not recognize the antigens on the surface of the next season's strain. When an antigenic shift occurs, the population will have little immunity to the new strain and an **epidemic** of influenza may result. Influenza vaccine is made from several different viral strains and is prepared each year by identifying the strains most likely to be prevalent. It is recommended mainly for the elderly or those with heart and chest disease who are most vulnerable. The vaccine provides reasonable protection against the selected strains but protection only lasts for about one year (Department of Health 1996).

HIV presents similar problems because when it replicates the **genome** is frequently copied inaccurately. Copies of the virus therefore vary slightly and make it difficult for the immune system to respond effectively.

Table 4.3 Types of vaccine in routine use

Type of vaccine	Examples
Live attenuated micro-organisms	Polio, measles, mumps, rubella, BCG
Killed organisms	Pertussis, cholera, typhoid
Viral proteins	Influenza
Capsule polysaccharide	Meningococcus, pneumococcus
Genetically engineered	Hepatitis B
Inactivated toxin	Diphtheria, tetanus

Administration of vaccines

Injection of a vaccine into an individual who has not previously been exposed to the infection induces a slow production of antibody, mostly IgM. The level rises to a peak within a few weeks and may then fall to undetectable levels. This is called the **primary response**. Further injections produce a more rapid response to a higher level, for longer; this is called the secondary response. The level of IgM produced is similar to the primary response but a much greater amount of IgG is produced (Fig. 4.10). After a full course of vaccine the level of antibody remains high for months or years. Another single dose of vaccine will increase the level of antibody rapidly because the immune system has been induced to make memory cells. Most immunizations require a course of at least three injections, although some vaccines of live-attenuated micro-organisms (e.g. MMR) produce a high level of antibody after one injection. In many cases, vaccination has been shown to confer protection for at least 15 years (e.g. rubella and BCG). Others may require a booster dose every few years (e.g. cholera).

Passive immunization

The immunity conferred by active immunization with vaccine takes several weeks to establish as it depends on the production of specific antibodies or immunoglobulins. In certain situations, where an individual has been exposed to an infection and is known to have no immunity to it, a more rapid protection against infection is required. The specific antibodies or immunoglobulins made after exposure to particular micro-organisms can be collected from people recently infected or who have high levels of antibody following immunization. If inoculated into another person, these specific immunoglobulins will protect against infection, although the protection will be only temporary as they will gradually be lost from the body.

This type of **immunization** can be used to protect against infection by hepatitis B following a needlestick injury and to protect **immunocompromised** individuals, who may develop serious illness, from chickenpox following exposure to the virus.

The impact of immunization programmes

Immunization is aimed at protecting individuals against a life-threatening or serious disease, a fetus (for example by the immunization of women against rubella) or the community as a whole through the principle of 'herd immunity'. If sufficient numbers of a population are immune to the disease the micro-organism is unable to find susceptible hosts in which to cause infection. For herd immunity to be effective a minimum of 60% of the population must be immune, and a higher level if the infection spreads rapidly and is highly **contagious**.

It is rare for an infection to be completely eradicated through immunization alone. The smallpox eradication programme was started in 1959 by the World Health Organization and not completed until the last case (outside of a laboratory) occurred in 1977. Its success depended on an effective vaccine, an easily identifiable disease with no animal or environmental reservoir, and an intensive worldwide surveillance and immunization programme.

It is essential that high rates of immunization are maintained. In instances when diphtheria immunization has been relaxed, resurgence of the disease has occurred rapidly. Following fears in the mid 1970s about brain damage associated with the pertussis vaccine, the rate of immunization fell from over 80% to 30%. As a result the number of cases of whooping cough increased from around 2400 in 1973 to over 100 000 in 1977–79 (Fig. 4.11).

As with all medicines, vaccines carry some risk but, even with the pertussis vaccine, the risk is extremely small and less than that of the risk of serious complications from the disease itself.

In the UK, the Department of Health recommends a schedule of immunization from early childhood and the primary healthcare services are responsible for its implementation (Table 4.4). Detailed information

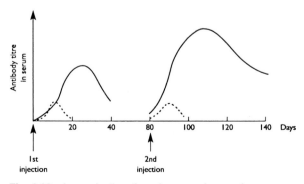

Fig. 4.10 Immunization: the primary and secondary response. Small amounts of IgG (–) and IgM (---) are formed after the first injection but disappear fairly rapidly. After the second injection IgG reaches a higher level and persists in the serum for much longer.

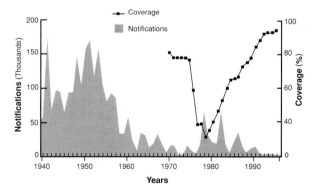

Fig. 4.11 Pertussis notifications (1940–1995) and the effect of immunization uptake (Department of Health 1996).

Table 4.4 Schedule for routine immunization

Vaccine	Age	
Diphtheria, tetanus, pertussis (DTP)	2 months	1st dose
polio, *Haemophilus influenzae* (Hib)	3 months	2nd dose
	4 months	3rd dose
Measles, mumps, rubella (MMR)	12–15 months	1st dose
Diphtheria, tetanus, polio, MMR	4–5 years	Booster 2nd dose
BCG	10–14 years or infancy	
Tetanus, diphtheria, polio	13–18 years	Booster

about all aspects of vaccines is available in the Department of Health publication *Immunisation Against Infectious Disease* (DoH 1996).

THE DAMAGED IMMUNE SYSTEM

Individuals vary widely in their ability to resist infection and this depends on many factors, including age, general health, state of nutrition, previous exposure to infection and vaccination. Young children have an immature immune system and are more likely to succumb to infection until they have developed a range of specific memory cells. The elderly also have a diminished immune response, particularly by the T lymphocytes, and are more susceptible to infection.

Physical or emotional stress, for example multiple traumatic injury or major surgery, can affect the immune response through the release of anti-inflammatory hormones such as **prostaglandin** from damaged tissue and corticosteroids from the adrenal glands. In major burns, **immunosuppression** occurs through the loss of white blood cells and immunoglobulins and reduced phagocytic function. Poor nutrition impairs phagocytosis and reduces the production of white blood cells and antibodies (Conry 1982).

These factors should be taken into account when assessing a patient's risk of acquiring an infection. The immune system of a patient who is malnourished or under stress will be less able to destroy bacteria that invade wounds, intravenous cannula, etc. Planning the care of patients towards improving the activity of their immune system is essential if infection is to be prevented. Risk assessment is discussed in more detail in Chapter 3.

Disease associated with immune deficiency

Impairment of the immune response occurs as a result of a variety of genetic disorders, autoimmune disease, chemotherapy and certain viral infections, notably HIV.

The most serious genetic disorder is severe combined immune deficiency disorder in which there is a failure of the bone marrow stem cells to differentiate into **B** and **T cells**, and as a result lymphocytes are not produced. It can be treated by bone marrow transplantation but the children often die from infection at a few months of age, before the diagnosis has been made.

Autoimmune disorders occur as a result of a malfunction of the body's mechanism for the recognition of cells as 'self', resulting in antibodies being made against host tissue. The damage to the tissue or the deposition of antibody–antigen complexes in joints, blood vessels or kidney causes the symptoms of the disease (see Table 4.5).

In rheumatic fever, antibodies formed against *Streptococcus pyogenes* infection in the throat cross-react with tissue on the heart valves that has very similar receptors. The antibodies recognize the heart valves as an antigen, and the resulting damage is called endocarditis.

Chemotherapy can have profound immunosuppressive effects. Cytotoxic drugs interfere non-specifically in cell division but because bone marrow cells divide very frequently, about once every 12–30 h, the drugs have a major effect on bone marrow and the production of blood cells. Some antibiotics inhibit **cellular**

Table 4.5 Autoimmune diseases

Autoimmune disease	Self-antigen recognized
Pernicious anaemia	Gastric parietal cells
Juvenile insulin-dependent diabetes	Pancreatic islet cells
Multiple sclerosis	Central nervous system myelin
Lupus erythematosus	DNA, red blood cells, lymphocytes, platelets

immunity (e.g. chloramphenicol, tetracycline). Steroids have long-term effects on the production of immunoglobulins and interfere with the inflammatory response.

Leukaemias are a group of malignant diseases affecting the white cell precursors in the bone marrow. Susceptibility to infection is increased through the overproduction of immature or abnormal white blood cells and the suppression of normal cell production.

Aplastic anaemia is a severe depression of the bone marrow which causes depletion of red blood cells, white blood cells and platelets. There are a variety of causes of aplastic anaemia, including exposure to drugs (e.g. chloramphenicol), chemicals (e.g. benzene) or ionizing radiation.

Acquired immune deficiency syndrome (AIDS)

The human immunodeficiency virus (HIV) attaches to and invades cells that carry a particular protein called CD4. Several cells involved in the immune response carry CD4, including the T helper lymphocytes (T4 cells) and macrophages. HIV depletes circulating T4 cells sited in the lymph nodes and gradually damages the immune system. The lymph nodes appear to be the site of greatest viral replication and their eventual destruction has devastating effects on the immune response (Greene 1993).

The main effect of T4 cell depletion is a diminished response to organisms that cause intracellular infection, for example tubercle bacilli and salmonella, protozoa such as toxoplasma and cryptosporidium, and viruses, in particular cytomegalovirus. Susceptibility to other organisms, which would not normally cause serious infection in an immune-competent host, is also increased (e.g. *Pneumocystis carinii*, herpes simplex, *Candida albicans*). Certain malignant tumours that would normally be destroyed by T cells may also develop, for example B cell lymphomas and Kaposi's sarcoma (a cancer of endothelial cells).

HIV has an RNA genome, which is converted to DNA before transcription by an enzyme called reverse transcriptase. This enzyme tends to copy inaccurately, so HIV tends to accumulate mutations rapidly; this reduces the chance of it being recognized by memory lymphocytes.

Hypersensitivity reactions

Sometimes the immune system responds in an excessive way to an antigen. This is called a hypersensitivity reaction. The reaction may be mild, for instance hay fever induced by allergy to pollen, or severe systemic anaphylactic reactions that are sometimes fatal (e.g. insect stings in a highly sensitized person).

Hypersensitivity reactions are caused by the rapid release of vasoactive amines from mast cells. These are triggered rapidly when exposed to the antigen for a second time, and result in local vascular permeability and oedema. If excessive amounts are released into the bloodstream, hypotensive shock, cardiac and respiratory failure may occur.

Delayed hypersensitivity reactions are mediated by T lymphocytes and occur 24–48 h after exposure to an intracellular pathogen. This reaction is the basis of the Heaf test used to determine immunity to *Mycobacterium tuberculosis*.

Organ transplants

It is now possible to treat many illnesses by replacing diseased organs or tissue with healthy tissue from another person, for example kidney, heart, lung and bone marrow. One of the major obstacles to successful organ transplantation is the rejection of the new or 'grafted' material by the recipient's immune system. The surface markers on the foreign tissue cells are recognized as 'non-self' and the foreign material is gradually destroyed, primarily by the T lymphocytes of the cellular immune system. This response is called 'graft versus host disease' or GVHD. Successful transplantation therefore depends on tissue typing, the selection of donor material that is closely related to that of the recipient and less likely to be destroyed, and the use of immunosuppressant drugs that interfere with the activity of T lymphocytes.

One of the most useful of these drugs was originally derived from a fungus and is called cyclosporin A. It blocks the production of lymphokines and therefore affects the immune response to new antigens but not the response by memory cells to previously encountered antigens. Another commonly used drug, azathioprine, inhibits the synthesis of **nucleic acids** and therefore prevents cell division. It has a preferential effect on T cells, but also affects cells in the bone marrow and intestine.

PREVENTING INFECTION IN THE IMMUNOCOMPROMISED PATIENT

Individuals who have a severely damaged immune system are at particular risk of life-threatening infection acquired either **endogenously** or **exogenously** whilst in hospital. They are more likely to be exposed to infection by contact with other patients, staff and through invasive procedures that bypass their defences against micro-organisms.

The immunocompromised host

The expression 'compromised host' is a vague term used to describe an individual who has a severely impaired immune system. Damage to the immune system renders these individuals particularly susceptible to infection, even by 'opportunists', micro-organisms that are not usually able to cause serious infection, for example *Pneumocystis carinii, Candida albicans.*

The type of infection associated with immunodeficiency depends on the part of the immune system that is affected. If the cellular or T cell response is reduced, those microbes that cause **intracellular** infections predominate. Examples are salmonella, listeria, cryptococcus, pneumocystis, and viruses that persist in a latent form, such as herpes virus and cytomegalovirus. If the humoral or B lymphocyte response is affected, protection against bacterial pathogens such as *Staphylococcus aureus* and pneumococcus is reduced. The phagocytic cells or **granulocytes** are important for both the B and T lymphocyte responses; therefore, a reduction in the number of these cells increases susceptibility to a wide range of infections, particularly **Gram-negative** bacteria, *Staphylococcus epidermidis* and *S. aureus.* Neutrophils account for the largest proportion of granulocytes, and in immunocompromised patients the number of neutrophils circulating in the blood is an important indicator of susceptibility to infection. Granulocytopenic patients are most vulnerable to infection from opportunistic pathogens amongst their own microbial flora. However, they are also more susceptible to infection from inhaled or ingested pathogens, micro-organisms introduced to the tissue via invasive devices such as intravenous cannulas, or transferred by equipment or on the hands of staff (Remington and Schimpff 1981, Schimpff et al 1978).

The most severe granulocytopenia occurs in patients receiving bone marrow transplants, who may have less than 1000 neutrophils per microlitre of blood for several weeks after the procedure and are at significant risk of acquiring infection (Bodey et al 1966, Tablan et al 1994). These patients are susceptible to opportunistic pathogens such as aspergillus. The spores of this fungus are carried in the air and, if inhaled, can cause invasive pulmonary aspergillosis, a serious infection associated with a high mortality rate. The infection may also disseminate to other organs via the bloodstream. Patients most at risk are those who have severe, prolonged granulocytopenia, and outbreaks of aspergillosis have been reported in bone marrow transplant units associated with contamination of hospital ventilation systems and high spore levels as a result of construction work (Tablan et al 1994).

Patients receiving solid organ transplants such as heart or kidney are usually less severely immunosuppressed because cyclosporin enables successful transplantation with minimal immune suppression. Patients receiving chemotherapy or with leukaemia are also immunosuppressed, but to a lesser degree than patients undergoing bone marrow transplantation.

Simple protective isolation

Complex methods of preventing infection in immunocompromised patients have been recommended, including the use of sterile equipment, masks, gowns, gloves and overshoes. However, such extensive precautions are expensive, increase the emotional deprivation of the patient and family, and there is evidence that they are no more effective in preventing infections than more simple methods (Garner 1996, Nauseef & Maki 1981).

The following simple precautions are based on routine infection control measures (see Ch. 7). They are recommended as an effective and practical method of minimizing the risk of infection in most severely immunocompromised patients and are summarized in Fig. 4.12.

Accommodation Most immunocompromised patients are as likely to acquire infection in single room as in a ward with other patients (Nauseef & Maki 1981). However, a single room can act as a reminder that special precautions are required.

There is evidence that patients in **protective isolation** are able to cope better with the experience than those isolated because of an infectious disease. This may be because the immunocompromised are involved in the decision to isolate and prepared for the experience (Collins et al 1989). However, isolation can cause patients to become demanding and irritable, and these behaviours should be recognized as a response to isolation (Denton 1986). Psychosocial care of the patients is important to help them through the period of isolation but is frequently overlooked (Gaskill et al 1997, Knowles 1993) (see Table 14.2). It should form part of the holistic care of all isolated patients.

Immunocompromised patients do not usually require segregation from other patients provided that simple precautions are taken to avoid contact with infectious diseases (e.g. chickenpox, respiratory tract infection). Common upper respiratory infection such as respiratory syncytial virus can also cause serious illness in undergoing bone marrow transplantation patients. Early identification and isolation of infected patients and restriction of infected visitors and staff are important to prevent transmission (Garcia et al 1997). Nauseef & Maki (1981) demonstrated that patients

Indication

Patients with a severely compromised immune system

Aims

- To reduce the risk of an immunologically compromised patient acquiring infection
- To give psychological support and reassurance to the patient whilst in isolation
- To ensure all staff (including domestic staff) are aware of the correct precautions to take

Equipment

- A single room with a washbasin
- The room must be clean before the patient is isolated

Inside room: soap
paper towels
washbowl
sphygmomanometer
alcohol handrub
disposable clean gloves
plastic aprons

- Display a protective isolation card at the entrance to the room

Practice	Rationale
Patient – explain reason for isolation and give reassurance	To reduce anxiety and gain the patient's cooperation
Apron – put on a plastic apron before contact with the patient and between dirty and clean procedures	To prevent transmission of organisms from clothing to patient
Gloves – not necessary except for aseptic procedures and contact with blood and body fluids. Discard immediately after use	To prevent contamination of vulnerable sites and cross-infection from one site to another
Masks – not necessary	
Hands – always wash hands before entering the room. Repeat before handling invasive devices or contact with susceptible sites	To remove transient micro-organisms
Staff – exclude staff with infections. Staff who are nursing patients with infections should avoid nursing patients in protective isolation during the same span of duty	To minimize the risk of transferring micro-organisms
Equipment – clean thoroughly with detergent and water before use.	To remove micro-organisms
Crockery – use normal utensils and wash in the normal way	The risk of cross-infection is minimal. Washing in hot water and detergent is sufficient
Visitors – instruct to wash hands on entering room; exclude those with infections	To remove potential pathogens

Practice	Rationale
Other department – should be notified in advance and where possible the patient seen on the ward	To enable appropriate arrangements to be made
Cleaning – ensure that a high standard of cleaning is maintained. Explain the precautions to domestic staff	Dust may harbour micro-organisms. Regular cleaning will remove them
Food – always wash hands and put on a plastic apron before handling food. Food must be served without delay and meals must not be retained for reheating later	These patients are more susceptible to illness from pathogenic bacteria in food. Bacteria multiply in food unless stored at above 65°C or below 5°C
If a microwave is used ensure that the instructions on the packet are followed precisely	To ensure the food reaches an even temperature throughout
The following food should be avoided: salads, 'take-away' foods (including delicatessen), soft-boiled eggs, soft ripened cheeses (e.g. Brie)	Soft cheese and ready-to-eat meals may be contaminated with listeria
Fruit should be washed and peeled	
Fresh tap water and fresh pasteurized milk are permissible	

Fig. 4.12 Policy for the protective isolation of immunocompromised patients.

with granulocytopenia in a ward with other patients were no more likely to acquire infection than those in single rooms. Filtered air systems may be indicated in some situations (Box 4.2), for example for wound dressings on patients with extensive burns or in specialized bone marrow transplant units where patients have severely depleted T cells and outbreaks of airborne fungal infections may occur (Ayliffe & Lilly 1985, Rogers & Barnes 1988).

Handwashing Handwashing is probably the most important method of protecting the immunocompromised patient. Hands should be washed thoroughly with soap and water before contact with the patient to prevent the transfer of micro-organisms from other patients. Hands should also be washed immediately before direct contact with vulnerable sites on the patient such as intravenous cannulae, urethral catheters and wounds. An alcohol handrub is a useful, quick alternative to soap and water when hands are not visibly soiled (see Ch. 7).

Protective clothing Protective clothing should be used to prevent micro-organisms from other patients in the ward and from the patient's own flora gaining access to vulnerable sites. Gloves and aprons should be used for contact with body fluids and changed before

---

Box 4.2 Air filtration systems

There are two types of air filtration: plenum and laminar flow. In plenum ventilation, air is filtered and drawn into the room through vents in the ceiling and out of the room through vents in the walls. In laminar flow, filtered air flows horizontally across the bed area and leaves on the opposite side of the room. It is highly effective in removing micro-organisms from the air but is costly to install and maintain. High-efficiency particulate air (HEPA) filters are used to remove particles of 0.5 μm or more. Doors and windows must be well sealed and the room air pressure maintained above that of the corridor to ensure that unfiltered air does not flow into the room from the outside.

Trexler isolators are plastic tents with built-in 'suits' that enable staff to administer care from outside the tent (Trexler et al 1975). They provide an absolute barrier to micro-organisms from the environment and staff, but they are expensive, often of no benefit, and are now rarely used.

---

contact with wounds, cannulas, catheters or drains. If used appropriately, they can minimize the risk of micro-organisms gaining access to vulnerable sites on the patient. Sterile protective clothing is unnecessary as it is an unlikely source of infection. There is little evidence that masks provide protection against respiratory pathogens (Nauseef and Maki 1981, Taylor 1980). Staff with upper respiratory tract infections should be excluded from direct contact with these patients as this is a safer means of protecting the patient from respiratory pathogens than masks. The use of unnecessary protective clothing should be avoided as this may increase the patient's sense of isolation.

Visitors Visitors should be asked to wash their hands before seeing the patients, but excluded from contact only if they have an infection. Visitors do not have contact with invasive devices or other susceptible sites on the patient and therefore do not need to wear protective clothing.

Equipment In general, there is no reason to treat equipment differently. Low-risk equipment used only on intact skin should be processed in the usual way (e.g. linen, bedpans, crockery). However, some equipment is easily contaminated and often not cleaned thoroughly (e.g. commodes, washbowls). It is therefore preferable to allocate one of these items for use only by the patient and to clean each item thoroughly with detergent and water after each use. There is little value in autoclaving a wide range of items used by immunocompromised patients, especially newspapers, toys and books. The only equipment that needs to be sterile are items used for invasive procedures.

Cleaning Dust harbours micro-organisms and should be removed regularly from all horizontal surfaces where it collects. Disinfection of surfaces is of no value. Dry floors and surfaces are an unlikely source of infection and contamination is removed only temporarily by **disinfectants** (Ayliffe et al 1967).

Food Food normally contains micro-organisms that are not harmful provided they are present in low numbers. Hospital food often contains Gram-negative bacilli (Remington & Schimpff 1981, Shooter et al 1969), which can cause serious infection in an immunocompromised host. Whilst it is impractical to sterilize food, particularly as the process may significantly alter the taste, every effort must be made to ensure that food is hygienically prepared and handled (see Ch. 12). Meat should be cooked thoroughly, fruit and vegetables should be washed and peeled before consumption, and hospital-prepared salads should be avoided. Cooked food, opened tins and jars should always be stored in the refrigerator

and discarded after 24 h, before micro-organisms have the chance to multiply. Reheating of meals should be avoided, except 'ready-to-eat' meals, which should be heated exactly as described by the manufacturer's instructions.

The main foods to avoid are soft cheeses, patés and freshly cut salads which may contain listeria, and cold meats, which are easily contaminated during handling (Jones 1990, Lund et al 1989). Eggs are sometimes contaminated with salmonella and should be thoroughly cooked before eating (De Louvois 1993). Food that contains raw egg (e.g. mayonnaise) should be avoided. Tap water from a drinking supply usually contains very few micro-organisms and is probably safe to drink provided it is fresh from the tap. Ice made in ice-making machines can be more hazardous because the water supplied to the machine may be contaminated, the ice may be present for considerable periods, and ice in the machine may be contaminated by patients or staff using it. Outbreaks of infection caused by Gram-negative bacteria and cryptosporidium have been associated with ice-making machines (Medical Devices Directorate 1993, Ravn et al 1991). Immunocompromised patients should not use ice from ice-making machines and, where machines are in use, they should be properly connected and maintained (Medical Devices Directorate 1993). Ice should not be removed by hand and vessels used to remove or store the ice should be washed with detergent and water after each use. Bottled water may contain large numbers of bacteria, although probably no more than may be consumed on food. Bottled water should be stored in the refrigerator once opened and drunk within 3 days. It should not be drunk directly from the bottle as this may contaminate the water (Hunter 1993).

Invasive procedures Probably the most important aspect of the care of the immunocompromised patient is rigorous attention to the care of intravenous cannulas. Nauseef & Maki (1981) suggest that a higher rate of **bacteraemia** observed when patients were isolated in a single room was related to the reduced attention to intravenous lines afforded to these patients. Total parenteral nutrition, in particular, increases the risk of infection associated with intravenous therapy. The recommended care for intravenous cannulae and urethral catheters is outlined in Chapters 9 and 10.

REFERENCES

Ayliffe GAJ, Lilly HA (1985) Cross-infection and its prevention. *J. Hosp. Infect.*, **6** (Suppl. B): 47–57.

Ayliffe GAJ, Collins BJ, Lowbury EJL et al (1967) Ward floors and other surfaces as reservoirs of hospital infection. *J. Hyg.*, **65**: 515–36.

Bodey GP, Buckley M, Sathe YS et al (1966) Quantitative relationships between circulating leukocytes and infection in patients with acute leukaemia. *Ann. Intern. Med.*, **64**: 328–40.

Collins C, Upright C, Aleksich J (1989) Reverse isolation: what patients perceive. *Oncol. Nurs. Forum*, **16**(5): 675–9.

Conry K (1982) Anergy: the hidden danger. *Heart Lung*, **11**: 85.

Denton P (1986) Psychological and physiological effects of isolation. *Nursing*, **3**(3): 88–91.

De Louvois J (1993) Salmonella contamination of eggs. *Lancet*, **342**: 367–8.

Department of Health (1996) *Immunisation Against Infectious Disease*. HMSO, London.

Garcia R, Raad I, Abi-Said D et al (1997) Nosocomial respiratory syncitial virus infections: prevention and control in bone marrow transplant patients. *Infect. Control Hosp. Epidemiol.*, **18**: 412–16.

Garner JS (1996) Guideline for isolation precautions in hospital. *Infect. Control Hosp. Epidemiol.*, **17**: 53–80.

Gaskill D, Henderson A, Fraser M (1997) Exploring the everyday world of the patient in isolation. *Oncol. Nurs. Forum.*, **24**(4): 695–700.

Greene WC (1993) AIDS and the immune system. *Sci. Am.*, **Sept**: 67–73.

Hunter P (1993) The microbiology of bottled natural mineral waters. *J. Appl. Bacteriol.*, **74**: 345–52.

Jones D (1990) Foodborne listeriosis. *Lancet*, **336**: 1171–4.

Kinmouth AL, Fulton Y, Campbell MJ (1992) Management of feverish children at home. *BMJ*, **305**: 1134–6.

Knowles HE (1993) The experience of infectious patients in isolation. *Nursing Times*, **89**(30): 53–6.

Lund BM, Knox MR, Cole MB (1989) Destruction of *Listeria monocytogenes* during microwave cooking. *Lancet*, **i**: 218.

Mackowiak PA (1994) Fever: blessing or curse? A unifying hypothesis. *Ann. Intern. Med.*, **120**: 1037–40.

Medical Devices Directorate (1993) Ice cubes: infection caused by *Xanthomonas maltophilia*. *Hazard*, **93**: 42.

Nauseef WM, Maki DG (1981) A study of the value of simple protective isolation in patients with granulocytopenia. *N. Engl. J. Med.*, **304**(8): 448–52.

Ravn P, Lundgren JD, Kjaeldgaard P et al (1991) Nosocomial outbreak of cryptosporidiosis in AIDS patients. *BMJ*, **302**: 277–9.

Remington JS, Schimpff SC (1981) Please don't eat the salads. *N. Engl. J. Med.*, **304**: 433–5.

Rogers TR, Barnes RA (1988) Prevention of airborne fungal infection in immunocompromised patients. *J. Hosp. Inf*, **11** (Suppl. A): 15–20.

Schimpff SC, Hahn DM, Brouillet MD et al (1978) Comparison of basic infection prevention techniques with standard room reverse isolation or with reverse isolation plus added air filtration. *Leuk. Res.*, **2**: 231–40.

Styrt B, Sugarman B (1990) Antipyresis and fever. *Arch. Intern. Med.*, **150**: 1589–97.

Tablan OC, Anderson LJ, Arden NH et al (1994) Guideline for the prevention of nosocomial pneumonia. *Am. J. Infect. Control*, **22**: 247–92.

Taylor L (1980) Are face masks necessary in operating theatres and wards? *J. Hosp. Infect.*, **1**: 173–4.

Trexler PC, Spiers ASD, Gaya H (1975) Plastic isolators for treatment of acute leukaemia patients under germ-free conditions. *BMJ*, **iv**: 549–52.

FURTHER READING

Bodey GP, Vartivarian S (1989) Aspergillosis. *Eur. J. Clin. Microbiol. Infect. Dis.*, **8**(5): 413–37.

Campbell K (1996) The principles of bone marrow and stem-cell transplantation. *Nursing Times*, **92**(48): 34–6.

Johnson HM, Bazer FW, Szente BE et al (1994) How interferons fight disease. *Sci. Am.*, **May**: 40–7.

Keithley J (1983) Infection and the malnourished patient. *Heart Lung*, **12**: 23.

Lindgren PS (1983) The laminar air flow room – nursing practices and procedures. *Nurs. Clin. North Am.*, **18**(3): 553–61.

Mackowiak PA, Bartlett JG, Borden EC et al (1997) Concepts of fever; recent advances and lingering dogma. *Clin. Infect. Dis.*, **25**: 119–38.

Mooney BR, Reeves SA, Larson E (1993) Infection control and bone marrow transplantation. *Am. J. Infect. Control*, **21**: 131–8.

Nowak MA, McMichael AJ (1995) How HIV defeats the immune system. *Sci. Am.*, **August**: 42–9.

Roitt IM (1997) *Essential Immunology*, 9th edn. Blackwell Scientific, Oxford.

Roitt I, Broscroff J, Male D (1996) *Immunology*, 4th edn. Times Mirror Publishers International, London.

Scientific American (1993) September issue.

Van Boehner H, Kisielow P (1991) How the immune system learns about self. *Sci. Am.*, **Oct**: 50–9.

Watson R (1998) Controlling body temperature in adults. *Nursing Standard*, **12**(20): 49–53.

Weir DM, Stewart J (1993) *Immunology*, 7th edn. Churchill Livingstone, Edinburgh.

5

A guide to antimicrobial chemotherapy

INTRODUCTION

Effective treatment of infection involves the elimination of the invading micro-organism whilst, at the same time, not harming the cells of the host. Modern drugs used for antimicrobial chemotherapy affect characteristic features of **procaryotic** cells that are not found in the **eucaryotic** cells of humans.

The recognition of bacteria as the cause of fever and infection was soon followed by the search for substances that could destroy them. Chemicals such as carbolic acid and iodine, known to kill bacteria cultured in the laboratory, formed the basis of the antisepsis in surgery used by Lister in the late nineteenth century. Other chemicals that destroyed bacteria (e.g. mercury) were used to treat infection but invariably caused as much harm to the patient as to the microbe. Ehrlich first perceived that what was required was an agent that was selectively toxic to microbes. In 1904, he succeeded in curing trypanosomiasis (sleeping sickness) with a dye called trypan. He continued his work using a variety of compounds based on arsenic. Then, in 1935, Domagk found that streptococcal infections could be treated with a dye called prontosil. This chemical was actually broken down in the body to form the effective compound, sulphonilamide. Other antimicrobial sulphonilamides were developed and widely used in the treatment of infection.

The ability to treat infections was revolutionized by the discovery by Sir Alexander Fleming of the first naturally occurring antimicrobial substance. In 1928, Fleming noticed that colonies of *Staphylococcus aureus* were 'dissolved' where they occurred close to a mould, *Penicillium notatum*, which had inadvertently contaminated the plate. He then grew the same fungus in a broth and found that the broth had marked inhibitory effect on many types of bacteria. The antibacterial substances were difficult to purify and were unstable, but after extensive work by Florey in the 1940s sufficient penicillin could be made for the treatment of patients.

Commercial production of penicillin began during the Second World War and the search continued for new antimicrobials from a range of micro-organisms living in natural environments. In the 1940s streptomycin, chloramphenicol and tetracycline were isolated from soil organisms, and cephalosporin from a fungus found in a sewage outlet. Erythromycin and rifampicin were discovered in the 1950s, and gentamicin and fucidin in the 1960s, all from soil organisms.

The term **antibiotic** was used to describe these naturally occurring substances produced by one microbial species and capable of inhibiting the growth of another species. In the laboratory, small alterations to the chemical structure of naturally occurring antibiotics were found to alter the range of microbes against which the drug was effective, the absorption by the body and the duration of action. There are now over 100 antimicrobial drugs available. Many are similar compounds but, with minor modifications, affect different species of bacteria.

Some people use the term antibiotic to refer only to the naturally occurring drugs made by bacteria or fungi, and the term antimicrobial agents to describe the whole range of antibacterial drugs now available, many of which are modifications of naturally occurring substances or are synthesized in the laboratory. Such a distinction is rather academic and for the purposes of this text the term antibiotic will be used for all drugs that are capable of destroying bacteria.

Most antibiotics cannot be used to treat fungal infections, and only a few drugs are available that destroy these more complex eucaryotic cells. Viruses are also not affected by antibiotics, as they do not have the cell structures targeted by these drugs.

CLINICAL APPLICATION OF ANTIMICROBIAL AGENTS

Considerable skill and knowledge is necessary to make the best use of the wide range of antibiotics that is available. In the UK, advice on antibiotic therapy is provided by a medical microbiologist, who is a doctor with a specialist knowledge and training in microbiology. Although nurses are not responsible for the prescription of antimicrobial therapy, they do have an important role to play in administering and monitoring the drugs prescribed and in discussing the treatment with the doctor when therapy seems unnecessary or unsuccessful.

Some of the characteristics of antibiotics that need to be taken into account when choosing an appropriate antibiotic to treat an infection are discussed below.

Indication for treatment

Specific signs and symptoms, for example a fever or cough, indicate the presence of infection. These need to be assessed to determine whether treatment with antimicrobial agents is required. The isolation of micro-organisms does not necessarily indicate infection. Some sites, in particular the skin and respiratory tract, are colonized by many bacteria and treatment with antibiotics is not required if signs of infection are not present. Antimicrobial therapy is usually not indicated for the treatment of upper respiratory tract infections, which are mostly caused by viruses, and gastrointestinal infections.

Micro-organism causing the infection

In most infections, the help of the microbiology laboratory is required to identify the causative organism and establish the antibiotics to which it is susceptible. The organisms may be more difficult to detect once treatment has commenced and microbiological specimens should therefore be collected as soon as the infection becomes apparent. Sometimes the signs and symptoms of the infection are sufficiently characteristic to indicate the probable causative organism; if the organism is likely to be susceptible to a specific antibiotic, treatment can be started immediately. This may be important for serious infections such as meningococcal meningitis where treatment with high doses of penicillin early in the course of the infection improves the chances of recovery.

Spectrum of activity

The term spectrum is used to describe the range of organisms against which an antibiotic is effective. Some antibiotics kill only a few different bacteria (e.g. only Gram-positive bacteria) and are said to have a narrow spectrum of activity. Penicillin is a narrow-spectrum antibiotic because it acts mainly on Gram-positive bacteria; the aminoglycosides are also narrow-spectrum because they are active mainly against Gram-negative bacteria, whereas metronidazole destroys only **anaerobic** bacteria and some **protozoa**.

The modern cephalosporins, quinolones, aminoglycosides, tetracycline and ampicillin are broad-spectrum antibiotics; that is, they are effective against a wide range of Gram-negative and Gram-positive bacteria. Broad-spectrum antibiotics are useful when the cause of the infection is unknown and action against a wide variety of organisms may be necessary. Unfortunately, they kill not only the pathogen but also bacteria that make up the **normal flora** of the body. These organisms play an important role in protecting against invasion by harmful species and, if destroyed, superinfection by other bacteria or fungi may occur. *Clostridium difficile* is an organism that multiplies in the gut if other normal gut flora are destroyed by antibiotics. It causes a bowel infection called **pseudomembranous colitis**, which can be serious and is sometimes life threatening (see p. 105).

Broad-spectrum antibiotics may also encourage the survival and multiplication of **strains** of bacteria that are resistant to antibiotics. When the cause of the infection is known, it is preferable to use an antibiotic that will destroy the **pathogen** only.

Drug combinations

Sometimes it is preferable to treat an infection with a combination of antibiotics, particularly where the cause of the infection is unknown. Some drug combinations enhance each other's activity (e.g. penicillin and gentamicin), this is known as synergy. Others interfere with one another (e.g. penicillin and tetracycline) or encourage the development of resistant strains (e.g. ampicillin and cloxacillin). Some antibiotics (e.g. rifampicin) encourage the rapid emergence of strains resistant to the antibiotic and should usually be used with another drug, to ensure resistant organisms are destroyed.

If resistance to a particular antibiotic is likely to develop during treatment, more than one type of drug will need to be given as pathogens are unlikely to develop resistance to both at the same time. This is particularly important for antituberculosis therapy, where a combination of three drugs is usually prescribed.

Drugs sometimes interact with each other to alter the therapeutic effect or induce toxicity. Adverse reactions are particularly common where drugs are administered in intravenous fluids, and this should be avoided where possible.

Pharmacodynamics

The pharmacodynamics of a drug relate to what happens to it in the body, whether it is absorbed from the intestine, how long it remains in the blood, what organs or tissues it reaches and how it is excreted. These factors influence the efficacy of a drug.

Absorption from the gut occurs mostly by passive diffusion, but may be delayed or enhanced by the presence of food in the stomach, or by its pH. Some drugs are better absorbed with food because of the accompanying delay in stomach emptying and increase in blood flow (e.g. nitrofurantoin). The absorption of erythromycin is reduced by the presence of food because the process is affected by the change in pH. The acid in the stomach alters some drugs and these have to be protected by a capsule that dissolves only in the small intestine.

Intravenous or intramuscular routes of administration are often preferred for antimicrobial agents because of the variability of oral absorption. Some antibiotics can also be administered topically as creams, ointments and drops, or absorbed through the rectal mucosa from suppositories.

The distribution of a drug through the body depends on whether it is lipophilic or hydrophilic. Lipophilic drugs, such as ciprofloxacin, pass readily through plasma membranes and therefore diffuse widely into the tissues. Hydrophilic or highly charged compounds such as aminoglycosides are restricted to the blood and fluid surrounding cells. Plasma proteins (e.g. albumin) play a part in the distribution of drugs. They bind to compounds, transporting them around the body and affect the rate at which a drug is excreted (Kitteringham & Park 1997).

Most antibiotics do not readily pass through the blood–brain barrier and, although they may reach a higher concentration in the brain when the meninges are inflamed, many cannot be used to treat meningitis successfully.

There are two main routes by which drugs are excreted from the body: via the biliary tract into the faeces and via the kidneys into urine. Many drugs are altered, or metabolized, to enable secretion. In particular, lipophilic compounds have to be charged in order to prevent their re-adsorption in the kidneys.

Antibiotics are eliminated from the body at different rates. Those that are eliminated fairly rapidly must be given in frequent doses, while others that are excreted slowly can be administered twice a day.

Duration of therapy

Antibiotics should be given for long enough to ensure complete eradication of the bacteria, but not for too long because this may encourage the development of resistant strains. Usually treatment should be given for 7 days, but for serious or **systemic infection** prolonged therapy may be necessary.

Prophylaxis

Antibiotics can be used to protect patients in situations that markedly increase their vulnerability to infection. These include surgery involving a part of the body heavily colonized with bacteria (e.g. bowel surgery), procedures where subsequent infection could have very serious consequences (e.g. valve or joint replacement) and treatment for people with abnormal heart valves who are at risk of developing endocarditis. Sometimes prophylaxis is indicated to protect intimate contacts of someone who has developed an infectious disease (e.g. meningococcal meningitis). The prophylactic antibiotic selected should be effective against the bacteria most likely to cause infection. For example, patients undergoing surgery of the large intestine will be most at risk from infection caused by **aerobic** coliforms and anaerobes of the gut flora. Prophylactic treatment should therefore include metronidazole to kill the **anaerobes** and gentamicin or a cephalosporin to kill the Gram-negative aerobes. It should be given close to the time of incision to ensure that the level of drug is adequate during the procedure. This may be achieved with a single dose, unless the procedure is prolonged or associated with heavy blood loss (Taylor 1997). Prophylactic therapy should not be continued for more than 24 h.

Antibiotic policy

More than half the hospitals in the UK have a policy for antimicrobial therapy (BSAC Working Party 1994). These policies are intended to discourage the indiscriminate use of antibiotics, to minimize the development of antibiotic-resistant strains and to reduce the costs of antibiotic prescribing. These controls are becoming increasingly important as problems with resistance increase and the cost of drug development reduces the rate at which new products are introduced. The policy will provide guidelines on the use of a range of antibiotics and limit others unless advised by the microbiologist or infectious disease consultant. To be effective, such policies need to be thoroughly implemented and subject to an ongoing audit. Nurses can play a key role in monitoring the prolonged or inappropriate use of antibiotics. Feedback of information to those prescribing the drugs appears to be an important factor in achieving adherence to the policy (Feely et al 1990).

HOW ANTIBIOTICS WORK

There are many species of bacteria and it is therefore to be expected that antibiotics affect each species differently. The effect may be **bactericidal**, that is, cause the destruction of the bacterial cell, or **bacteriostatic**, that is, prevent replication of the cell, enabling it to be destroyed by the host's immune defences. There are a number of different mechanisms of antimicrobial action.

Interference with cell wall synthesis

Bacteria differ from human cells in having a cell wall and this is a useful target for antibiotics. A number of different aspects of **cell wall** synthesis can be affected; for example, penicillin binds to enzymes involved in making **peptidoglycan** whereas vancomycin prevents the cross-linkage process. The inhibition of cell wall synthesis affects the ability of the cell to withstand osmotic pressures; it therefore swells and eventually breaks open. **Gram-negative** bacteria contain much less peptidoglycan in their cell walls and are therefore much less susceptible to penicillin than the **Gram-positive** bacteria.

Interference with protein synthesis

Several antibiotics inhibit protein synthesis by binding to bacterial **ribosomes**. They are unable to bind on to the much larger eucaryotic cell ribosomes, and therefore selectively affect bacteria. Protein synthesis either occurs abnormally or is completely prevented. Some substances do not bind permanently to the ribosome and their action is therefore bacteriostatic (e.g. tetracycline, chloramphenicol). Aminoglycosides affect both protein synthesis and the permeability of the membrane.

Inhibition of nucleic acid synthesis

Nucleic acid synthesis can be affected in numerous ways. The sulphonamides and trimethoprim prevent the synthesis of folic acid, an essential coenzyme in the synthesis of **nucleotides**. Human cells also use folic acid but, because they do not synthesize it and depend on a dietary source, they are not affected by these antibiotics. Bacteria that are able to use preformed folic acid are also resistant to these antibiotics.

Metronidazole inhibits an **enzyme** involved in nucleic acid production, and rifampicin inhibits the transcription of **DNA** into **RNA**.

The quinolones (e.g. ciprofloxacin) affect an enzyme called gyrase, which controls coiling and uncoiling of DNA strands.

Disruption of the cell membrane

Polymyxins selectively damage the cell membrane of bacteria, causing the cell to swell and burst. Agents such as amphotericin and nystatin disrupt membranes that contain cholesterol and cause the cell to lyse. Fungal cell membranes are particularly rich in cholesterol but, because human cell membranes also contain some cholesterol, many of these agents are toxic and some can only be used topically.

MAIN GROUPS OF ANTIMICROBIAL AGENTS

Penicillins

The penicillins bind to an enzyme involved in the production of peptidoglycan and, as a result, prevent cell wall synthesis. They are bactericidal. The original, naturally occurring penicillins (e.g. benzylpenicillin, penicillin V) have a narrow spectrum of activity and are mainly active against Gram-positive bacteria (e.g. streptococci). However, a large number of different penicillin antibiotics have been synthesized, which have the same basic β-lactam ring structure but, by modification of the side-chain molecules, are able to affect a wider range of bacterial species (Fig. 5.1). Alterations to the side-chains can also influence the pharmacology of the drugs; for example, benzylpenicillin is destroyed by gastric acid and so must be given intravenously, whereas ampicillin is acid-stable and can therefore be given orally (Table 5.1).

Penicillins are very useful antibiotics; they can infiltrate most sites of infection and they are usually used for initial treatment of infection until sensitivity testing indicates that an alternative drug is necessary.

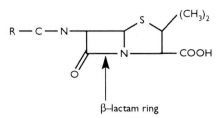

Fig. 5.1   The structure of penicillin.

The penicillins are virtually non-toxic and can therefore be given in very high doses. Their main adverse effect is a **hypersensitivity** reaction, which can range from minor rashes to severe **anaphylaxis**.

Resistance to penicillin was reported within a few years of its introduction and in certain species is widespread. For example, 90% of *Staphylococcus aureus* isolates in hospitals are resistant to penicillin. Resistant bacteria produce an enzyme, penicillinase (β-lactamase), which breaks open the β-lactam ring and destroys the activity of the antibiotic. Pharmaceutical manufacturers are constantly searching for side-chain modifications that prevent attack by β-lactamases. Flucloxacillin, a β-lactamase-resistant antibiotic, was introduced in the 1960s and is of considerable value for the treatment of *S. aureus* infections. Methicillin is a

Table 5.1   Penicillins

Antibiotic	Spectrum of activity and principal uses
Natural penicillins	
Benzylpenicillin (Penicillin G)	Effective against Gram-positive bacteria and neisseria (meningococcal meningitis, gonorrhoea). Used to treat a wide variety of infections by IM or IV route
Penicillin V	Same spectrum of activity as benzylpenicillin but used to treat mild tissue infections (e.g. otitis media, tonsillitis). Administered orally
Broad-spectrum penicillins	
Ampicillin Amoxycillin	Effective against Gram-positive bacteria, enterococci and *Haemophilus influenzae*. Used to treat urinary and middle ear infections, and some serious infections in combination with other drugs. Penetrates sputum well and is therefore used to treat respiratory infections. Administered orally or IV
Co-amoxiclav (Augmentin)	A combination of amoxicillin and clavulanic acid. The clavulanic acid binds with penicillinases. Used for urinary tract, respiratory or soft tissue infections resistant to amoxicillin
Penicillinase-resistant penicillins	
Flucloxacillin Oxacillin Methicillin	Same spectrum of activity as penicillin G but also active against penicillinase producers such as *Staphylococcus aureus*. Mainly used to treat staphylococcal infection. Flucloxacillin better absorbed from gut Methicillin is not used clinically
Antipseudomonal penicillins	
Mezlocillin Piperacillin Azlocillin	Derivatives of benzylpenicillin. Used to treat serious Gram-negative and anaerobic infections, usually in combination with aminoglycosides. Azlocillin is particularly effective against *Pseudomonas aeruginosa*

β-lactamase-resistant antibiotic introduced at the same time but, as it is associated with toxicity, is now used only in the laboratory to detect resistance to beta-lactams.

Cephalosporins

The cephalosporins have a similar chemical structure to the penicillins. They have a β-lactam ring, an additional side ring and different side-chains. They also kill bacterial cells by preventing cell wall synthesis. The first cephalosporin, cephalothin, was obtained from a fungus in the mid 1960s. These early, or first generation, cephalosporins had a similar spectrum to ampicillin, and some are still commonly used today (e.g. cephradine) (Table 5.2). Susceptibility to β-lactamases limited their use until the second generation of β-lactamase-resistant cephalosporins was introduced in the 1970s. These drugs are more potent and are active against a wider range of bacteria. They are used for prophylaxis in major surgery and in the treatment of penicillin-resistant strains of bacteria such as gonococcus and haemophilus. The third-generation cephalosporins, introduced in the early 1980s, are more active against Gram-negative bacteria, but less active against *S. aureus* and pneumococci. They are expensive and subject to widespread misuse in situations where a cheaper, narrower spectrum antibiotic would be more appropriate. Their use has been linked to pseudomembranous colitis caused by toxogenic strains of *Clostridium difficile*, and to increased resistance in pseudomonas, enterobacteria and serratia.

Recently, fourth-generation cephalosporins have become available. These are broad-spectrum and β-lactamase resistant.

The main side-effect of cephalosporins is **hypersensitivity**. About 10% of penicillin-allergic patients have some cephalosporin allergy as well.

Other β-lactams

There are a variety of antibiotics that have a β-lactam ring as part of their structure. One group, the monobactams (e.g. imipenem) are particularly useful as they are very potent and effective against a range of Gram-positive and Gram-negative bacteria. They also do not cause hypersensitivity reactions in patients who are sensitive to penicillin. The carbapenems are very broad spectrum, active against most bacteria including anaerobes, and are used to treat serious infections caused by resistant bacteria.

Aminoglycosides

The aminoglycoside antibiotics interfere with protein synthesis by binding to bacterial ribosomes and preventing accurate reading of the **messenger RNA**. They are bactericidal and active against many Gram-negative, aerobic bacteria and some Gram-positive bacteria. They are often used in combination with another antibiotic to provide activity against a broad range of organisms. Aminoglycosides are not absorbed from the gut and so must be administered parenterally. The concentration of the drug in the blood must be moni-

Table 5.2 Cephalosporins

Antibiotic	Spectrum of activity and principal uses
First generation Cephradine Cephalexin Cefaclor	Active against a wide range of Gram-negative and Gram-positive bacteria (although not pseudomonas, streptococcus or pneumococcus). Similar spectrum to ampicillin. Not usually used as first choice of treatment for serious infections
Second generation Cefuroxime Cefamandole	Active against a wide range of Gram-positive and Gram-negative bacteria (including *Haemophilus influenzae*) and resistant to action of β-lactamases. Used to treat severe systemic infection and for prophylaxis against infection
Third generation Cefotaxime Ceftazidime Ceftizoxime	Better activity against Gram-negative organisms, including pseudomonas and acinetobacter. Less effective against Gram-positive bacteria. Used to treat serious sepsis, but prone to encourage superinfection by resistant organisms
Fourth generation Cefepime Cefpirome	Broad spectrum of activity against Gram-positive and Gram-negative organisms. Less susceptible to β-lactamases

tored closely as aminoglycosides tend to accumulate in the tissues where they can cause damage, particularly the kidney and ear. Resistance to aminoglycosides through the production of enzymes that can modify the molecule is becoming increasingly common.

The main aminoglycoside antibiotics are listed in Table 5.3.

Tetracyclines

The name tetracyclines is derived from their structure of four rings fused together. They bind to bacterial ribosomes and block protein synthesis by preventing **transfer RNA** from attaching to **messenger RNA**. The attachment to the ribosomes is reversible and their effect is therefore bacteriostatic rather than bactericidal. Within the group there are natural products such as oxytetracycline and tetracycline, and semi-synthetic derivatives such as methacycline and minocycline. Their main side-effect is gastrointestinal disturbance, especially following large doses (2 g or more). Irritation to the gastric mucosa causes nausea and vomiting, and disruption of the normal bowel flora may result in diarrhoea. Tetracyclines are also deposited in developing bones and teeth, causing the teeth to stain yellow. They are therefore contraindicated in pregnant women and children aged under 12 years.

Tetracyclines are effective against a broad range of Gram-positive and Gram-negative bacteria. They should not be given intramuscularly as this causes considerable pain.

Bacteria that acquire resistance to tetracycline are able to prevent the drug from entering the cell. Increased resistance to tetracyclines has resulted in a decline in their use. However, they remain an important treatment for sexually transmitted diseases (e.g. Chlamydia).

Macrolides

These drugs inhibit bacterial protein synthesis by binding to the ribosome. They are bacteriostatic as the attachment to the ribosome is reversible. The first of this group of drugs, erythromycin, was isolated from a streptomyces. The naturally occurring macrolides are active against most Gram-positive organisms, neisseria, haemophilus and a range of anaerobes. They are also effective against intracellular pathogens such as chlamydia and rickettsia. Their activity against a number of emergent pathogens such as toxoplasma, legionella and helicobacter has recently stimulated interest in the group, and a range of synthetic macrolides is now being developed (e.g. clarithromycin).

Erythromycin has been commonly prescribed for patients who are allergic to penicillin, although many *S. aureus* and group A streptococci are resistant. Serious side-effects are rare, but gastrointestinal disturbances (nausea, vomiting, abdominal pain) may occur, especially when erythromycin is given in high doses. The new macrolides are less likely to cause these effects.

Quinolones

These drugs are rapidly bactericidal. They inhibit DNA gyrase, the enzyme responsible for supercoiling microbial DNA molecules. They are synthetic antibiotics, first used in 1962 when naladixic acid was introduced. This drug is active against a wide range of Gram-negative bacteria, except pseudomonas, and is used to treat urinary tract infections, although resistance often develops during treatment.

The addition of a fluorine molecule into the compound was found to increase both its potency and spectrum of activity, and a new range of compounds, the fluoroquinolones, was subsequently produced (e.g. ciprofloxacin, norfloxacin, ofloxacin). These drugs are effective against pseudomonads, staphylococci (including methicillin-resistant strains) and intracellular pathogens such as chlamydia and mycobacteria. As they distribute widely into tissue and bone, they can be used to treat a wide range of

Table 5.3 Aminoglycosides

Antibiotic	Spectrum of activity and principal uses
Gentamicin Tobramycin Amikacin	Broad spectrum of activity against a range of Gram-negative and Gram-positive bacteria. Potent antibiotics used to treat serious infection, especially Gram-negatives, often in conjunction with other antibiotics. Must be given IM or IV. Blood levels should be checked regularly to avoid ototoxicity or nephrotoxicity
Neomycin	Only for topical use; toxic if absorbed. Used to treat otitis externa
Streptomycin	Used to be used more widely but largely replaced by gentamicin. Important drug for treatment of tuberculosis in combination with other drugs

infections in almost any part of the body. However, to ensure that they retain their usefulness they should only be used to treat infection caused by pathogens resistant to conventional treatments (Brown & Reeves 1997). Resistance to fluoroquinolones is associated with prolonged treatment of chronic infections and excessive prescribing. They can cause gastrointestinal disturbances, but such side-effects are uncommon.

Glycopeptides

These compounds were originally obtained from actinomyces found in soil. Vancomycin was the only clinically useful glycopeptide until teicoplanin was introduced in the 1980s. Glycopeptides interfere with the synthesis of peptidoglycan, inhibiting the formation of bacterial cell walls. They are poorly absorbed from the gut and vancomycin given by the intramuscular route is painful, so is usually only administered intravenously. Glycopeptides are active against Gram-positive organisms, in particular staphylococci. Their main use is in the treatment of serious staphylococcal infection, including methicillin-resistant strains. Oral preparations can be used to treat *Clostridium difficile* colitis. Vancomycin may be nephrotoxic and ototoxic, and can cause a reversible neutropenia. Serum levels must be monitored carefully to avoid these side-effects. Teicoplanin is more potent than vancomycin and does not cause significant side-effects.

Until recently, resistance to glycopeptides was very rare. However, strains of vancomycin-resistant enterococci (VRE) have been causing outbreaks of infection since the early 1990s (see p. 96) and vancomycin-resistant strains of *S. aureus*, although at present unusual, have been reported (see p. 93).

Other antimicrobial agents

Chloramphenicol

This drug was originally derived from a streptomyces, but is now made synthetically. It is bacteriostatic, preventing protein synthesis by binding reversibly to bacterial ribosomes. It is active against a wide range of bacteria including unusual ones such as rickettsia, spirochaetes, chlamydia and mycoplasma. Its most important side-effect is bone marrow suppression, and on rare occasions it may cause aplastic anaemia. It is therefore not used systemically except for life-threatening infections, but can be used safely as a topical preparation for eye infections.

Sulphonamides

These are synthetic chemicals that interfere with para-amino benzoic acid (PABA), an enzyme involved in the production of folic acid, which is an essential ingredient for the production of nucleic acids. Sulphonamides were the first antimicrobials found to be effective against bacteria whilst not harming the patient. Introduced in the 1930s, they are still available today, although resistance and toxicity now restrict their use. They still provide a useful treatment for urinary tract infection when used in combination with trimethoprim (co-trimoxazole). Silver sulphadiazine is a topical preparation used to prevent colonization of burns, especially with pseudomonas.

Trimethoprim

Trimethoprim also affects folic acid synthesis and, because it enhances the activity of sulphonamides, is often used in the combined form of co-trimoxazole. As this drug is excreted in the urine, it is a useful treatment for urinary tract infection. It can also be used to treat chronic bronchitis, *Pneumocystis carinii*, toxoplasmosis and intracellular infections (e.g. typhoid).

Metronidazole

Metronidazole was originally introduced as a treatment for protozoal infections such as trichomonas and giardia. These are anaerobes and their specialized enzymes used for energy production convert metronidazole into toxic substances, which then destroy the cell. Anaerobic bacteria use the same enzymes, and metronidazole has now become the main treatment for infections caused by anaerobes (e.g. bacteroides). It is also used as prophylaxis before operation on the bowel or uterus, and in combination with other drugs in the treatment of *H. pylori*.

Metronidazole is distributed throughout the tissues, and adverse reactions and resistance are rare, although it should not be taken with alcohol.

Clindamycin

This drug is similar in activity to the macrolides, but penetrates bone well and is a useful treatment for osteomyelitis.

Fusidic acid

This is a steroid-like substance produced as a product of fermentation by a fungus; it interferes with protein synthesis in bacteria. Fusidic acid is used mainly for the treatment of staphylococcal infections, particularly those involving bone. It can also be used topically for treating skin infections. Using it in combination with penicillin discourages the emergence of resistance.

Rifampicin

This is a synthetic derivative of an antibiotic produced by a streptomyces which inactivates RNA polymerase and is bactericidal. It is used mainly for the treatment of tuberculosis, but is also given to eliminate throat carriage of *Neisseria meningitidis* in outbreaks of meningococcal meningitis.

Antituberculosis therapy

Tuberculosis is a difficult infection to treat because the mycobacteria grow very slowly and may be protected in cavities in the lungs and in macrophages. A combination of antibiotics must be used to kill both multiplying and intracellular mycobacteria and to prevent resistant bacteria from emerging. The main drugs used are isoniazid, rifampicin, ethambutol and pyrazinamide. Prolonged therapy is given: three drugs together for the first 8–10 weeks, followed by two drugs for about 4 months (Table 5.4).

The prolonged nature of therapy affects compliance with the treatment regimen. Recently, shorter courses of therapy, with doses given once or twice a week under supervision, have been developed to address this problem. Therapy using too few drugs or incomplete courses of treatment encourages resistance to emerge. Although resistance to antituberculous drugs is very rare in the UK, resistance rates as high as 30% to one or more drugs has been reported in other parts of the world (Uttley & Pozniak 1993) (see p. 97).

Patients with acquired immune deficiency syndrome are particularly susceptible to an atypical mycobacterium, *Mycobacterium avium intracellulare*. These bacteria are usually highly resistant to antituberculous drugs and treatment of the infection can be extremely difficult (Lewis 1989).

ANTIFUNGAL THERAPY

Fungi may cause a variety of infections, ranging from superficial infections of the skin and mucous membranes to serious systemic infection which may be fatal, and are usually associated with immune suppression. The eucaryotic cells of fungi are not susceptible to antibiotics, and specific antifungal agents are required to treat the infections they cause. Some of these agents disrupt the cell membranes by altering their sterol content (e.g. amphotericin); others affect cell formation (e.g. griseofulvin), disrupt protein synthesis by substituting a nucleic acid (e.g. flucytosine), or interfere with cell wall synthesis (e.g. imidazoles). A range of topical preparations is available to treat superficial infections of the skin and mucous membranes. Far fewer drugs are available for the treatment of systemic fungal infections and, because they affect eucaryotic cells, many are associated with toxicity (Table 5.5).

Table 5.4   Antituberculous agents

Agent	Indication
First-line drugs	
Isoniazid	Used only for the treatment of tuberculosis. Highly effective, although resistant strains common. Peripheral neuritis and hepatitis may occur at high doses
Rifampicin	Most potent of the antituberculous drugs. Causes failure of low-dose oestrogen contraceptive pill, colours urine and tears red; may cause liver damage
Pyrazinamide	Good penetration of tissues and meninges; useful for treatment of tuberculosis meningitis. Hepatotoxic
Second-line drugs	
Ethambutol	Reserved for treatment of resistant strains and atypical mycobacteria. May cause visual impairment
Streptomycin	Effective, but has to be used parenterally
Cycloserine	Used only when resistant to several first-line drugs
Thiacetazone	Rarely used in developed countries

Table 5.5   Major antifungal agents

Antifungal agent	Indication
Polyenes	
Nystatin	Superficial candidiasis, too toxic for parenteral use
Amphotericin B	Broad antifungal spectrum, main form of treatment for deep mycoses. Nephrotoxic
Flucytosine	Active against yeasts (e.g. candida, cryptococci); can be used to treat systemic infections. Blood levels need to be monitored to avoid neutropenia and thrombocytopenia
Imidazoles	
Clotrimazole	Superficial candidiasis (e.g. vaginal thrush)
Miconazole	Second-line treatment for systemic candidiasis. Adverse reactions common
Fluconazole	Treatment of, and prophylaxis against, systemic candidiasis and cryptococcus. Minimal toxicity
Itraconazole	Treatment of systemic infections including aspergillus
Griseofulvin	Concentrates in the skin and therefore used for treatment of ringworm
Allylamine	
Terbinafine	New antifungal, active against candida and aspergillus

ANTIVIRAL THERAPY

Viruses are intracellular parasites that use the structures of the host cell to replicate themselves. Antiviral agents must be able to target the virus without damaging the host cell. Alick Isaacs, a British virologist, discovered the first antiviral agent, interferon, in 1956. Interferons are proteins produced by lymphocytes and other cells infected by a virus. They cause cells to become resistant to invasion by viruses by preventing the translation of messenger RNA, and also have a range of effects on the immune system and inflammatory response (see p. 63). They can now be produced commercially using recombinant genetic techniques in *Escherichia coli*. The severe side-effects associated with the use of interferon, 'flu-like symptoms, lymphocytopenia, gastrointestinal disturbances and bone marrow suppression, have limited their use. However, they are used to treat chronic hepatitis B and C infections, hairy cell leukaemia and Kaposi's sarcoma. They can also be applied topically to treat herpes simplex eye infections.

Because many viral infections are self-limiting and laboratory techniques are frequently too slow to produce results in time to influence the management of the infection, until recently there has been little interest in the development of new antiviral agents. However, the need to find effective treatments for human immunodeficiency virus (HIV) and other chronic viral infections (e.g. hepatitis) has stimulated research. A number of stages in viral replication are now recognized as potential targets for antiviral agents whilst not interfering with the host cell (Box 5.1). The development of rapid diagnostic methods for identifying viruses has also increased the value of antiviral therapy.

The majority of antiviral agents currently available are analogues of nucleotides which block the production of nucleic acids (e.g. acyclovir). Other important antiviral drugs include foscarnet, a phosphonic acid that inhibits the RNA and DNA polymerases of a number of viruses (e.g. herpes simplex, varicella, hepatitis B and influenza). Zidovudine (ZDV) or azidothymidine (AZT) is a thymidine analogue that binds to HIV reverse transcriptase and stops the construction of the DNA strand. ZDV is a highly effective inhibitor of HIV replication, but resistant strains emerge after several months of treatment, although this is less likely where it is used in combination with other antiviral drugs. Side-effects of treatment are anaemia, neutropenia and gastrointestinal disturbances.

Other drugs effective against HIV have now been developed. Protease inhibitors, such as saquinavir, target an enzyme unique to retroviruses, and there are

---

Box 5.1   Potential targets for antiviral agents

- Inactivating virus before attachment
- Blocking attachment to cell membrane receptors
- Blocking penetration of the cell
- Preventing virus from uncoating
- Preventing integration into host genome
- Blocking transcription of viral genome
- Blocking translation of viral genome
- Interfering with viral assembly
- Interfering with viral release

Table 5.6 Major antiviral agents

Antiviral agent	Indication
Idoxuridione (IDU)	Herpes skin or corneal infection. Too toxic to use systemically
Amantadine	Can be used prophylactically to prevent infection with influenza A virus
Acyclovir	Herpes simplex, including ocular, skin, mucous membrane, genital infections and encephalitis. Also effective against varicella zoster virus. Requires prompt administration to be effective and does not destroy latent virus
Ganciclovir	Similar to acyclovir, but more effective against cytomegalovirus, especially in immunosuppressed patients. May induce neutropenia
Vidarabine	Has been used IV for varicella zoster virus in the immunosuppressed, and for herpes simplex (e.g. corneal lesions). Low toxicity
Ribovirin	Blocks viral RNA production. Used to treat Lassa fever and, as an aerosol, severe respiratory syncytial virus in children
Foscarnet	Inhibits DNA polymerases in herpes viruses and reverse transcriptase in retroviruses. Used to treat severe cytomegalovirus infection
Zidovudine (ZDV) (AZT)	Inhibits DNA polymerases; slows down viral replication and progression of disease in people infected with HIV. Nausea and vomiting common; toxic to bone marrow, causing anaemia and neutropenia
2',3'-Dideoxycytidine	Inhibits DNA polymerases in a similar way to AZT. Less bone marrow toxicity but can cause peripheral neuropathy
Sequinavir Ritonavir Indinavir	Protease inhibitors that affect an enzyme in retroviruses. Key component of combination therapy against HIV
Nevirapine Efavirenz Delavirdine	Reverse transcriptase inhibitors (not nucleotide analogues) used to treat HIV

also other reverse transcriptase inhibitors (e.g. nevirapine), which unlike ZDV are not nucleotide analogues. It is now recognized that treatment of HIV with a combination of three or four drugs achieves maximum viral suppression and reduces the risk of resistance emerging. This approach is called highly active antiretroviral treatment (HAART) (Pillay 1998). The main antiviral drugs are listed in Table 5.6.

RESISTANCE TO ANTIMICROBIAL AGENTS

Micro-organisms are not all intrinsically sensitive to all antibiotics. The terms sensitive and resistant to antibiotics are used to distinguish between those antibiotics that will or will not destroy a micro-organism. On a simple level, bacteria can be described as *sensitive* to a particular antibiotic if their growth is inhibited or they are killed by a concentration of the drug that could be achieved by the usual dose regimen. *Resistant* bacteria

are not inhibited or killed by this concentration of the drug. However, in practice, it is not always possible to make a clear distinction between sensitive and resistant strains: treatment with a particular antibiotic may still be effective if given at a higher dose. Determining the minimum inhibitory concentration (MIC) of the antibiotic will assess the sensitivity of a particular micro-organism. If the MIC is high, the organism is resistant and unlikely to be affected by treatment with the antibiotic; if it is low, then treatment is likely to be effective provided the antibiotic is able to penetrate the site of infection (Fig. 5.2).

Bacteria may have a *natural resistance* to certain antibiotics because the drug cannot penetrate their cells or because they do not possess the protein to which the drug attaches. Some bacteria are naturally resistant to many antibiotics (e.g. *Pseudomonas aeruginosa, Staphylococcus epidermidis*).

Resistance by selection occurs when one or two cells in a population of bacteria are naturally resistant to the

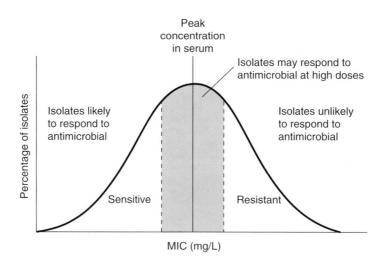

Fig. 5.2   Relationship between sensitive, intermediate and resistant bacterial isolates and minimum inhibitory concentration (MIC) of an antimicrobial agent.

antibiotic. On exposure to the antibiotic these cells are able to survive and multiply, and eventually the sensitive cells are replaced by resistant ones. This type of resistance develops rapidly when sulphonamides are used and is also a problem with antituberculous drugs.

Inherently sensitive bacteria can *acquire resistance* to antibiotics by means of one or more of the following mechanisms:

- the permeability of the cell membrane changes so that the drug cannot enter the cell (e.g. resistance to tetracycline)
- the site with which the drug reacts is altered and the drug is unable to affect the cell (e.g. resistance to trimethoprim)
- the bacterium produces enzymes that inactivate the antibiotic (e.g. β-lactamases which destroy penicillins, cephalosporins)
- the drug may be actively expelled from the cell

Acquired resistance to antibiotics has been evident since antibiotics were first widely used. It may occur as a result of a mutation in the chromosome or the acquisition of new DNA. Mutational resistance usually involves the substitution of one or more amino acids in a target protein; for example, rifampicin resistance in *Mycobacterium tuberculosis* is due to a mutation in RNA polymerase. This type of resistance may be induced during therapy.

The transfer of antimicrobial resistance frequently occurs on plasmids, small molecules of DNA independent of the chromosome, which can be replicated and transferred between cells by conjugation, transforma-

tion or transduction (see p. 10). Plasmids provide a highly effective means of spreading resistance genes, both within a species and to other species.

Resistance genes may also be carried on transposons. These are specific sequences of DNA that can insert into both plasmids and chromosomes, and transfer, or jump, between them. They can carry genes encoding for resistance to a wide variety of antibiotics, and play a key role in the dissemination of antibiotic resistance, particularly where species develop resistance to more than one drug. *Multiple drug resistance* is a term used to describe bacteria that have developed resistance to several, unrelated antibiotics, for example Gram-negative bacilli that are resistant to both streptomycin and the sulphonamides. These multiresistant bacteria often have one plasmid or transposon that carries several genes conferring resistance to several antibiotics.

The ability of microbes to acquire resistance to antibiotics was recognized soon after the first drugs were introduced in the 1940s. Initially, the steady supply of new drugs was able to combat the problem. However, although modifications to existing drugs have been made, no new classes of antimicrobial agents have been introduced for 15 years. The costs of development and controls on usage to limit resistance affect the economic viability of producing new antimicrobial drugs (Neu 1992). The development of vaccines has provided some solutions; for example, the vaccination of children against *Haemophilus influenzae* has helped to resolve the problem of emerging resistance in this pathogen. However, vaccines are unlikely to help combat resistance amongst commensal organisms such as enterococci. There is increasing interest in bacteriophages, viruses that destroy specific bacteria, although their use is associated with practical problems such as selecting an appropriate phage and delivery to the site of infection (Barrow & Soothill 1997). Probiotics are harmless commensal micro-organisms which can be used to displace pathogens from certain sites on the body, although their usefulness is limited.

Factors contributing to the emergence of resistance

Although much of the evidence is circumstantial, there are a number of factors considered to play a key role in the development of antimicrobial resistance (Box 5.2).

Use of antimicrobial agents

There is considerable evidence to connect heavy use of antimicrobial agents with the emergence of resistance (Department of Health 1999). The extent of the problem varies considerably between countries. The USA and Japan consume large quantities of antimicrobial agents and have correspondingly high levels of resistance. In Japan, 70% of *S. aureus* isolates are resistant to methicillin, compared with less than 1% in Scandinavia where antimicrobial usage is much lower. In some countries, particularly South-East Asia and Latin America, problems of over-usage are aggravated by poor controls over supplies. Drugs can be purchased without a prescription and as single, low-dose tablets, which are highly likely to encourage resistance to develop. The use of single-dose therapy for the treatment of gonorrhoea has resulted in the progressive selection of resistant strains, so that around 50% of *Neisseria gonorrhoea* in developing countries is now resistant to penicillin (Department of Health 1999).

Unnecessary prescribing of antimicrobial agents

Many studies have shown that unnecessary use of antimicrobial agents is widespread. In countries where these drugs can be obtained without a prescription, the problem may be endemic. For example, in Mexico people commonly use antibiotics to treat diarrhoea, for which they are both ineffective and unnecessary (Bojalil & Calva 1994). However, even in the UK inappropriate prescribing is a major problem. Of the 50 million antibiotic prescriptions dispensed annually in the UK, 80% originate from community practice (general practitioners and dentists). Half of these agents are prescribed for the treatment of minor, upper respiratory tract infections, such as sore throat, otitis media, sinusitis or coughs and wheezes, most of which are caused by viruses, and treatment with antibiotics is unnecessary (Del Mar et al 1997).

In hospitals, antimicrobial agents are frequently given for unnecessarily prolonged periods. Commensal micro-organisms, particularly those in the gut, play an important role in the selection and spread of resistance. Prolonged antimicrobial therapy favours the growth of resistant strains, which may then become pathogenic, particularly in hospital patients whose defence mechanisms are impaired. When used for prophylaxis in surgery, a single dose of antibiotic is usually adequate, unless evidence of infection is found at the time of operation (see p. 162). Box 5.3 illustrates some simple principles of good practice in antimicrobial therapy that should be used to help prevent the emergence of resistance.

Transmission of resistance

In many circumstances, the emergence of resistant strains is followed by their spread by cross-infection. Such transmission is particularly likely to occur in hospitals where invasive devices and underlying illness make patients more vulnerable to infection.

Box 5.2 Factors encouraging the emergence of antimicrobial resistance

- Unnecessary use of antimicrobial agents to treat trivial infections caused by viruses
- Use of antimicrobial agents as growth promoters or prophylactics in agriculture
- Uncontrolled sale of antimicrobial agents without prescription
- Inappropriate use of antimicrobial agents (e.g. incorrect agent, dose, duration)

Box 5.3 Good practice in antimicrobial therapy

- Do not give for trivial reasons
- Use for prophylaxis only when the risk of infection is high
- Use good infection control to prevent infection rather than use antibiotics
- Take an appropriate specimen as soon as infection is suspected
- Use antibiotics only when clinically indicated by signs of infection, not just because of a positive laboratory report
- Use an antibiotic that has a specific action against the infecting organism rather than one that affects a wide range of organisms
- Administer the correct dose for an adequate period, but stop at the end of the course or if there is no obvious clinical response

Resistant strains are spread to other hospitals when patients are transferred, and transmission of strains between countries is also frequently reported (Soares et al 1993). Patients from countries with no reasonable controls on antimicrobial consumption are more likely to be infected or colonized by resistant micro-organisms.

Antimicrobial usage in agriculture

Some 50% of antimicrobial agents used in the UK are given to animals, not humans. They are used for three reasons: the treatment of disease, prophylaxis against disease to contain the spread of a particular infection, and as growth promoters. The latter practice is highly controversial. In some countries it has been banned (e.g. Sweden), whereas in others (e.g. the USA) common human antibiotics such as penicillin and tetracycline are still used as growth promoters. In the UK the use of antibiotics as growth promoters is restricted, but the phasing out of their use has been recommended (Department of Health 1999).

Strategies for preventing antimicrobial resistance

Although reductions in the use of antimicrobial agents have been followed by a decrease in incidence of resistant pathogens (Arason et al 1996), the effect is by no means automatic and may take a long time. Selection of resistant strains may continue because several resistance genes may be carried on one plasmid and ongoing use of one antibiotic maintains resistance to the others. Resistance is particularly difficult to eliminate where it is carried by many strains of the same species, rather than by only one epidemic strain, and improvements in prescribing practice may prevent only a deterioration of the situation rather than a reduction in current levels of resistance. In 1999, the House of Lords Science and Technology Committee reviewed the problem of resistance to antimicrobial agents. Later the same year, the Standing Medical Advisory Committee (SMAC) of the Department of Health responded to the concerns raised by this review in a report called 'The Path of Least Resistance' (Department of Health 1999). Key recommendations include measures to change public expectations and attitudes to antibiotics, education of clinicians (especially general practitioners and junior doctors) to improve their awareness of resistance and good prescribing practice, surveillance of resistance and the development of therapy guidelines.

Hospital antibiotic policies

Written policies are commonly used to control the indiscriminate use of antimicrobial agents in hospitals (McGowan 1994). These policies may include recommended treatment and prophylaxis regimens and restricted access to some drugs. The microbiology laboratory will encourage appropriate use by reporting only a limited number of antibiotic sensitivities and may indicate when organisms are likely to be colonizing rather than causing infection. The consultant microbiologist has a key role to play in educating and advising doctors in the appropriate use of antimicrobial agents and, together with the pharmacy, may monitor the effectiveness of the policy and the incidence of antibiotic resistance.

CLINICAL PROBLEMS ASSOCIATED WITH ANTIMICROBIAL RESISTANCE

Before the introduction of the first antibiotics death from sepsis was commonplace, especially amongst hospital patients (Simpson 1869). Until recently, it seemed that new drugs could be found to cope with emerging problems of resistance to antimicrobial agents. However, it is now apparent that this is not the case and widespread resistance amongst major pathogens is seriously threatening our ability to treat some infections.

Hospitals provide a particularly fertile breeding ground for resistant micro-organisms. Antimicrobial usage exerts a selective pressure on commensal micro-organisms, seriously ill patients are particularly vulnerable to infection, and resistant strains can spread easily between patients on contaminated hands or equipment. This section reviews the key pathogens for which antimicrobial resistance presents significant problems in the UK.

Methicillin-resistant *Staphylococcus aureus* (MRSA)

Staphylococci are an important cause of infection. For example, *S. aureus* is responsible for more than one-third of surgical wound infections (Public Health Laboratory Service 2000a). Staphylococci have a remarkable capacity to adapt to the presence of antibiotics in their environment by developing resistance (Box 5.4). β-Lactamase-producing strains of *S. aureus*, resistant to penicillin, appeared very soon after the antibiotic came into use. Now approximately 90% of strains in hospitals and about 50% of strains in the community are resistant to penicillin.

Box 5.4   The development of antibiotic resistance in *Staphylococcus aureus*

1960	Methicillin introduced
1961	Methicillin-resistant *S. aureus* first reported
1970	5% of *S. aureus* isolates methicillin resistant
1976	*S. aureus* resistant to gentamicin and methicillin reported
1980	New penicillins and cephalosporins introduced. Epidemic strain of MRSA reported in London
	Incidence of MRSA increases
1990	MRSA affecting most parts of the UK. Many different strains identified

Modifications to the β-lactam ring were made to prevent attack by β-lactamases, and in 1960 methicillin, a penicillin resistant to β-lactamases, was introduced. It could be administered only **parenterally** and was therefore replaced by a similar drug, flucloxacillin, which could also be given orally. Flucloxacillin soon became established as the drug of choice for the treatment of staphylococcal infection, since resistance to other penicillins was widespread. Methicillin is now used only in the laboratory for sensitivity testing.

Soon after the introduction of methicillin, resistant strains of *S. aureus* (MRSA) were reported. The incidence of MRSA increased until the 1970s and caused many serious outbreaks of infection in hospitals. During the 1970s outbreaks of MRSA diminished but, unfortunately, this was not the end of the problem; in the early 1980s, the third-generation cephalosporins and new penicillin derivatives were introduced and this coincided with increased reports of MRSA. Epidemics of MRSA first occurred in London in the mid 1980s. Sporadic outbreaks of MRSA have continued to be reported throughout the country and several distinct strains have been identified (Marples & Reith

1992). Most are resistant to many other antibiotics, including erythromycin and ciprofloxacin, seriously limiting options for the treatment of infection. Usually the only drugs to which MRSA is reliably sensitive are vancomycin and teicoplanin. Since the early 1990s two new epidemic strains have emerged, EMRSA-15 and EMRSA-16. The former is particularly associated with colonization of chronic wounds and urine, the latter with invasive infections such as pneumonia (Cox et al 1995). The number of hospitals affected by these strains has increased significantly in the past 5 years (Communicable Disease Report 1997) (Fig. 5.3). The extent of the problem is also reflected in laboratory reports of bacteraemia. The proportion of *S. aureus* bacteraemias resistant to methicillin has increased from less than 2% in the early 1990s to 19% in 1998 (Communicable Disease Report 1999). Recent data from the Nosocomial Infection National Surveillance Scheme in England suggest that 50% of *S. aureus* causing surgical wound infections are resistant to methicillin (Public Health Laboratory Service 2000a).

MRSA occurs worldwide and the importation of strains of MRSA from other countries remains a problem.

Vancomycin-resistant *S. aureus*

The glycopeptides are the main antibiotic available to treat serious infection caused by MRSA and, should resistance to these agents emerge, such infections could become effectively untreatable. With the emergence of vancomycin-resistant enterococci (VRE), the risk of resistance transferring to staphylococci has become a real possibility. So far, only strains of *S. aureus* with a degree of resistance to vancomycin (vancomycin-intermediate *S. aureus* or VISA) have been reported (Hood et al 2000) and there is no evidence that the resistance has been acquired from enterococci (Communicable Disease Report 1997).

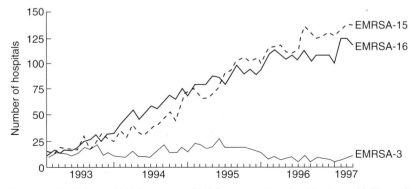

Fig. 5.3   Hospitals affected by EMRSA-3, EMRSA-15 and EMRSA-16 strains of epidemic methicillin-resistant *Staphylococcus aureus*, 1993–1997. Source: Communicable Disease Report Weekly (1997) **7**(22): Front page.

Virulence and epidemiology

S. aureus causes a variety of infections ranging from mild infection of the skin (boils and abscesses) to serious systemic infection, **septicaemia, pneumonia** and major wound infection. MRSA causes the same type of infection as sensitive strains of *S. aureus* and most studies suggest that it has equal pathogenicity (French et al 1990), although a higher incidence of septic shock in critically ill patients has been reported (Coello et al 1997). In addition to causing infection, *S. aureus* is a part of the normal flora of the skin, especially in axillae, groins, perineum and nose. Some people are heavily colonized with *S. aureus* and areas of damaged skin are especially prone to colonization (e.g. wounds, cannula sites). MRSA may replace sensitive strains of *S. aureus* on the skin, which it will colonize without causing infection but provide a reservoir from which it may spread to other patients or staff (Muder et al 1991).

Hospitalization is a major risk factor for the acquisition of MRSA; exposure to antibiotics encourages resistant strains to emerge and the presence of wounds or invasive devices facilitates colonization. Patients in some specialties are more at risk than others (Box 5.5). In long-term care settings, whilst the risk of transmission and serious infection is lower, patients may act as a reservoir of MRSA, bringing the organism into hospital when they are admitted (Fraise et al 1997).

Serious staphylococcal infection usually occurs in people made more vulnerable by an underlying illness or medical intervention. Healthy people are unlikely to develop infection, although they may become colonized. Although most patients lose the resistant strain after discharge from hospital, some may remain colonized for many weeks (Hicks et al 1991).

Box 5.5 High-risk hospital settings: patients vulnerable to colonization or infection with MRSA

- intensive care units
- neonatal and special care baby units
- burns units
- transplant units
- cardiothoracic units
- orthopaedic and trauma wards
- vascular surgery
- general surgery
- urology
- gynaecology and obstetrics
- dermatology

Source: Taylor (1997), with permission

MRSA is spread in the same way as sensitive strains of *S. aureus*. The most important route of transmission is on the hands of staff who acquire the organism through direct contact with infected or colonized skin and, if **carriage** is not removed by handwashing, will deposit it on patients (Mortimer et al 1966). Heavily contaminated uniforms, equipment or surfaces could potentially transmit infection. Airborne spread is theoretically possible and commonly cited, but there is little direct evidence that it occurs. It is probably not a significant route of transmission unless patients are shedding excessive amounts of skin scales or the standard of cleaning is very low (Barrett et al 1993, Mylotte 1994).

Although many strains of MRSA do not spread from person to person easily, some have a particular propensity to transmit and are often referred to as **epidemic** strains. It is not unusual for such epidemic strains of MRSA to colonize and infect several patients on one ward, and they may spread throughout a hospital if left unchecked. Patients colonized with MRSA have an increased risk of developing serious infection, which may be extremely difficult to treat (Coello et al 1997).

Treatment of colonization

Colonized patients or staff provide a reservoir from which resistant bacteria can be spread to other patients. *S. aureus* can be removed from colonized sites by topical treatment with antistaphylococcal solutions and creams. The most effective of these is mupirocin applied to skin lesions or to the nose for 5 days, three times a day, and this is usually sufficient to eliminate MRSA. Unfortunately, resistance to mupirocin has already been reported although, so far, infrequently (Cookson 1990). Mupirocin should not be applied to central vascular catheters as it may damage the material (Medical Devices Agency 1995). Recently, tea tree oil has been suggested as a topical treatment for the eradication of MRSA. There is some evidence that it is effective, although this has not yet been demonstrated by clinical trials and little is known about potential toxicity or other side-effects (Carson et al 1995, Chang & London 1998). Antiseptic skin disinfectant solutions (e.g. chlorhexidine handwash) can also be used to eliminate *S. aureus* and should be used daily for washing and twice weekly on the hair. The treatment of MRSA-colonized staff is usually arranged by the occupational health department.

Colonization of staff

Staff may acquire MRSA in the nose and on damaged skin, and may contribute to the spread of the organism.

However, the probability of staff becoming colonized is low and usually related to the extent of contact with infected or colonized patients. More importantly, carriage is usually transient and the organism will generally disappear after a few hours (Cookson et al 1989). None the less, the screening of staff for MRSA colonization during outbreaks may be necessary to help control the spread.

Control of MRSA in hospitals

Although there is considerable debate about the efficacy of measures to prevent the spread of MRSA, many argue that not controlling it is very costly (BSAC Working Party 1998). The guidelines recommended by the working party recommend different approaches to control depending on the clinical area affected, and emphasize the importance of risk assessment when selecting a level of control. A high standard of routine infection control is also important to minimize the risk of spread from patients not known to be colonized or infected with MRSA (see Ch. 7). Box 5.6 outlines the important principles of MRSA control in hospitals.

Control of MRSA in community settings

The risk of MRSA transmission in residential care homes, where residents are generally more healthy and have fewer invasive devices than hospital patients, is much lower. Spread of MRSA between residents may occur, but is usually associated with colonization rather than infection. Isolation of residents

---

Box 5.6   Important principles for controlling methicillin-resistant *Staphylococcus aureus* in hospitals

Isolation
- Colonized or infected patients should be nursed in a single room, where available
- Gloves and aprons should be used for contact with the patient and discarded after use. They should also be changed between procedures
- Hands should be washed after contact with patients or their environment

Cohorting
- A group of several affected patients can be isolated together in a designated part of the ward. This can help to reduce workload for staff and improve adherence to the control measures

Cleaning
- Isolation rooms should be kept clean during use, especially the horizontal surfaces where dust may settle and bacteria accumulate
- Rooms should be cleaned with detergent and water after isolation has been discontinued to remove micro-organisms remaining in the environment

Treatment of affected patients
- Apply antistaphylococcal cream to open skin and intranasally (mupirocin, three times per day for 5 days; naseptin, four times a day for 7 days). To prevent resistance to mupirocin emerging, no more than two courses of treatment should be given in any one admission
- Bathe daily for 5 days using antiseptic detergents (e.g. chlorhexidine) to eliminate skin colonization
- Wash hair with antiseptic detergent to eliminate colonization
- Isolation can be discontinued when three sets of negative swabs from all previously positive sites have been obtained
- Clinical infections will require treatment with antibiotics, usually vancomycin or teicoplanin

Readmission
- Previously colonized or infected patients should be rescreened on readmission to hospital as the resistant strain may persist in small numbers
- Notes can be labelled and records flagged in computer-held records to indicate patients who have had MRSA

Screening of other patients
- Other patients may need to be sampled for MRSA carriage by taking swabs from the nose, perineum or groin, skin lesions and invasive device insertion sites. This can enable early identification, isolation and treatment of MRSA carriers and help to limit spread
- The extent of screening will depend on the type of clinical area and the number of patients affected

Screening of staff contacts
- This is usually necessary only in high-risk areas, such as the intensive care unit, or where the organism continues to spread despite the control measures and a staff carrier may be contributing to transmission
- Swab nose and skin lesions of staff in contact with affected patients
- Staff who are colonized with MRSA should be treated with mupirocin. In high-risk wards, exclusion from work for 48 hours may be necessary

with MRSA is not necessary and they should be able to use communal areas with other residents. They may share a room, provided neither occupant has open lesions, invasive devices or catheters. Routine infection control precautions such as handwashing and the use of disposable gloves and apron for contact with body fluids, dealing with wounds or invasive devices should be sufficient to prevent spread (see Ch. 7). Such precautions are also sufficient for district nurses visiting the homes of patients infected or colonized with MRSA. In community hospitals the risk may be slightly greater as other residents may have open wounds and devices; precautions similar to those used in hospitals are therefore more appropriate (BSAC Working Party 1995).

Colonization with MRSA should not interfere with the admission of a patient into either a hospital or a residential home (Department of Health 1996). Good communication between staff in hospitals, residential homes and the community is essential. The hospital or community infection control nurse (ICN) can help to evaluate the risk to other residents and provide advice on control measures.

Glycopeptide-resistant enterococci (GRE)

Enterococci are normal commensals of the gut and until recently were not a common cause of nosocomial infection. However, during the last two decades their intrinsic resistance to many antibiotics, such as the cephalosporins and quinolones, has enabled them to emerge as major nosocomial pathogens with *Enterococcus faecium* and *E. faecalis* responsible for most of the infections. During this time they have acquired resistance to most other antibiotics, for example tetracyclines, macrolides, trimethoprim and aminoglycosides. *E. faecium* is intrinsically resistant to penicillin and therefore the glycopeptides have provided the only effective treatment for infections caused by this organism.

Enterococci take advantage of seriously ill or immunocompromised patients and invasive devices. They can cause septicaemia, endocarditis, urinary tract infection and peritonitis associated with continuous ambulatory peritoneal dialysis (CAPD), and are usually associated with specialized units such as intensive care, renal, liver and haematology (Gray & George 2000, Morrison et al 1996, Sanyal et al 1993). Acquired resistance to vancomycin was first reported in enterococci in 1988 (Uttley et al 1988) and since then GRE have been reported in many hospitals both in the UK and elsewhere in the world. In England, recent data from the Nosocomial Infection National Surveillance Scheme has found 26% of *E. faecium* and 4% of *E. faecalis* to be glycopeptide resistant (Public Health Laboratory Service 2000b). Resistant strains are selected following exposure to glycopeptides, and resistance can then be spread to other strains and species on plasmids. There are virtually no antimicrobial agents currently available to treat infections caused by these highly resistant pathogens, and there is also a serious risk that resistance will be transmitted to other important pathogenic bacteria.

Outbreaks of infection have demonstrated that transmission between patients occurs. The organism is probably readily transmitted on the hands of staff in contact with colonized or infected patients, and the environment is also thought to play a role (Weber and Rutala 1997). Enterococci can survive for several days on surfaces and a particularly high level of environmental contamination has been reported where a patient has diarrhoea (Bonilla et al 1995, Boyce et al 1994, Noskin et al 1995). A variety of medical equipment has also been implicated in transmission, including fluidized beds, thermometers and defective bedpan washers (Weber & Rutala 1997, Chadwick et al 1996).

Patients whose intestines become colonized with GRE and are otherwise asymptomatic are less likely to contaminate the environment than those who are colonized or infected with GRE at another site or have symptomatic gastrointestinal infection (Gray & George 2000). The latter group of patients should be isolated in a single room to minimize the extent of environmental contamination. Gloves and aprons should be used for contact with the patient or their immediate environment, and these should be changed between procedures, particularly after handling material likely to be heavily contaminated with GRE (e.g. stool) and before leaving the room. Hands must also be washed after any contact with these patient or their environment. Equipment such as commodes, stethoscopes and thermometers should be dedicated for use by the isolated patient (Hospital Infection Control Practice Advisory Committee 1995). Where patients have asymptomatic colonization of the gut, gloves and aprons need be worn only for contact with urine and faeces (Gray & George 2000). Where clusters of cases of GRE occur, other patients in the affected unit may need to be screened for GRE carriage by the collection of stool or rectal swabs. As with MRSA, marking medical records of infected or colonized patients and isolation precautions on readmission to hospital is recommended, as the resistant organisms may be carried in the bowel for prolonged periods. High standards of cleanliness are important to minimize environmental contamination and to reduce the risk of transmission between patients (George et al 1998).

Multidrug-resistant tuberculosis

Resistance to antituberculous drugs was recognized as a problem when streptomycin was first used in the 1940s. Unlike other bacteria, antimicrobial resistance in mycobacteria is not associated with transmissible plasmids or transposons. Instead, resistance is due to mutation in single chromosomal genes; for example, resistance to rifampicin is due to a mutation in the gene encoding for RNA polymerase. These mutations occur spontaneously at a low rate within a population of mycobacteria but, if exposed to therapy with a single drug, resistant organisms will eventually predominate. The chances of mycobacteria developing more than one spontaneous mutation that confers resistance to more than one drug are very low. Therapy regimens involving more than one drug were therefore devised to ensure that mutants resistant to one drug would be destroyed by a second drug. However, in populations of mycobacteria already resistant to one drug, mutants to a second drug will be selected by a treatment regimen involving both drugs. Strains resistant to isoniazid and rifampicin, the two most important drugs, are called multidrug-resistant tuberculosis (MDRTB). Once resistant populations of mycobacteria have emerged in one person, they may then be transmitted to others, who will develop a primary drug-resistant infection.

In many parts of the world poor treatment regimens, inadequate supplies of drugs and non-adherence to prescribed therapy has resulted in the widespread emergence of strains resistant to one or more drugs. In a recent study by the World Health Organization 10% of cases were found to be resistant to at least one drug. Levels of resistance were particularly high in parts of the former USSR, South America and Africa. In some countries, over 15% of cases were resistant to all four antituberculous drugs, and over 50% were resistant to isoniazid and rifampicin (Pablos-mendez et al 1998). Treatment options for MDRTB are extremely limited and the mortality rate is high, especially in patients who are HIV positive (Telzak et al 1995).

In the UK, systems for the diagnosis, treatment and surveillance of *Mycobacterium tuberculosis* have been in place for many years, and levels of resistance are relatively low. In 1995 just over 6% of cases were resistant to isoniazid and 1.6% to isoniazid and rifampicin. However, there has been a gradual increase in the level of drug resistance during the 1990s (Interdepartmental Working Group 1998). None the less, there are prob-

lems with non-adherence with therapy (Morse 1996), and in a recent outbreak of MDRTB poor antituberculous treatment, notably the addition of a single drug to a failing treatment regimen, resulted in the emergence of MDRTB in the index case (Breathnach et al 1998).

HIV-related drug-resistant tuberculosis

Individuals with HIV are especially vulnerable to *M. tuberculosis*. Although probably no more likely to acquire infection if exposed, infection is much more likely to become active and latent infections are also likely to reactivate. Treatment of tuberculosis in HIV-positive patients is complicated by poor absorption of drugs, interaction with other drugs, and a high risk of recurrence. HIV is also a major risk factor for MDRTB (Albino & Reichman 1997). Many outbreaks of tuberculosis amongst patients with HIV nursed together in hospital have been reported. Unfortunately, many of these have involved MDRTB (Frieden et al 1996, Interdepartmental Working Group 1998). In 1998, an outbreak of MDRTB occurred in the UK. The index case did not have HIV, but was nursed on the same ward as patients with HIV, seven of whom subsequently acquired MDRTB and two of which died (Breathnach et al 1998). This outbreak highlighted the importance of adhering to clearly defined infection control policies. Factors that contributed to the spread of infection were an isolation room with airflow directed into the ward and inadequate isolation of suspected cases.

Recent guidance issued by the Interdepartmental Working Group in 1998 recommends that hospitals have a tuberculosis control plan which includes assessment of the risk of transmission in all patient areas and identifies an appropriate level of isolation facilities to cope with the risk. Systems should be in place to ensure that precautions are taken, with all patients suspected to have tuberculosis until non-infectiousness is proven, and that they are not placed in the same ward as patients with HIV. Patients with suspected or confirmed MDRTB require isolation in a room with negative pressure ventilation (Box 5.7). As they are likely to have mycobacteria in their sputum for months, prolonged isolation is likely to be necessary (Interdepartmental Working Group 1998).

Other problem species

Streptococcus pneumoniae is an important cause of community-acquired pneumonia, otitis media in children, and meningitis. In the past it was highly sensitive to penicillin, which is useful treatment because of its ability to penetrate the meninges.

> **Box 5.7** Key infection control measures for patients with multidrug-resistant tuberculosis
>
> - Nurse in a negative-pressure isolation room and ensure the efficiency of air handling is monitored regularly
> - Ensure the patient remains in the room with the door closed
> - Restrict the number of staff involved in care of the patient
> - Limit visitors to those who have been in close contact before the diagnosis of MDRTB
> - Only perform aerosol-generating procedures (e.g. sputum induction) in a room with local exhaust ventilation
> - Teach patients to cover their mouth and nose with a tissue when coughing or sneezing
> - Ask patients to wear a mask during transportation to other areas
> - Staff should wear a mask in the isolation room
>
> Source: Interdepartmental Working Group (1998)

Resistance to penicillin began to be reported in the 1970s. In some countries levels of resistance are now extremely high, for example in Spain where 44% of isolates are resistant, probably related to the inappropriate treatment of viral infections in children. In the UK, the rates of resistance are relatively low at around 7.5%, but increasing (Department of Health 1999).

Antibiotic resistance amongst hospital-acquired Gram-negative pathogens is gradually increasing. Resistance to a wide range of antimicrobial agents is readily transmitted between different Gram-negative species on plasmids, although chromosomal mutation also plays a part (e.g. ciprofloxacin resistance). Resistance amongst enteric pathogens such as salmonella and campylobacter is also emerging and thought to be related to the use of antibiotics as animal growth promoters and in veterinary practice (Department of Health 1999).

The key to successful control is good isolation techniques, especially rigorous attention to handwashing by all members of staff who have contact with patients **infected** or colonized with MRSA. The aim should be to eliminate infection or colonization as rapidly as possible and ensure the patient's period of isolation is kept to a minimum.

The infection control team will coordinate the management of outbreaks of MRSA among hospital patients and work closely with the occupational health department to monitor and treat colonized staff.

REFERENCES

Albino JA, Reichman LE (1997) Multi-drug resistant tuberculosis. *Curr. Opin. Infect. Dis.*, **10**: 116–22.

Arason VA, Kristinsson KG, Sigurdson JA et al (1996) Do antimicrobials increase the carriage rate of penicillin resistant pneumococci in children? Cross sectional prevalence study. *BMJ*, **313**: 387–91.

Barrett SP, Teare EL, Sage R (1993) Methicillin-resistant *Staphylococcus aureus* in three adjacent health districts of South-East England 1986–91. *J. Hosp. Infect.*, **24**: 313–25.

Barrow P, Soothill J (1997) Bacteriophage therapy and prophylaxis; rediscovery and reviewed assessment of potential. *Trends Microbiol*, **5**: 268–71.

Bojalil R, Calva JJ (1994) Antibiotic misuse in diarrhoea. A household survey in a Mexican community. *J. Clin. Epidemiol.*, **47**: 147–56.

Bonilla HF, Zervos MJ, Kauffman CA (1996) Long-term survival of vancomycin-resistant *Enterococcus faecium* on a contaminated surface. *Infect. Control Hosp. Epidemiol.*, **17**(12): 770–1.

Boyce JM, Opal SM, Chow FW et al (1994) Outbreak of multi-drug resistant *Enterococcus faecium* with transferable vanB class vancomycin resistance. *J. Clin. Microbiol.*, **32**: 1148–53.

Breathnach AS, de Ruiter A, Holdsworth GMC et al (1998) An outbreak of multidrug resistant tuberculosis in a London teaching hospital. *J. Hosp. Infect.*, **39**(2): 111–18.

Brown EM, Reeves DS (1997) Quinolones. In *Antibiotics and Chemotherapy. Anti-infective Agents and their Use in Therapy*, 7th edn, Ch. 32 (F O'Grady, HP Lambert, RG Finch, eds). Churchill Livingstone, London.

BSAC Working Party (1994) Hospital antibiotic control measures in the UK. *J. Antimicrob. Chemother.*, **34**: 21–42.

BSAC Working Party (1995) Guidelines on the control of methicillin-resistant *Staphylococcus aureus* in the community. Report of a combined working party of the British Society for Antimicrobial Chemotherapy and the Hospital Infection Society. *J. Hosp. Infect.*, **31**: 1–12.

BSAC Working Party (1998) Revised guidelines for the control of methicillin-resistant *Staphylococcus aureus* in hospitals. Combined working party of the British Society for Antimicrobial Chemotherapy, Hospital Infection Society and Infection Control Nurses Association. *J. Hosp. Infect.*, **39**(4): 253–90.

Carson CF, Cookson BD, Farrelly HD et al (1995) Susceptibility of methicillin resistant *Staphylococcus aureus* to the essential oil of *Melaleuca alternifolia*. *J. Antimicrob. Chemother.*, **35**: 421–4.

Casewell MW, Desai N (1983) Survival of multiply-resistant *Klebsiella aerogenes* and other Gram-negative bacilli on finger-tips. *J. Hosp. Inf.*, **18** (Suppl.): 23–8.

Chadwick PR, Chadwick CD, Oppenheim BA (1996) Report of a meeting on the epidemiology and control of glycopeptide-resistant enterococci. *J. Hosp. Infect.*, **33**(2): 83–92.

Chang CH, London KW (1998) Activity of Tea Tree Oil on methicillin-resistant *Staphylococcus aureus* (MRSA). *J. Hosp. Infect.*, **39**(3): 244.

Coello R, Glynn JR, Gaspar C et al (1997) Risk factors for developing clinical infection with methicillin-resistant

Staphylococcus aureus strains among hospital patients initially colonised with MRSA. *J. Hosp. Infect.*, **37**: 39–46.

Communicable Disease Report (1997) Epidemic methicillin resistant *Staphylococcus aureus*. *CDR*, **7**(22): 191.

Communicable Disease Report (1999) Methicillin resistance in *Staphylococcus aureus* isolated from blood in England and Wales: 1994 to 1998. *CDR Weekly*, **9**(8): 65.

Cookson BD (1990) Mupirocin resistance in staphylococci. *J. Antimicrob. Chemother.*, **25**: 497–503.

Cookson BD, Peters B, Webster M et al (1989) Staff carriage of epidemic methicillin resistant *Staphylococcus aureus*. *J. Clin. Microbiol.*, **27**(7): 1471–6.

Cox RA, Conquest C, Mallghan C et al (1995) A major outbreak of methicillin-resistant *Staphylococcus aureus* caused by a new phage-type (EMRSA 16). *J. Hosp. Infect.*, **29**: 81–106.

Del Mar C, Glasziou P, Hayem M (1997) Are antibiotics indicated as initial treatment with acute otitis media. A meta-analysis. *BMJ*, **314**: 1526–9.

Department of Health (1996) Methicillin-resistant *Staphylococcus aureus* in community settings. PL(CMO)96. Department of Health, London.

Department of Health (1999) Standing Medical Advisory Committee. Subgroup on antimicrobial resistance. *The Path of Least Resistance*. Department of Health, London.

Feely YJ, Chan P, Cocoman L et al (1990) Hospital formularies: need for continuous intervention. *BMJ*, **300**: 28–30.

Fraise AP, Mitchell R, O'Brien SJ et al (1997) Methicillin-resistant *Staphylococcus aureus* (MRSA) in nursing homes in a major UK city: an anonymised point prevalence survey. *Epidemiol. Infect.*, **118**: 1–5.

Freiden TR, Sherman LF, Maw KL et al (1996) A multi-institutional outbreak of highly drug-resistant tuberculosis. *JAMA*, **276**: 122–35.

French GL, Cheng AFB, Ling JML et al (1990) Hong Kong strains of methicillin-resistant and sensitive *Staphylococcus aureus* have similar virulence. *J. Hosp. Infect.*, **15**(2): 117–26.

George RH, Cox P, Hobbs PM et al (1998) An outbreak of vancomycin-resistant enterococci (VRE) infection on a paediatric intensive care unit (PICU). *J. Hosp. Infect.*, **40** (Suppl. A): 3.2.7.

Gray JW, George RH (2000) Experience of vancomycin-resistant enterococci in a children's hospital. *J. Hosp. Infect.*, **45**: 11–18.

Hicks NR, Moore EP, Williams EW (1991) Carriage and community treatment of methicillin-resistant *Staphylococcus aureus*. What happens to colonized patients after discharge. *J. Hosp. Infect.*, **19**(1): 17–24.

Hood J, Cosgrove B, Curran E et al (2000) Vancomycin-resistant *Staphylococcus aureus* in Scotland. Abstracts of the Centers for Disease Control Fourth Decennial Conference on Nosocomial and Healthcare Associated infections. Abstract S-Th-02.

Hospital Infection Control Practices Advisory Committee (1995) Recommendations for preventing the spread of vancomycin resistance: recommendations of the Hospital Infection Control Practices Advisory Committee (HICPAC). *Am. J. Infect. Control*, **23**: 87–94.

Humphries H, Duckworth G (1997) Methicillin-resistant *Staphylococcus aureus* (MRSA) – a re-appraisal of control measures in the light of changing circumstances. *J. Hosp. Infect.*, **36**(3): 167–70.

Interdepartmental Working Group on Tuberculosis (1998) *The Prevention and Control of Tuberculosis in the United Kingdom. Guidance on the Prevention and Control of Transmission of 1. HIV Related Tuberculosis 2. Drug-resistance, Including Multiple Drug-resistant Tuberculosis.* Department of Health Stores, Wetherby, UK.

Kitteringham NR, Park BK (1997) Pharmacokinetics. In *Antibiotics and Chemotherapy. Anti-infective Agents and their Use in Therapy*, 7th edn, Ch. 4 (F O'Grady, HP Lambert, RG Finch, eds). Churchill Livingstone, London.

Lewis MJ (1989) Mycobacterial disease. In *Antimicrobial Chemotherapy*, pp. 279–88 (D Greenwood, ed.) Oxford Medical Publications, Oxford.

McGowan JE (1994) Do intensive hospital antibiotic control programs prevent the spread of antibiotic resistance? *Infect. Control Hosp. Epidemiol.*, **15**(7): 478–83.

Marples RR, Reith S (1992) Methicillin-resistant *Staphylococcus aureus* in England and Wales. *CDR*, **2** (Review 3): R25–9.

Morrison D, Woodford N, Cookson B (1996) Epidemic vancomycin-resistant *Enterococcus faecium* in the UK. *Clin. Microb. Infect.*, **1**(2): 146.

Morse DI (1996) Directly observed therapy for tuberculosis. *BMJ*, **312**: 719–20.

Mortimer EA, Wolinsky E, Gonzaga AJ et al (1966) Role of airborne transmission in staphylococcal infections. *BMJ*, **1**: 319–22.

Muder RR, Bennan C, Wagner MN et al (1991) Methicillin-resistant staphylococcal infection colonisation and infection in a long-term care facility. *Ann. Intern Med.*, **114**: 107–12.

Mylotte JM (1994) Control of methicillin-resistant *Staphylococcus aureus*: the ambivalence persists. *Infect. Control Hosp. Epidemiol.*, **15**: 73–7.

Neu HC (1992) The crisis in antibiotic resistance. *Science*, **257**: 1064–73.

Noskin GA, Stosor V, Cooper I et al (1995) Recovery of vancomycin-resistant enterococci on fingertips and environmental surfaces. *Infect. Control Hosp. Epidemiol.*, **16**: 577–81.

Pablos-mendez A, Raviglione MC, Laszlo A et al (1998) Global surveillance for antituberculosis drug resistance. *N. Engl. J. Med.*, **338**: 1641–9.

Péchere JC (1994) Antibiotic resistance is selected primarily in our patients. *Infect. Control Hosp. Epidemiol.*, **15**: 472–7.

Pillay D (1998) Emergence and control of resistance to antiviral drugs in herpes viruses, hepatitis B virus and HIV. *Commun. Dis. Pub. Health*, **1**(1): 5–13.

Public Health Laboratory Service (2000a) *Surveillance of Surgical Site Infection in English Hospitals, 1997–1999*. Nosocomial Infection National Surveillance Scheme, London.

Public Health Laboratory Service (2000b) *Surveillance of Hospital-acquired Bacteraemia in English Hospitals, 1997–1999*. Nosocomial Infection National Surveillance Scheme, London.

Sanyal D, Williams AJ, Johnson AP et al (1993) The emergence of vancomycin resistance in renal dialysis. *J. Hosp. Infect.*, **24**(3): 167–74.

Simpson JY (1869) Some propositions on hospitalisation. *Lancet*, **16 Oct.**, 535–8.

Soares S, Kristensson KG, Musser JM et al (1993) Evidence for the introduction of a multiresistant clone of serotype 6B *Streptococcus pneumoniae* from Spain to Iceland in the late 1980s. *J. Infect. Dis.*, **168**: 158–63.

Taylor EW (1997) Abdominal and other surgical infections. In *Antibiotics and Chemotherapy. Anti-infective Agents and their Use in Therapy*, 7th edn, Ch. 42 (F O'Grady, HP Lambert, RG Finch, eds). Churchill Livingstone, London.

Taylor L (1997) Nursing update: MRSA. *Nursing Standard*, **27**(11).

Telzak EE, Sepkowitz K, Alpert P et al (1995) Multidrug resistant tuberculosis in patients without HIV infection. *N. Engl. J. Med.*, **333**: 907–11.

Uttley AHC, Pozniak A (1993) Resurgence of tuberculosis. *J. Hosp. Infect.*, **23**(4): 249–54.

Uttley AHC, Collins CH, Naidoo J et al (1988) Vancomycin resistant enterococci. *Lancet*, **i**: 57–8.

Weber DJ, Rutala WA (1997) Role of environmental contamination in the transmission of vancomycin-resistant enterococci. *Infect. Control Hosp. Epidemiol.*, **18**: 306–9.

World Health Organization (1983) Control of antibiotic resistant bacteria. *Bull WHO*, **61**: 423–33.

FURTHER READING

Boyce JM (1991) Should we vigorously try to contain and control methicillin-resistant *Staphylococcus aureus? Inf. Control Hosp. Epid.*, **12**: 46–54.

Boyce JM (1996) Preventing staphylococcal infections by eradicating nasal carriage of *Staphylococcus aureus*: proceedingwith caution. *Infect. Control Hosp. Epidemiol.*, **17**: 775–9.

Cohen ML (1992) Epidemiology of drug resistance. Implications for a post-antimicrobial era. *Science*, **257**: 1050–5.

Cooksey S (1995) Managing chemotherapy for tuberculosis. *Nursing Times*, **91**(35): 32–3.

Greenwood D (1995) *Antimicrobial Chemotherapy*, 3rd edn. Oxford University Press, Oxford.

Greenwood D (1995) Sixty years on: antimicrobial drug resistance comes of age. *Lancet*, **346** (Suppl.): 1.

O'Grady F, Lambert HP, Finch RG (eds) (1997) *Antibiotics and Chemotherapy. Anti-infective Agents and their Use in Therapy*, 7th edn. Churchill Livingstone, London.

McGowan JE (1995) Editorial: preventing nosocomial tuberculosis – progress at last. *Infect. Control Hosp. Epidemiol.*, **23**: 141–5.

Murray BA (1990) The life and times of the enterococcus. *Microbiol. Rev.*, **3**(1): 46–65.

Walters J (1988) How antibiotics work: *Prof. Nurse*, **3**(7): 251–4.

Walters J (1989) How antibiotics work: the cell membrane. *Prof. Nurse*, **4**(10): 508–10.

Walters J (1990) How antibiotics work: nucleic acid synthesis. *Prof. Nurse*, **5**(12): 641–3.

Wilson J, Richardson J (1996) Keeping MRSA in perspective. *Nursing Times*, **92**(19): 58–60.

6

Micro-organisms and their control

INTRODUCTION

There are many different **species** of bacteria, types of virus and other micro-organisms, but only a very small proportion are able to infect a human or animal host and cause disease. This chapter provides a brief outline of some pathogenic bacteria, fungi, protozoa and viruses commonly encountered in the healthcare environment. It focuses on the infection control implications of each organism and the precautions that may be required when caring for a patient with the infection.

PATHOGENIC BACTERIA

Gram-positive cocci

There are four main groups of bacteria, distinguished by their shape and response to the Gram stain (see p. 18): Gram-positive cocci and bacilli, and Gram-negative cocci and bacilli (Plate 2.1). Other important groups include acid-fast bacilli, spirochaetes and atypical bacteria.

Staphylococci

The staphylococci are differentiated into 'coagulase positive' and 'coagulase negative' species, depending on whether they produce the **enzyme coagulase**, which clots **plasma**.

 Staphylococcus aureus *Staphylococcus aureus* is a coagulase-positive staphylococcus. It is both a commensal of humans, as well as an important pathogen. It causes a range of superficial infections of the skin (Plate 6.1) such as septic spots, boils, abscesses and impetigo, and can also cause more serious infections including osteomyelitis, septicaemia, endocarditis and pneumonia. *S. aureus* is responsible for between 40% and 50% of surgical wound infections (Public Health Laboratory Service 2000a) and is the second most common cause of hospital-acquired infection (Emori & Gaynes 1993). *S. aureus* may colonize normal skin, particularly of the axillae, groins and perineum, but is most commonly found colonizing the nasal mucosa. Some 20–35% of people persistently carry the organisms in their nose, and a further 30–70% carry it intermittently (Williams 1963). Organisms from the nose are then easily transferred to other sites, and there is considerable evidence to show that nasal carriers are at increased risk of developing staphylococcal infection, particularly surgical wound infection (Kluytmans et al 1995, Wenzel & Perl 1995). Nasal carriage may also increase the risk of infection in patients undergoing haemodialysis (Glowacki et al 1994).

A variety of toxins are produced by different strains of *S. aureus*. Some produce a toxin that attacks cells in the skin, causing it to split and desquamate. Infections sometimes occur in neonates where they cause 'scalded skin syndrome', characterized by large, red, weeping areas where the skin has desquamated. Another toxin is responsible for toxic shock syndrome, associated with retained sanitary tampons. This can cause severe disease, with hypotension, fever, diarrhoea, and desquamative skin rash. Other strains produce an enterotoxin which interferes with electrolyte transfer in the gut and causes acute gastroenteritis if eaten with food.

S. aureus is particularly adept at developing resistance to antibiotics (see p. 89). Most isolates are now resistant to penicillin. Methicillin-resistant strains, which are resistant to many other antibiotics used to treat staphylococcal infection, emerged in the 1980s and are now a frequent cause of infection throughout the world (Voss & Doebbeling 1995). Methicillin-resistant *S. aureus* (MRSA) is mainly a problem amongst hospital patients and, although most cases are not associated with serious infection, the incidence is increasing. A recent survey reported that nearly 30% of *S. aureus* isolates from blood cultures were MRSA (Morgan et al 1999). Residents of nursing homes may also acquire the organism, often following a period of hospitalization (Fraise et al 1997). Strains of *S. aureus* with partial resistance to vancomycin, the antimicrobial agent used to treat infections caused by MRSA, have also recently been reported (Edwards & Hood 1999).

Staphylococcus epidermidis   *S. epidermidis* is a coagulase-negative staphylococcus. It colonizes the skin and used to be considered as non-pathogenic but is increasingly recognized as a major cause of infection acquired in hospital. It produces extracellular slime which enables it to adhere to and multiply on plastics and metals (Fig. 6.1). It is therefore able to cause infections associated with invasive plastic or metal devices,

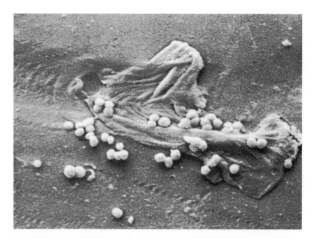

Fig. 6.1   *Staphylococcus epidermidis* adhering to a plastic intravenous cannula.

including peritoneal dialysis catheters, arterial grafts, cardiac prosthetic valves and prosthetic orthopaedic joints. It is also frequently responsible for bloodstream infections associated with intravenous devices (Public Health Laboratory Service 2000b). Immunocompromised patients are particularly vulnerable and the natural resistance of *S. epidermidis* to many antibiotics makes the infections it causes difficult to treat (Hamory & Parisi 1987).

Infection control precautions   Staphylococci present on skin and nasal mucosa are able to gain access to, and cause infection in, damaged skin sites such as wounds and cannula insertion sites. Although patients frequently provide a reservoir of *S. aureus*, staff may act as both a source of *S. aureus* themselves and a means by which organisms are transferred to others. Outbreaks of infection caused by *S. epidermidis* and *S. aureus* have frequently been reported (French et al 1990, Hamory & Parisi 1987). Staphylococci are most frequently transmitted on the hands and clothing of staff, as the classical experiments of Mortimer et al (1966) eloquently demonstrated. Aseptic technique should always be used to handle invasive devices, which are particularly vulnerable to invasion by both coagulase-negative and coagulase-positive staphylococci. Occasionally outbreaks of surgical wound infection are caused by a member of staff in the operating theatre who is heavily colonized with staphylococci and releases large numbers of organisms into the air on skin scales. Identification and treatment of the member of staff is necessary to prevent further spread. Staphylococci released on skin scales will collect in dust, where they may survive for several hours (Skaliy et al 1964). Regular cleaning will reduce the risk of dissemination. Outside the operating theatre, airborne spread on skin scales is possible, but probably overestimated as a route of transmission (Mylotte 1994, Reybrouck 1983).

Handwashing is the most important measure to prevent cross-infection of staphylococci. Elimination of nasal carriage with *S. aureus* has been shown to reduce the risk of postoperative infection and infections associated with continuous ambulatory peritoneal dialysis (CAPD) (Kluytmans et al 1996, Perez-Fontan et al 1993). Mupirocin is usually used to eradicate nasal carriage, but its widespread use for prolonged periods should be avoided, or resistance is likely to emerge rapidly (Boyce 1996).

Patients with *S. aureus* infection do not usually require isolation unless a large area of open wound is involved. However, special precautions are necessary where a patient is colonized or infected with antibiotic-resistant strains of *S. aureus*. The management of antibiotic-resistant strains of *S. aureus* is discussed in more detail in Chapter 5.

Streptococci

Streptococci are divided into more than 20 different types, called Lancefield groups. Many pathogenic species produce toxins called haemolysins, which lyse red blood cells and, when grown on blood agar, produce a characteristic change in appearance of the agar around the colony (Plate 2.5). Streptococci that cause complete haemolysis are called β-haemolytic, those that cause incomplete haemolysis are described as α-haemolytic. The most pathogenic species in humans is *Streptococcus pyogenes*. This group A streptococcus causes pharyngitis, skin infections and puerperal sepsis. It produces a range of toxins which help it to spread through tissue. These include streptokinase, an enzyme that dissolves fibrin, and streptodornase which breaks DNA into small fragments. Streptococci can invade damaged skin, surgical wounds, burns, ulcers, and cause invasive infections of the skin (e.g. impetigo, erysipelas (a spreading infection of subcutaneous tissues; Plate 6.2) and cellulitis (inflammation of connective tissues). In scarlet fever, an erythrogenic toxin causes the characteristic rash.

Puerperal sepsis is a septicaemia that originates from the uterus infected by *S. pyogenes* during childbirth. It was a frequent complication of childbirth before the introduction of antibiotics and a more hygienic approach to delivery. Now it is an uncommon, but still serious, infection.

Occasionally, acute rheumatic fever or glomerulonephritis occurs after a group A streptococcal infection caused by a hypersensitivity reaction. Antibodies formed against the streptococcus recognize and destroy tissue in the heart muscle, valves or kidneys by mistake. Subsequent streptococcal infection is likely to reactivate rheumatic fever and prophylaxis against infection is required to prevent this.

A particular cell surface protein, the M protein, confers resistance to phagocytosis and is an important virulence factor. The antigenic structure of the M protein varies and some types, such as M1 and M3, are associated with a particularly serious form of streptococcal infection called necrotizing fasciitis. This is a serious infection of soft tissue characterized by tissue necrosis. The disease progresses extremely rapidly, probably as a result of the diffusion of toxins through the skin. There is some evidence that strains of *S. pyogenes* that cause necrotizing fasciitis have a particular toxin (SpeA) introduced on a bacteriophage (Cartwright et al 1995). Tissue necrosis is accompanied by systemic toxaemia, with hypotension and damage to kidney function and blood coagulation. Necrotizing fasciitis is extremely rare, but the fatality rate is high, with 25% of patients dying as a result of the infection. Only one cluster of cases has been reported in the UK in this century (Cartwright et al 1995). In this outbreak, six cases occurred over a 3-month period, with two thought to be transmitted from a carrier amongst staff in the operating theatre.

Although frequently associated with *S. pyogenes*, mixtures of other bacteria, notably bacteroides and coliforms, may also cause necrotizing fasciitis.

Group B streptococci (*Streptococcus agalactiae*) are normal inhabitants of the intestine and sometimes the vagina. They can cause **meningitis** and septicaemia in the neonate who is exposed to the bacteria in the vagina during delivery. Risk factors for group B streptococcal infection in the newborn include prematurity, prolonged rupture of membranes and evidence of infection in the mother (Bignardi 1999).

Group C and G streptococci are similar to the group A streptococci and, although associated with less serious infection, can cause skin infections, tonsillitis and septicaemia.

The viridans group of streptococci are α-haemolytic and include at least five species that are prevalent amongst the normal flora. *Streptococcus mutans* is responsible for dental caries and can cause endocarditis. This occurs when bacteria lodge on an endocardium previously damaged by rheumatic fever, surgery or congenital defect. The body reacts to their presence by forming a layer of white blood cells and fibrin, which protects the bacteria from the immune system. Endocarditis is therefore a difficult infection to treat. Patients at risk of endocarditis should be given prophylactic antimicrobial therapy before dental treatment.

Streptococcus milleri forms part of the normal flora of the mouth and gastrointestinal tract but, if it gains access to the bloodstream, may cause abscesses, for example in the abdomen or brain.

Streptococcus pneumoniae   These bacteria are also known as pneumococci and are characterized by the arrangement of their cells into pairs (diplococci) rather than the chains normally associated with streptococci. Pathogenic strains have capsules made from polysaccharides which protect the cell from phagocytosis. There are many different types of capsule, which are distinguished by antigenic reactions. Non-capsulated strains of pneumococcus are normal inhabitants of the respiratory tract, whilst capsulated strains cause pneumonia, bronchitis, otitis media, sinusitis and meningitis.

Resistance to infection amongst the general population is high but is reduced by underlying heart or lung disease, influenza or **immunodeficiency**, and **epidemics** may occur in overcrowded conditions. Pneumococcal pneumonia is transmitted by respiratory droplets or by contact with oral secretions, and several episodes of cross-infection amongst elderly or immunocompromised patients have been described (Denton et al 1993). Penicillin is the antibiotic of choice for pneumococcal infection, but penicillin-resistant *S. pneumoniae* now accounts for around 3% of serious pneumococcal infection in the UK (Laurichesse et al 1998).

Infection control precautions   Reports of outbreaks of infection in hospital due to streptococci A, B, C and G have been described (Burnett & Norman 1990, Denton 1993, Efstratiou 1989, Ramage et al 1996). The bacteria may be acquired on the hands of staff by contact with colonized or infected wounds and skin, and transferred to vulnerable sites on other patients. Isolation of patients with streptococcal infection is therefore recommended until the patient has received appropriate antibiotic therapy for 48 h (see Ch. 14). Longer periods of isolation may be necessary for infections in chronic wounds where the organism is more difficult to eradicate.

Equipment has also been implicated in transmission. Dowsett & Willson (1981) reported an outbreak of infection associated with poor cleaning of baths and damaged enamel surfaces, and Takahashi et al (1998) described an outbreak caused by a contaminated bed covering.

Patients with penicillin-resistant strains of *S. pneumoniae* should be isolated, especially in a ward with a high proportion of elderly or **immunocompromised** patients (Pallett & Strangeways 1988, Ridgeway et al 1991).

Enterococcus

The main pathogens in the **genus** are *Enterococcus faecalis* and *E. faecium*, which are normal inhabitants of the bowel but are increasingly reported as a cause of hospital-acquired infection (Korten & Murray 1993). They mostly cause urinary tract and wound infections, especially in seriously ill patients. Occasionally they cause meningitis in neonates and pneumonia.

Enterococci are intrinsically resistant to many antibiotics, and the glycopeptides are usually used to treat serious infection. Glycopeptide-resistant strains first emerged in the late 1980s and have been reported as causing a number of outbreaks (Johnson 1998) with spread both within and between hospitals (see p. 96).

Infection control precautions   Until recently, it was thought that enterococci were acquired from the patient's own bowel flora. It is now recognized that they can be spread from patient to patient on the hands of staff and that environmental contamination and other reservoirs of the organism, such as electronic thermometers, may be involved (Gray & George 2000, Livornese et al 1992, Weber & Rutala 1997). Outbreaks are particularly likely to occur in intensive care, bone marrow transplant, renal and liver units. Control measures include isolation of infected or colonized patients, stringent handwashing, high standards of cleaning and identification of potential environmental reservoirs (see p. 96).

The emergence of multiresistant strains can be discouraged by the prudent use of antibiotic therapy.

Gram-positive bacilli

Bacillus

These are **aerobic** bacteria which form **spores**. They are widely distributed in soil, water and dust. The main pathogen is *Bacillus anthracis*, which causes anthrax, an infection of animals, especially sheep and cattle, and occasionally affects people whose work brings them into contact with animals or animal carcasses. It is spread by spores which can survive in soil for many years, but decontamination of hides and other animal products has made it an uncommon disease in the UK.

Bacillus cereus causes food poisoning and is usually associated with foods that have been kept for prolonged periods (e.g. rice), although infections associated with dietary supplements prepared in hospital have been reported (Rowan & Anderson 1998). *B. cereus* has occasionally been reported as a cause of surgical wound infections in association with unusual reservoirs of infection (e.g. linen) (Barrie et al 1992,

Stansfield and Caudle 1997). It can also cause a severe endophthalmitis following traumatic injury or insertion of contaminated contact lens. Orsi et al (1999) reported an outbreak of endophthalmitis associated with inadequate decontamination of irrigation equipment, and Gray et al (1999) described an outbreak of respiratory tract infection in a neonatal unit associated with inadequate decontamination of ventilator circuits.

Clostridia

The clostridia are **anaerobic** bacteria which form spores. They are mostly found in soil where they play an important role in the decomposition of **organic** materials, and many species are normal commensals of the gut. The pathogenic species cause disease by producing potent toxins that have profound effects on the host.

Clostridium tetani *Clostridium tetani* is present in the intestinal tract of herbivores and in soil. Tetanus occurs when a wound is contaminated by *C. tetani* spores and the conditions in the tissues are sufficiently anaerobic for them to germinate, multiply and produce toxin. The toxin stimulates motor nerve cells and causes convulsive muscle contractions, beginning near to the site of the wound but spreading progressively throughout the body.

Tetanus is most likely to occur in wounds contaminated with soil or a foreign body, in deep puncture wounds or those with extensive tissue damage. It is associated with a high incidence and mortality rate in countries without **immunization** programmes or anti-tetanus prophylaxis treatment. In the UK all children should receive immunization and a single booster of toxoid vaccine will protect immune individuals who are at risk of tetanus infection from a potentially contaminated wound. Elderly people are less likely to have been immunized and are at greater risk of acquiring tetanus. Tetanus is not spread from one person to another.

Clostridium perfringens *Clostridium perfringens* is a normal commensal of the gut but may also cause food poisoning and infection of the soft tissues. Food poisoning occurs when spores of *C. perfringens* contaminating raw meat or poultry survive the cooking process. If ingested, they sporulate and release a toxin that causes abdominal pain and watery diarrhoea. *C. perfringens* is frequently recovered from wounds, but rarely causes the serious infection called gas gangrene, characterized by muscle destruction, release of gas into the tissues and toxaemia. Gas gangrene occurs only when wounds are contaminated by soil or street dust, or intestinal organisms. It is most likely to develop where there is extensive tissue damage or an impaired blood supply, creating the anaerobic conditions necessary for the organism to multiply. Cases are usually associated with crush injuries, road accidents or underlying vascular disease.

Gas gangrene is not infectious and does not spread from patient to patient. The organism is acquired **endogenously** from the gut or the environment, and gas gangrene develops only if the conditions in the wound are favourable for its multiplication. It may also be caused by other species of clostridia.

Clostridium difficile *C. difficile* is commonly found in the human intestine where it is carried asymptomatically. It was not recognized as a cause of disease until the late 1970s when it was identified as a cause of hospital-acquired gastrointestinal infections, the symptoms of which range from mild diarrhoea to a severe and sometimes fatal pseudomembraneous colitis.

The incidence of infection has increased significantly over the last decade. Patients over 65 years of age are particularly vulnerable, as are those with chronic illness who are frequently admitted to hospital (e.g. renal and oncology patients) (Bignardi 1998, Djuretic et al 1999). The infection usually occurs when the normal gut flora is altered by antibiotic therapy, especially ampicillin, clindamycin and cephalosporins (Kelly and Lamont 1998). *C. difficile* multiplies in the absence of competition from other organisms, producing toxins that are responsible for the symptoms and cause necrosis of the lining of the gut and loss of fluid from the mucosa. The diagnosis is confirmed by the presence of the organism and its toxin in faeces, but asymptomatic carriage of *C. difficile* is not uncommon. Recurrence of symptoms after treatment is common and probably associated with the persistence of spores in the gut. Affected patients may continue to excrete the organism for prolonged periods.

A number of outbreaks of *C. difficile* have been reported, particularly amongst elderly patients, and it is clear that the organism can be transmitted between patients (Cartmill et al 1994). The main route of transmission is probably on the hands of staff but spores, disseminated in high numbers from infected patients, may survive for several months in the environment. In outbreaks of infection extensive contamination of the environment has been implicated as an important factor in its spread, and *C. difficile* has been recovered from toilets, bedpans, bedding and mops (Fekerty et al 1981, Hoffman 1993).

Infection control precautions Patients with toxin-producing stains of *C. difficile* in their faeces should be isolated while they have diarrhoea. Protective clothing should be used to handle excreta. Excreta should be discarded promptly into bedpan washer, macerator or toilet, and hands washed after any contact with the patient. Regular cleaning with detergent and water should reduce the number of spores present in the environment of affected patients. There is no evidence that disinfectants are more effective (DoH/PHLS Joint Working Group 1994).

The standard of cleaning should be closely monitored and spillages of excreta promptly removed and the area cleaned thoroughly (Worsley 1993). Equipment such as commodes and mattress covers should also be cleaned thoroughly before use by another patient.

Admission may need to be restricted to units affected by an outbreak. Measures to control antibiotic usage, such as the use of narrow-spectrum drugs and early discontinuation of antimicrobial therapy, are important to prevent *C. difficile* disease amongst hospital patients (DoH/PHLS Joint Working Group 1994).

Corynebacteria

Many species are commensals that colonize the upper respiratory tract, mucous membranes and skin, and are usually referred to as diphtheroids or coryneform bacilli. They occasionally cause serious postoperative infections following cardiac surgery or other infections in immunocompromised patients. The main human pathogen is *Corynebacterium diphtheriae*, the cause of diphtheria. *C. diphtheriae* can be carried asymptomatically in the nose or throat of a healthy person, although not all strains are toxogenic. In susceptible individuals, the organism infects the pharynx and larynx, forming a membrane that may obstruct the airway.

Infection is transmitted by respiratory droplets. Powerful exotoxins cause damage to distant nerves, resulting in paralysis of the soft palate, eye and extremities. The muscles of the heart are also affected. Treatment reverses these effects, although patients remain infectious for several weeks after the symptoms have resolved.

In the UK, routine immunization of children has ensured that cases of diphtheria are now extremely rare. Where a case of diphtheria is suspected, the patient should be isolated.

Listeria

Listeria monocytogenes is the main pathogen of this genus and is commonly found in soil and in the faeces of a variety of animals. It usually causes a mild influenza-like illness. However, infection during pregnancy can cause premature delivery, septicaemia and meningitis in the neonate. Cross-infection in neonatal units has been reported and extensive environmental contamina-

tion may occur following the delivery of an infected baby (Schlech 1991). Serious infections may also occur in immunocompromised patients. The incidence of infection is low with around 130 cases reported annually (Newton et al 1992). It may be acquired through contact with live animals and raw meat, but most infections are acquired by consumption of contaminated food. Soft cheese, coleslaw, fruit, vegetables, ice-cream and salami have all been associated with outbreaks of infection (Jones 1990). Listeria has been found in a variety of chilled foods and can survive and even multiply below normal refrigeration temperatures.

Infection control precautions Immunocompromised patients or pregnant women are most at risk of listeriosis and they should eat fresh and well-cooked or thoroughly reheated food. Food likely to contain listeria should be avoided (e.g. soft cheese, paté and coleslaw; DHSS 1989). Isolation of infected patients is necessary only in neonatal units.

Mycobacteria

Mycobacteria, although **Gram-positive** bacteria, are characterized by their unusual staining properties. They are termed acid-fast **bacilli** (AFB) because, unlike most bacteria, their waxy cell walls retain the stain after treatment with strong acids. There are many different species; some are found in animals and birds, others in soil and water. The main human pathogens are *Mycobacterium tuberculosis* and *M. leprae*, which cause tuberculosis and leprosy respectively.

Mycobacterium tuberculosis

The usual site of infection of this micro-organism is the lungs, where it causes pulmonary tuberculosis. In the past over 90% of children living in cities would develop tuberculosis, although in most the infection would resolve spontaneously with no long-term adverse effects. The incidence of the infection declined during the last century as a result of the improvement in living conditions and the introduction of effective chemotherapy (Fig. 6.2). In the early 1950s, 50 000 cases were reported every year. Now, only about 5000 cases are reported annually, with more than half occurring in people who were born outside the UK (Communicable Disease Report 1999e). Since the mid 1980s the rate of decline has begun to slow and the incidence is now increasing. Some of this increased incidence may be related to improved reporting of cases, but socioeconomic conditions, overcrowding and migrants from parts of the world where tuberculosis is endemic are all thought to be important underlying factors (Bhatti et al 1995, Mangtani et al 1995).

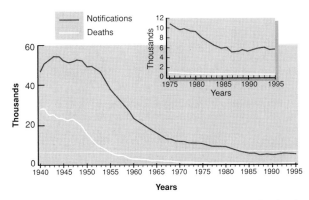

Fig. 6.2   Notification of tuberculosis and deaths in England and Wales. From Department of Health (1996).

Tuberculosis is a chronic, progressive infection which begins as an inflammatory reaction at the point in the lung where inhaled mycobacteria settle. The tubercle bacilli are unusual in that they are ingested by **phagocytic** cells but, instead of being destroyed, multiply within them. The body must therefore respond to the infection by **cell-mediated immunity** and by the production of specially activated **macrophages** that are able to kill the phagocytes containing the mycobacteria. The infected phagocytes move to the nearest lymph node, where another inflammatory reaction is initiated. Usually this primary infection resolves without causing disease, but leaves a characteristic calcified lesion in the lung visible on a chest radiograph. The tubercle bacilli remain dormant in these lesions but may eventually start to multiply, reactivating the disease. This is most likely to occur later in life as the efficacy of the immune system diminishes. About 10% of primary infections do not resolve but develop into active tuberculosis. The lesions enlarge to form cavities that fill with pus. When these spread to involve the bronchus, the tubercle bacilli in the cavities are coughed up in sputum. This condition is described as 'open tuberculosis'. The mycobacteria expelled from the respiratory tract may be inhaled by others and can be detected in sputum under the microscope. The expansion and spread of lesions may be brought under control by the immune system, but, if not, the patient will eventually die as a result of progressive destruction of lung tissue, haemorrhage from eroded arteries or secondary infection. The disease may also spread to other tissues, including skin, bones, central nervous system, kidney and intestine. Miliary tuberculosis occurs in the immunocompromised when tubercle bacilli are carried in the blood and produce small foci of infection – the size of millet seeds – throughout the body.

The vaccine against tuberculosis, Bacille Calmette–Guérin (BCG), is made from a live attenuated strain of *Mycobacterium bovis*. It causes a localized, non-progressive, primary infection that induces cellular immunity. It is considered to be 70–80% effective in protecting against tuberculosis, although transmission to previously immunized individuals may still occur (Department of Health 1996). In the UK children are vaccinated at 10–14 years of age. Immunization is also offered to immigrants from countries with a high prevalence of the disease and to babies born to them.

Tuberculin skin testing   The cellular immunity that develops following a primary infection forms the basis of the tuberculin skin tests (Heaf and Mantoux) used to establish whether an individual has active tuberculosis or is immune to infection. A small amount of protein derived from mycobacteria is inoculated under the skin. If, after a few days, the area is inflamed and blistered, the individual probably has active tuberculosis. A slight response to the tuberculin indicates immunity to tuberculosis, whilst no response indicates non-immunity (Joint Tuberculosis Committee 1990).

The risk of transmission to close contacts is relatively low, with 12% likely to acquire the infection if the index case has *M. tuberculosis* in the sputum. This risk is reduced to 1.5% if the contacts have been immunized with BCG (DoH Interdepartmental Working Group 1996).

The treatment for tuberculosis is prolonged and complex, and requires both specialist knowledge and close supervision. Inadequate or incomplete treatment is the main cause of relapse, and facilitates the emergence of multidrug-resistant strains (see p. 97).

Outbreaks of infection in hospital have been reported and infection is particularly likely to spread amongst immunocompromised patients (George et al 1986). The very young, elderly or people with human immunodeficiency virus (HIV) infection are at greater risk of developing tuberculosis. The impairment of the immune system caused by HIV infection enables dormant *M. tuberculosis* to reactivate (Watson 1991). Large outbreaks of multidrug-resistant strains have occurred amongst patients with HIV infection in the USA and have also been reported in the UK (Breathnach et al 1998, Hannan et al 1996). The problems associated with multidrug-resistant tuberculosis and recommended control measures are discussed in Chapter 5.

Opportunistic mycobacteria

Other species of mycobacteria may infect the lungs of immunocompromised people or those with abnormal respiratory tracts. *Mycobacterium avium intracellulare* (MAI) is a complex of mycobacteria that cause infection in the immunocompromised, especially people with acquired immune deficiency syndrome (AIDS). It is acquired through the gastrointestinal tract, causes a severe infection affecting both the gastrointestinal tract and lung, and is frequently resistant to conventional antimicrobial therapy.

Infection control precautions   The control of tuberculosis depends on the early detection of cases, effective treatment and infection control measures whilst the patient is infectious (DoH Interdepartmental Working Group 1996). Special planning is required to protect immunocompromised patients as they are particularly vulnerable to acquiring tuberculosis even after brief exposure to an infected person (Breathnach et al 1998). The Interdepartmental Working Group on Tuberculosis (DoH 1998) has recently issued specific guidance on the protection of the immunocompromised and the control and prevention of drug-resistant *M. tuberculosis* infection. The working group recommends minimum levels of infection control precautions according to local circumstances (see Table 14.1).

Patients with 'open' tuberculosis (i.e. with sufficient numbers of *M. tuberculosis* in their sputum for bacteria to be seen under the microscope) are infectious. If the bacilli cannot be seen in three separate sputum specimens, the patient may still have tuberculosis but is not exhaling sufficient mycobacteria to be considered infectious. The non-pulmonary forms of tuberculosis are also not infectious.

Transmission occurs by the inhalation of tubercle bacilli in minute airborne droplets (droplet nuclei) expelled from the lungs of an infected person, although close, prolonged contact is usually required for transmission to healthy people to occur. Patients with open tuberculosis are usually treated at home but, if nursed in the hospital, should be segregated from other patients, preferably in a single room with a lower air pressure inside the room so that airflow is directed into the room from other patient areas (see Fig. 14.1). Such negative pressure isolation rooms are essential if multidrug-resistant tuberculosis is suspected or immunocompromised patients are present in the same ward. The door of the room should be kept closed and the patient should not visit communal areas of the ward. Visitors should be restricted to those who had already had close contact before the diagnosis was made.

Masks are not necessary in most situations, but should be worn by staff during procedures that involve direct exposure to sputum, for example cough induction, bronchoscopy or where a high-dependency patient requires prolonged periods of intensive care. The masks should be close fitting, dust-mist or high-efficiency particulate (HEPA) filtering masks able to filter out minute droplet nuclei. The patient should be encouraged to cough into tissues covering the mouth and to wear a mask if required to visit another department. Cough-inducing procedures should never be performed in an open ward area (DoH Interdepartmental Working Group 1996, 1998).

Precautions are required for the first 2 weeks of chemotherapy, and can then be discontinued provided that the patient's condition is improving and multidrug-resistant tuberculosis is not suspected.

The risk of healthcare workers acquiring infection from patients is extremely low and can be minimized by ensuring that all staff who have close contact with potentially infected patients or specimens are tuberculin tested and given vaccination where necessary by the occupational health department (Department of Health 1996).

The family and other close contacts of the patient should be investigated for the presence of active tuberculosis. This 'contact tracing' is coordinated by the local authority Proper Officer (usually the Consultant in Communicable Disease Control) and is initiated following notification of the disease (see p. 40).

All health authorities should have a written policy for tuberculosis prevention and control which describes the measures in place to coordinate the surveillance, diagnosis and treatment of cases; the infection control arrangements; contact tracing responsibilities; education of staff; and monitoring procedures. The policy should reflect local epidemiology and ensure the integration of services between hospital and community (DoH Interdepartmental Working Group 1996).

Mycobacterium bovis

This organism causes pulmonary tuberculosis in cattle. In humans, infection is usually acquired by drinking unpasteurized milk from cows with tuberculous mastitis. The disease usually involves the gastrointestinal tract, tonsils and related lymph glands, although farmers may acquire pulmonary tuberculosis through contact with infected cattle.

Gram-negative cocci

Neisseria spp.

Neisseria characteristically occur as pairs of cells called diplococci. There are a number of harmless species that form part of the normal flora of the mucous membranes, including the upper respiratory and genital tracts. The two main pathogens are *N. gonorrhoeae* (gonococcus) and *N. meningitidis* (meningococcus).

Neisseria gonorrhoeae This is a sexually transmitted disease which primarily affects the genito-urinary tract, but may also occur in the anal canal, throat and eyes. *N. gonorrhoeae* is a delicate organism that is susceptible to cold and lack of moisture and therefore unable to survive for long outside the body. Newborn infants may be infected from the mother's birth canal at the time of delivery and subsequently develop conjunctivitis, which damages the sight if not treated promptly. Infections may be asymptomatic, facilitating spread of the infection.

Until recently, the infection could be successfully treated with a single dose of penicillin, but penicillin-resistant strains are now becoming increasingly prevalent (see p. 91).

Neisseria meningitidis *N. meningitidis* colonizes the nasopharynx of about 10% of healthy people, from where it can be passed to other people on nasopharyngeal discharges or respiratory droplets. Rarely, the organisms in the nasopharynx invade the bloodstream to cause meningococcal septicaemia, which is accompanied by a characteristic petechial rash. From the blood, the bacteria may reach the meninges to cause meningococcal meningitis. Both infections may be rapidly fatal if not treated with antibiotics.

Septicaemia has the highest fatality rate of approximately 20% (PHLS Meningococcal Infections Working Group 1995b). Meningococcal disease is most common amongst children and young adults, and occurs most frequently in the winter months. In the UK, two-thirds of cases are caused by the group B strain, which mostly affects young children. The group C strain occurs less frequently and affects school-aged children (5–18 years) as well as children aged under five years. Other strains are rare in the UK (Jones & Kaczmarski 1995).

Most cases of meningococcal disease occur in isolation (termed sporadic) and not as part of an outbreak. However, outbreaks in which two or more related cases occur, sometimes affect schools, universities or other institutions housing large numbers of young people. The incidence of meningococcal disease in the UK has been increasing since 1995, and over 200 cases are reported annually (Communicable Disease Report 1999a) (Fig. 6.3). *N. meningitidis* does not survive for long outside the body and close contact, for example kissing within a household, is required for transmission to occur.

Although there is no vaccine against group B meningococcus, a new vaccine against group C strains has recently become available and a widespread vaccination programme has been initiated in the UK (Communicable Disease Report 1999b).

Infection control precautions In hospital, isolation of infected patients for the first 24 or 48 h of antibiotic therapy is usually recommended, although the risk of transmission is low. Prophylactic antibiotic therapy is recommended for all close contacts. Healthcare workers are at risk of infection only if they are intimately exposed to nasopharyngeal secretions (e.g. mouth-to-mouth resuscitation), and prophylactic antibiotics are rarely necessary (Benenson 1995).

Management of outbreaks of meningococcal disease in the community Cases of meningococcal disease frequently cause immense alarm within a community, and a careful and consistent approach to their management is essential. When an isolated case occurs, people living in the same household should be given antibiotic prophylaxis to eliminate meningococcal carriage and reduce the risk of invasive disease. In this situation prophylaxis is not recommended for other nursery or school children as the risk of carriage amongst these contacts is low and chemoprophylaxis may have the adverse effect of eradicating other protective strains of meningococcus from the respiratory tract.

If two or more cases of the same strain of meningococcal infection occur at the same school or other

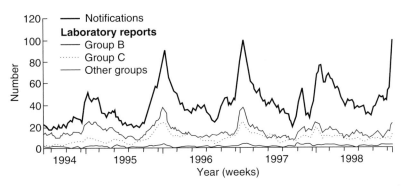

Fig. 6.3 Incidence of meningitis from 1994 to 1998. From Communicable Disease Report Weekly (1999) **9**(4): 29.

institution within a 4-week period, chemoprophy-laxis is likely to be offered to children and staff as well as close household contacts. The Consultant in Communicable Disease Control will be responsible for the management of outbreaks and will liaise closely with the Centres for Disease Surveillance and Control and the Regional Epidemiologist. It is particularly important to ensure that parents receive adequate information about the disease and how the situation is being managed (PHLS Meningococcal Infections Working Group 1995b).

Gram-negative bacilli

Enterobacteria

The coliforms Coliforms is a general term given to a broad group of organisms that are normal inhabitants of the gut called the enterobacteriaceae. They can survive in either aerobic or anaerobic environments under a wide range of different temperatures and are commonly associated with warm, moist environments.

The coliform bacteria primarily responsible for infections in hospital are *Escherichia coli*, klebsiella, serratia, proteus and enterobacter. They often colonize sites where the normal defence mechanisms are breached, for example intravenous cannulas, urinary catheters and endotracheal or tracheostomy tubes. They can also cause severe infections including **peritonitis**, wound infection and urinary tract infection especially in the seriously ill, **immunocompromised** or neonates. Many are resistant to a wide range of antibiotics and survive when antibiotic therapy is used to treat other micro-organisms. For example, *Klebsiella pneumoniae* often colonizes the respiratory tract when the normal flora is eradicated by antimicrobial therapy. Outbreaks of infection caused by antibiotic-resistant coliforms are commonly reported and are sometimes related to contaminated equipment such as portable suction and ventilator tubing (Davies and Blenkharn 1987, Gorman et al 1993, Krishnan et al 1991).

E. coli is a normal member of the gut flora, but some strains can cause gastroenteritis. Enterotoxogenic *E. coli* is foodborne, common in developing countries, and the usual cause of 'traveller's diarrhoea'. Enteropathogenic strains cause severe prolonged diarrhoea in children, especially in developing countries. They can be transmitted via contaminated food, baby milk and water, or on hands through contact with faeces. Verocytotoxin-producing *E. coli* (VTEC) causes a range of symptoms from mild diarrhoea to haemorrhagic colitis, with bloody diarrhoea and severe abdominal pain. Although the illness usually resolves within a few days, about one-third of cases require hospitalization

and 2–7% of cases develop haemolytic–uraemic syndrome (HUS), a form of renal failure associated with a high mortality rate. The strain that usually causes disease in humans is called O157. It is a normal inhabitant of animal intestines and outbreaks of infection have been linked to the ingestion of undercooked meat, bathing in contaminated water and handling animals (PHLS 1995a).

Infection control precautions The hands of staff are often implicated as the route of transmission of **Gram-negative** coliforms, and organisms can remain on hands for prolonged periods (Casewell & Desai 1983, Casewell & Phillips 1997). Colonized or infected patients may have the organism in their faeces and respiratory secretions, as well as in a variety of skin sites and wounds. The opportunity for transmission between patients is therefore high. Hands may also be contaminated by coliforms acquired from the environment, for example by handling towels, washbowls, bed linen and equipment in the sluice (Sanderson & Weissler 1992).

Transmission between patients should be prevented by the use of simple infection control precautions such as handwashing after contact with every patient or potentially contaminated equipment, and the wearing of gloves to handle body fluids. However, some antibiotic-resistant strains appear to spread readily and are not completely removed by handwashing with soap and water. Outbreaks of infection with these strains may need to be controlled by isolating infected or colonized patients. In some circumstances disinfectant solutions for handwashing may be recommended (Wade et al 1991).

Antibiotic-resistant strains are a particular problem in intensive care or neonatal units where the patients are more susceptible to infection and where frequent staff contact facilitates their spread. Ventilator circuits are prone to contamination from respiratory secretions, and hands should be washed after any contact (Gorman et al 1993).

Salmonella Salmonella are also enterobacteria. There are more than 2000 species, most of which live in the intestines of animals and cause food poisoning in humans. Two species, *Salmonella typhi* and *S. paratyphi*, are strictly human pathogens. They cause enteric fever (typhoid and paratyphoid), a severe illness with symptoms of septicaemia rather than gastroenteritis. The organism multiplies in the reticuloendothelial system, may be excreted in urine and faeces for prolonged periods, and sometimes colonize the gallbladder. Some people become chronic carriers and continue to excrete the organism intermittently for many years. Typhoid and paratyphoid are usually transmitted by food or water that has been contaminated by untreated sewage or a human carrier. Outbreaks have been associated with shellfish grown in polluted estuaries. In the UK most cases have been acquired abroad.

Other species of salmonella originate in animals but cause food poisoning if ingested. The illness may persist for several days but the organism is usually excreted in the faeces for only 1–2 weeks and long-term carriage is rare.

Infections are associated mainly with foods derived from poultry, which are frequently contaminated with salmonella. Infection occurs if the bacteria are not destroyed by adequate cooking. Infection can also occur if contaminated raw food cross-contaminates other food which is then eaten without further cooking. *S. enteritidis*, in particular, has been linked to the consumption of eggs (De Louvois 1993), particularly food containing raw shell eggs, for example mayonnaise or lightly cooked eggs. Salmonella are a common cause of outbreaks of gastroenteritis in both hospital and community settings (Evans et al 1998).

Infection control precautions Safe handling of food and strict attention to hygiene in the kitchen is essential to prevent transmission of salmonella on food. People who have a compromised immune system should only eat eggs cooked until the yolk is solid and avoid eating food containing raw eggs. The principles of food hygiene are discussed in greater detail in Chapter 12. Handwashing after defaecation and before handling food is an important measure to prevent transmission of infection.

Person-to-person transmission of salmonella may occur (Joseph & Palmer 1989) but can be prevented by the use of simple infection control measures such as handwashing and the use of protective clothing for direct contact with faeces. Patients with salmonella do not require isolation once they are asymptomatic. Affected individuals should not prepare food for others while they are still likely to be excreting the organism in faeces.

Shigella spp. These enterobacteria cause bacillary dysentery, a gastrointestinal infection of humans, characterized by bloody mucopurulent stools. Epidemics are associated with low standards of hygiene and are common in developing countries, where *S. dysenteriae* causes a severe disease associated with a high mortality rate. In the UK, most cases are caused by *S. sonnei* and the disease is relatively mild.

As very few organisms are necessary to cause infection, direct physical contact where hands have not been washed after defaecation is frequently responsible for spread of the disease. Transmission also occurs indirectly by the contamination of food, and flies may transfer the organism from faeces to food (Benenson 1995). Outbreaks amongst children in nursery schools are sometimes reported (Maguire et al 1998). Shigella is not usually associated with long-term carriage in the faeces after the acute infection.

Infection control precautions Prevention of transmission of infection requires the use of gloves and aprons to handle excreta and thorough handwashing after contact with the patient. Control of outbreaks in schools and nurseries is a particular problem because standards of hygiene amongst young children may be poor and personnel may have frequent, close contact with one another. Staff with shigella infection should not work in these establishments or handle food until they have stopped excreting the organism (about 4 weeks after infection).

Pseudomonas Pseudomonas is a strictly aerobic environmental organism commonly found in soil and water. The main pathogenic species is *P. aeruginosa*, which takes advantage of damaged host defences to establish infection in burns, wounds and the urinary tract. It has therefore become a major cause of hospital-acquired infection. *P. aeruginosa* is sometimes found in the bowel of healthy people but rapidly colonizes the gut of hospital patients. After a few weeks in hospital, up to 50% of patients will have the organism in their faeces (Olsen et al 1984). Pseudomonas is able to multiply in situations where very few nutrients are available such as moist equipment and solutions. Although commonly found in sinks and taps there is little evidence that organisms from these sources cause infection in patients (Levin et al 1984). Cross-infection has been reported in association with colonized pipework in whirlpool baths (Hollyoaks et al 1995).

Infection control precautions Many infections caused by pseudomonas are acquired from patients' own intestinal colonization, although cross-infection on equipment and the hands of staff may occur. Respiratory therapy equipment is prone to contamination and may present a major risk of infection if not decontaminated appropriately and stored dry. Outbreaks of infection have been associated with humidifiers, temperature probes and irrigation tubing (Kolmos et al 1993, Weems et al 1993).

Strains of pseudomonas resistant to aminoglycoside antibiotics may cause outbreaks of infection that are difficult to treat, especially in intensive care or burns units (Tassios et al 1997). Preventing the spread of these antibiotic-resistant strains may require the isolation of infected or colonized patients.

Haemophilus These organisms are commensals of the upper respiratory tract but may also cause infection. Strains with capsules (capsulate) cause serious infection in children (e.g. meningitis, pneumonia, epiglottitis, osteomyelitis, septic arthritis and septicaemia). Non-capsulate strains are particularly associated with chronic bronchitis and otitis media.

Cross-infection in paediatric wards has been reported and may also occur with *Haemophilus influenzae* pneumonia on adult wards (Howard 1991). Isolation of infected patients should be considered, particularly if the patient has contact with immunocompromised patients. A vaccine against the capsulate strain (serotype 6) is now given to infants and the incidence of infection has fallen as a result (Department of Health 1996).

Legionella There are several different species of legionella, but the main human pathogen is *Legionella pneumophila* which causes a severe respiratory illness called Legionnaires' disease. This usually affects the elderly, mostly men and those with other risk factors such as smoking, chronic bronchitis, emphysema or immunosuppressive treatment. The infection does not respond to conventional antimicrobial therapy and is associated with a high mortality rate. A similar, but milder, disease called Pontiac fever occurs in younger people.

The build-up of rust, biofilms or algae in water storage tanks, supply pipework or cooling towers can encourage the multiplication of legionella. Subsequent aerosolization of the water, for example in showers or air-conditioning vents, exposes people to the risk of legionella infection. Infections are often associated with exposure in large air-conditioned buildings such as hotels, factories and hospitals, but water supplies, spa baths and whirlpools have also been implicated as sources of infection. In the UK, less than 300 cases of Legionnaires' disease are reported annually, and many of these are acquired in hotels abroad (Joseph et al 1999). Contamination of the water system can be prevented by proper maintenance. This includes regular draining, cleaning and disinfection of tanks and cooling towers, ensuring that stagnant water is not allowed to collect in pipework, and maintaining the temperature of the hot water above 50°C to discourage the multiplication of the bacteria (NHS Estates 1993). Legionella normally live in water and infection is acquired by the inhalation of aerosols of contaminated water. Outbreaks of infection have been associated with water-cooled air-conditioning systems, humidifiers, showers and whirlpools (Communicable Disease Report 2000b, Hutchinson 1990). There is no evidence that the infection can transmit from person to person and therefore isolation of patients with Legionnaires' disease is not necessary.

Acinetobacter Acinetobacters are aerobic bacteria that are found widely in the environment and are also part of the normal flora of the skin. Like the coliforms they can cause a range of infections in susceptible patients, including pneumonia, meningitis, septicaemia and wound infection, and hospital strains are sometimes resistant to many antibiotics. They also have an affinity for warm, moist places and outbreaks of infection related to humidification equipment and damaged mattresses have been reported (Dealler 1998, Loomes 1988). Vegetables are commonly contaminated with acinetobacter and may provide a source of infection in vulnerable hospital patients (Berlau et al 1999). Acinetobacter is able to survive on dry surfaces for several days. Outbreaks of infection are increasingly reported in intensive care and burns units, where spread between patients on the hands of staff is the most likely route of transmission (Musa et al 1990). The same infection control precautions as those described for coliforms are required to prevent spread of acinetobacter.

Curved Gram-negative bacteria

Vibrio

These micro-organisms are commonly found in the environment. The most well-known species, *Vibrio cholerae*, causes cholera. It produces an enterotoxin that causes the severe symptoms of watery diarrhoea and abdominal cramps. Cholera is endemic in South-East Asia and parts of Africa, where it is spread by contaminated water and food. Cases in the UK are usually a result of infections acquired abroad.

Campylobacter

These organisms are found in the intestines of animals. The specialized techniques required to isolate campylobacter were not developed until the 1970s and *Campylobacter jejuni* is now recognized as a major cause of gastroenteritis in humans. Infection is commonly acquired by the ingestion of undercooked poultry. Only a few organisms are required to cause infection, as they multiply within the gastrointestinal tract. Outbreaks associated with milk or contaminated water have also been reported. The organism is not excreted in faeces for long and person-to-person spread is unusual. Routine infection control precautions are sufficient to prevent transmission in hospitals.

Helicobacter

These are spiral-shaped micro-organisms which, since improvement in diagnostic techniques, are now recognized as a cause of gastritis and ulcers. Some 95% of patients with duodenal ulcers are infected with *Helicobacter pylori* and the disease can be cured effectively with antimicrobial therapy (Cottrill 1996). Although the organism is readily destroyed by chemical disinfectants, there is some evidence that it can be transmitted to staff who perform endoscopies. Gloves should be worn during these procedures to minimize the risk of transmission (Williams 1999).

Anaerobic Gram-negative bacilli

These are strictly anaerobic bacteria with two genera of clinical importance.

Fusobacterium and bacteroides

These are normal inhabitants of the intestine, where they are present in considerable numbers, and are also found in the mouth and genital tract. The main pathogenic species are *Fusobacterium necrophorum* and *Bacteroides fragilis* which can cause appendicitis, pelvic inflammatory disease and puerperal sepsis. They may also be responsible for postoperative infection, usually in combination with other organisms, particularly following abdominal or gynaecological surgery. Infection occurs endogenously, rather than as a result of cross-infection.

Mycoplasma

Mycoplasma are very small bacteria that do not have cell walls and therefore do not have a consistent cell shape. They are resistant to a range of antibiotics, including penicillins, which exert their effect on bacterial cell walls. Some species of mycoplasma have been implicated as causes of non-specific urethritis. *Mycoplasma pneumoniae* causes respiratory tract infections which range from mild pharyngitis to pneumonia and **bronchitis**. Outbreaks of infection have been reported in crowded institutions and within families. Spread of infection occurs through close contact, and in hospitals the principal risk is the transmission of infection from staff to patients. Staff suffering from the infection should not work (Kleemola & Jokinen 1992).

Rickettsia

These are very small bacteria that cannot grow outside the cells of their host and, except for Q fever, are transmitted by insects. They cannot be cultured on conventional bacterial culture medium but are grown in the yolk sac of chick embryos. The diagnosis is usually based on serological tests.

Rickettsia prowazeki causes epidemic typhus and is transmitted by the human louse (see p. 268). *R. typhi* is transmitted by rat fleas and lice, and causes endemic typhus in urban areas with large rat populations. The microbe multiplies in the intestine of the louse and is excreted in the faeces on to the skin of a new host where it is introduced into the tissues by scratching. Typhus cannot be transmitted directly from person to person and epidemics are usually associated with unusual social conditions where the body louse is able to proliferate in the absence of regular washing of clothes, for example in wars and famines. Patients in hospital suffering with typhus do not require isolation.

Q fever is an atypical pneumonia caused by the inhalation of rickettsia from faeces, milk or the placenta of farm animals.

CHLAMYDIA

These are very small bacteria-like micro-organisms that cannot live outside the cells of their host. There are three main species. *Chlamydia trachomatis* is divided into several groups; one causes a severe blinding conjunctivitis called trachoma, common in South-East Asia, the Middle East and Africa. Other strains cause a sexually transmitted disease and are the most common cause of non-specific urethritis in males. Infants who acquire the organism from the mother's vagina during delivery may develop pneumonia.

C. psittaci is a parasite of parrots but is also found in other birds (e.g. pigeons, ducks, canaries). In humans it causes respiratory tract infection, which can range from a mild or asymptomatic infection to a severe pneumonia with a high fatality rate. Infection is acquired through the inhalation of infected dust and faeces, and usually occurs in people who have close contact with birds (e.g. bird breeders and pluckers). The risk of transmission of psittacosis to patients should be considered when parrots or other caged birds are kept as pets in clinical areas.

C. pneumoniae is associated with **community-acquired** upper and lower respiratory tract infection, including pneumonia. Outbreaks may occur in schools or other institutions.

FUNGAL INFECTIONS

There are over 70 000 species of fungi, of which only a few are pathogenic. Diseases include superficial infections of the mucosa (e.g. thrush caused by yeasts) or infection by filamentous fungi of the skin, nails and hair (e.g. ringworm). More importantly fungi can invade the body to cause serious widespread disease, which is often fatal (Bodey 1988). Patients who are immunocompromised and have had multiple courses of antibiotics are particularly vulnerable. The eradication of the normal flora enables fungi to establish infection in these patients (Flanagan & Barnes 1998). In the last few decades infections caused by fungi, particularly candida, have increased significantly (Lipman & Saadia 1997, Vincent et al 1995). In most cases, the source of micro-organisms is the gastrointestinal tract, where fungi are normal commensals. Infections are usually acquired endogenously, but transmission on the hands of healthcare staff also occurs (Pfaller 1996, Strausburgh et al 1994).

Candida

Most candida infections in humans are caused by *Candida albicans*, found in the normal flora of the mouth, intestinal tract and vagina. Superficial infection of mucous membranes or skin may occur, particularly in neonates and in debilitated adults or those who have received broad-spectrum antibiotic therapy which has destroyed the competing bacteria (Plate 6.3). **Systemic** infection may occur in people who are immunosuppressed, resulting in endocarditis and abscesses. Infections may also establish in invasive devices such as intravenous and urinary catheters. These infections can be difficult to treat (Flanagan & Barnes 1998). Although infection is usually **endogenous**, cross-infection may occur and the use of gloves for oral hygiene and handwashing after the procedure is important to prevent this (Burnie et al 1985, Fowler et al 1998).

Aspergillus

This saprophytic fungus occurs widely in the environment in dust and soil. It can cause infection in the lungs of people with underlying lung disease, for example cystic fibrosis, and a severe systemic infection in people who are immunocompromised, for example following organ or bone marrow transplant (Manuel & Kibbler 1998). Outbreaks of infection in susceptible patients are often associated with high spore levels in the air derived from environmental sources (e.g. building sites) rather than person-to-person spread (Humphries et al 1991).

Ice machines, nebulizers and food substances have also been associated with outbreaks of infection. The regular removal of dust and the use of air filtration has been recommended for the protection of highly immunocompromised patients (Barnes & Rogers 1989).

Cryptococcus

C. neoformans is a yeast that causes meningitis and brain abscesses but is extremely rare, usually occurring only in patients with severe immunodeficiency. The main source of the organism is probably soil, although it has been associated with pigeon droppings, and infection is acquired through inhalation of dust.

Dermatophytes (ringworm or tinea)

These are fungi that cause superficial infection of the skin, hair and nails, and are readily transmitted from person to person. They include species that cause athlete's foot and ringworm of the body or scalp. Outbreaks of ringworm in schools are difficult to eradicate as prolonged treatment of the infection is necessary and infected children are difficult to detect (Communicable Disease Report 1995).

Pneumocystis carinii

This organism used to be considered a protozoon but has recently been reclassified as a fungus. It is found colonizing the lungs of healthy people, but in the immunocompromised causes a severe pneumonia.

PROTOZOAL INFECTIONS

Protozoa are an unusual cause of infection in the UK although very common in other parts of the world. Amoeba and giardia cause gastrointestinal infections and are acquired by drinking water contaminated with faeces. Infections are usually associated with poor sanitation and in the UK cases are often acquired abroad. *Trichomonas vaginalis* is a parasite of the vagina which causes a sexually transmitted disease. Some protozoal infections have taken on a new significance because of their ability to cause serious disease in people with acquired immune deficiency syndrome (AIDS).

Toxoplasma

Toxoplasma gondii is a **parasite** of the cat family. It lives in the intestine of the cat and cysts are released in faeces. These can remain viable in soil for prolonged periods and may be ingested by humans or other animals. Once ingested, the protozoa reproduce asexually and circulate through the body establishing cysts in other tissue (e.g. brain, muscle and eye). In most cases the infection is mild and immunity develops rapidly.

Primary infection in early pregnancy can cause fetal death or brain damage and in the immunocompromised dormant cysts can be reactivated, resulting in large cerebral abscesses or retinitis. In the UK between 30 and 40% of the population has evidence of previous infection (Thomas 1988). Toxoplasma are not directly transmitted from person to person and therefore no special infection control precautions are indicated.

Infection is usually acquired by handling cat faeces or soil contaminated by cat faeces, and occasionally by ingesting eggs in raw or undercooked meat.

Cryptosporidium

C. parvum causes profuse watery diarrhoea lasting for 1–2 weeks. Oocysts are excreted in the faeces for several months following infection and person-to-person spread may occur (Benenson 1995). Oocysts from livestock excreta or human sewage can contaminate drinking water supplies. The oocysts are highly resistant to water treatment chemicals, and outbreaks of infection can sometimes occur as a result. These have been reported in association with contaminated drinking water and swimming pools (Communicable Disease Report 1999d, Willcocks et al 1998). In the immunocompromised the organism is not easily eradicated from the bowel and prolonged severe disease may result, which has a poor response to antimicrobial therapy.

Plasmodium

Several species of this protozoa are transmitted by mosquitoes and cause malaria. Once inside the human body the plasmodia replicate in the liver and red blood cells. The red cells rupture as a result, causing bouts of fever, anaemia and tissue hypoxia. Malaria does not occur in the UK, but around 2000 cases a year are seen in people returning from abroad. Travellers to areas where malaria is endemic should take antimalarial prophylaxis. However, because resistance to antimalarial drugs is becoming more prevalent, physical protection against mosquitoes is also essential (e.g. hats, insect repellents) (Communicable Disease Report 1997). In endemic areas the local population gradually develops immunity, which reduces the severity of the illness. This immunity diminishes once an individual leaves an endemic area.

VIRAL INFECTIONS

Most viruses cause self-limiting infections, the effects of the disease depending on the particular cells they infect. Table 6.1 lists some important viral pathogens, indicating those of greatest significance for infection prevention and control in clinical settings.

Herpes viruses

These DNA viruses include herpes simplex types 1 and 2, Epstein–Barr virus, varicella zoster virus and cytomegalovirus. An important feature of all herpes viruses is their ability to become **latent**, causing repeated episodes of infection when reactivated.

Herpes simplex virus (HSV)

There are two types of this virus. Initial infection with HSV-1 usually occurs in infancy or early childhood, often asymptomatically, but it can produce acute gingivostomatitis and ulcers on the gums and oral mucosa. It may also cause meningoencephalitis, a severe infection that is frequently fatal, and infections of the eye. The virus may remain dormant in local nerve cells, periodically reactivating to cause vesicles on the lip or recurrent eye infections. Herpatic whitlow sometimes affects healthcare workers and occurs when herpes virus contaminates abrasions on the fingers, particularly around the nail bed (Plate 6.4). HSV-2 mainly occurs in adults where it causes genital herpes lesions, affecting the penis in the male and vulva, labia and cervix in the female. There is a correlation between HSV infection of the cervix and cervical cancer, but HSV as a cause is not proven. Although the primary infection resolves after a few days, lesions recur when the virus is reactivated by fluctuations in hormone levels, immunity or infection.

The virus can be transmitted congenitally if the mother acquires the primary infection during pregnancy, or during delivery if active lesions are present in the genital tract. This is the reason for elective caesarian in these patients. In neonates HSV-2 causes encephalitis and has a high mortality rate.

Both viruses are transmitted by direct contact with lesions; HSV-1 by kissing or touching sores, genital herpes by sexual intercourse although it may also be carried asymptomatically in saliva. Infection with one type of HSV does not provide immunity against the other type.

Infection control precautions Transmission to healthcare workers or other patients may occur as a result of contact with active lesions. Gloves should be used routinely for contact with mucous membranes (e.g. mouth and vagina) and for contact with active herpes lesions such as cold sores or genital lesions. Care should be taken to prevent transmission from mothers with active genital lesions to their babies. The mother should be

Table 6.1 Some important viral pathogens

Virus group	Disease	Route of entry
Adenoviruses	Respiratory tract infection Conjunctivitis	Respiratory tract
Rhinoviruses	Common cold	Respiratory tract
Orthomyxoviruses Influenza A & B	Influenza	Respiratory tract
Paramyxoviruses Para-influenza Respiratory syncytial virus Mumps Measles	Para-influenza Bronchiolitis Mumps Measles	Respiratory tract Respiratory tract Respiratory tract Respiratory tract
Herpes viruses Herpes simplex 1 Herpes simplex 2 Varicella zoster Cytomegalovirus Epstein–Barr virus	Herpetic skin lesions Genital herpes Chickenpox, shingles Febrile illness Glandular fever	Skin, mucosa Sexual intercourse Respiratory tract, lesions Mucosa Mucosa
Enteroviruses Polio Coxsackie A Coxsackie B Hepatitis A Echoviruses Calicivirus	Polio Hand, foot & mouth disease Myo/pericarditis Hepatitis Meningitis Hepatitis A	GIT GIT GIT GIT GIT GIT
Papoviruses Papilloma	Warts, tumours	Skin
Reoviruses Rotavirus	Gastroenteritis	GIT
Hepatitis viruses	Hepatitis B, C, D	Blood, sexual intercourse
Retroviruses HIV1 & 2 HTLV I	Immune deficiency Leukaemia, lymphoma	Blood, sexual intercourse course

GIT, gastrointestinal tract.

advised to wash her hands before handling her baby (Valenti & Wehrle 1986). Staff with active HSV lesions should not care for immunocompromised patients; those with herpetic whitlow should not undertake any patient's care until the lesion has resolved.

Varicella zoster virus

This virus causes chickenpox as a primary infection, mainly in children (Plate 6.5). Although usually a mild illness in children, primary chickenpox in adults may be complicated by pneumonia which can cause serious disease. Immunocompromised people may also develop a severe disseminated infection which can be

fatal. Virus is secreted in the characteristic vesicles on the skin but it is primarily an infection of the respiratory tract and large amounts of virus are found in respiratory secretions which provide the main route of transmission. It is extremely infectious and in the UK around 90% of people will have had chickenpox by the time they reach adulthood (Department of Health 1996). The virus travels from the skin along sensory nerves and remains dormant in the ganglion for prolonged periods. If reactivated, it travels back along the sensory nerve and erupts on to the surface of the skin along the nerve pathways, appearing as vesicles. This is called shingles (Plate 6.6). It often causes severe, localized pain. Shingles cannot be caught from people with either shingles or chickenpox; it usually occurs in older adults or the immunosuppressed and represents a reactivation of the primary infection. The fluid from shingles vesicles contains varicella virus and therefore non-immune individuals can acquire chickenpox through contact with people with shingles.

Chickenpox acquired during the first 3 months of pregnancy may cause fetal abnormalities. A mother who acquires chickenpox a few days before delivery may transmit infection to her non-immune baby, who may subsequently develop severe illness (Cradock-Watson 1990).

Infection control precautions The main infection control problem presented by patients infected with chickenpox is the risk of transmission to immunocompromised patients (e.g. patients receiving immunosuppressive therapy, neonates, patients with HIV infection), who may develop serious and life-threatening disease (Stover & Bratcher 1998).

When a patient or member of staff develops chickenpox, the infection control team should be notified so that they can identify other patients who may be at risk of infection and who may need protection with specific **immunoglobulin** or prophylactic acyclovir if they are found to be non-immune. Immunity to chickenpox can be checked by looking for antibodies to the virus in blood. To minimize the risk of outbreaks of infection in high-risk areas such as maternity units, some occupational health departments routinely check the immunity of healthcare workers without a history of previous infection (Jones et al 1997).

Other herpes viruses

The Epstein–Barr virus (EBV) causes infectious mononucleosis (glandular fever) in teenagers and young adults. The virus invades B lymphocytes and causes fever, sore throat and enlarged lymph nodes. Most cases are mild but the symptoms may be persistent. EBV is transmitted by saliva and may be excreted for a long time after the symptoms have resolved. In parts of Africa EBV is associated with Burkitt's lymphoma and nasopharyngeal cancer.

Cytomegalovirus (CMV) causes a mild disease, similar to glandular fever. It establishes a persistent latent infection which may be periodically reactivated throughout life, resulting in virus being shed in urine and other body fluids. It is a very common infection and 80% of the population have been infected by late middle-age (Tookey & Peckham 1991). More serious infection occurs in the immunosuppressed, often as a result of the reactivation of the latent virus. Infection, either primary or reactivation, during pregnancy does not usually cause harm to the fetus but around 1% die or have severe congenital defects.

The virus is excreted in large amounts in saliva and urine and is transmitted by close contact and kissing; most patients excreting the virus will be asymptomatic.

Infection control precautions Most healthcare workers will be immune to primary CMV infection but may experience reactivation of a latent infection. There is no evidence that healthcare workers are more likely to acquire the virus at work. The routine use of gloves for handling body fluids and handwashing after the removal of gloves, minimizes the risk of CMV transmission and additional precautions are not recommended, even for pregnant staff caring for infected patients (Health and Safely Executive 1990, Tookey & Peckham 1991).

Adenoviruses

There are many different types of these DNA viruses. Most cause mild respiratory illness and establish persistent, latent infection in the adenoids and tonsils. Other types cause outbreaks of conjunctivitis and respiratory tract infection, particularly amongst children. The main infection control problem associated with adenovirus is in neonatal intensive care units where they can cause severe viral pneumonia and may spread easily between babies (Piedra et al 1992). The spread of eye infections can be prevented by strict hygiene during eye examinations and the sterilization of equipment (e.g. tonometers).

Other respiratory viruses

There are a number of other viruses commonly encountered in hospitals which, although not related, spread from person to person by respiratory droplets and by respiratory secretions carried on hands (Ansari et al 1991). Respiratory syncytial virus is one of the most important causes of respiratory tract infection in children and can be extremely severe in babies, causing bronchiolitis, croup and pneumonia. Although most people are infected as children, the antibodies formed do not protect against subsequent infection. Adults may therefore acquire the infection and, although the effects are usually mild, it can cause serious, often fatal, infections in the elderly (Crowcroft et al 1999). Outbreaks of infection may occur in paediatric, haematology or bone marrow transplant units. Infected patients should therefore be isolated whilst symptomatic (Jones et al 2000, Madge 1992). Measles (Plate 6.7), mumps and rubella are also sometimes seen in paediatric units, although the incidence of all of these childhood diseases has declined since the introduction of the combined MMR **vaccine** in 1988 and around 90% of children now receive the vaccine (Department of Health 1996). Measures to reduce the spread of infection should be taken because a proportion of those infected may develop serious complications especially if they are immunocompromised, for example mumps meningitis and encephalitis, otitis media and pneumonia associated with measles. If possible, infected patients should be discharged home and those that remain should be cared for by staff known to be immune to the infection to avoid secondary spread.

Influenza is caused by orthomyxoviruses. The illness can be serious, especially in the elderly or debilitated, and some people succumb to a secondary bacterial pneumonia. These viruses are easily transmitted by respiratory droplets and outbreaks of infection are common, particularly amongst the elderly (Communicable Disease Report 1998). Influenza vaccines are prepared annually to protect against the prevalent strain of the virus. Although not completely protective, they reduce the severity of the disease. Vaccination is recommended for residents of nursing homes for the elderly and other vulnerable groups (Department of Health 1996).

Enteroviruses

Enteroviruses are a large group of viruses that usually infect the gut but then establish infection in lymphoid tissue and spread to other parts of the body in the bloodstream.

Polio viruses

There are three distinct types of polio virus which are transmitted by contact with faeces and pharyngeal secretions. They generally cause a mild febrile illness but in a few cases cause meningitis. In less than 1% of cases the virus invades the spinal cord or brainstem and the resulting damage to motor neurons causes paralysis. In some countries, where standards of hygiene are low, the population overcrowded and there is no vaccination programme, the virus is **endemic** amongst children aged under 5 years. In the UK, about 90% of children are vaccinated and less than three cases are reported annually.

Approximately two cases of the vaccine strain of poliomyelitis a year are reported in association with polio vaccination. The **live-attenuated** virus is excreted in the faeces for up to 6 weeks after vaccination and people who have been recently vaccinated should wash hands thoroughly after defaecation (Department of Health 1996). People born before 1958 when routine vaccination was introduced may not be immune and may acquire the virus from immunized children.

Coxsackie viruses

Coxsackie A virus causes 'hand, foot and mouth' disease where vesicles erupt on the mouth, hands and feet. Coxsackie B virus causes a **myocarditis** and **pericarditis** from which most patients completely recover. Infection is mainly spread through contact with faeces and respiratory secretions. Outbreaks occasionally occur in neonatal units.

Hepatitis A and E

Hepatitis A is a gastrointestinal infection that spreads to the liver. It is characterized by nausea and abdominal pain followed after a few days by jaundice. It is generally a mild illness, often asymptomatic in children, lasting 1–2 weeks and not associated with any long-term adverse effects. The infection is spread by contact with faeces and is sometimes associated with poor sanitation. The virus is excreted in the faeces for 1 week to 10 days before symptoms develop, and for several days afterwards. Hepatitis A can also be transmitted in food and water, particularly sandwiches and salads, and molluscs cultivated in contaminated water (Benenson 1995). Hepatitis E is caused by a calicivirus but results in a similar infection to hepatitis A. It is spread by water contaminated with faeces and from person to person via the faecal–oral route. Although rare in developed countries, it is endemic in South-East Asia and Africa.

Infection control precautions Outbreaks of infection sometimes occur in schools and nurseries. The transmission of infection can be prevented by the use of gloves to handle faeces or change nappies and by strict attention to hand hygiene after using the toilet by both staff and children. During outbreaks of infection in residential institutions or child day-care centres, protection of staff by vaccination or with immunoglobulin may be considered necessary.

Other gastrointestinal viruses

Several other viruses cause gastrointestinal illness in both children and adults and may cause outbreaks of infection in hospital patients (Mitchell et al 1989). Infections are of greatest concern amongst the very young or the elderly, who easily become severely dehydrated. Rotavirus causes a severe gastroenteritis associated with vomiting, watery diarrhoea and fever usually in children under 5 years, in whom it can cause severe dehydration. Most people acquire the infection during childhood and develop immunity to further infection; however, immunity may diminish with age and outbreaks of rotavirus amongst the elderly also occur (Benenson 1995). Other viruses associated with outbreaks of gastrointestinal illness in hospitals include the small round structured viruses (Norwalk group of viruses), some adenoviruses, astroviruses and caliciviruses. Outbreaks usually develop gradually and can spread extensively to both patients and staff (Reid et al 1990). Virus present in vomit may contribute to the spread of infection and virus is also frequently excreted in faeces for several days after the illness has resolved, particularly in the immunosuppressed (Benenson 1995, Chadwick & McCann 1994).

Infection control precautions Outbreaks of infection should be controlled by isolation of patients until at least 48 h after symptoms have resolved. Virus may be particularly easily acquired on the hands through contact with excreta, vomitus, bedding and nappies. Rigorous handwashing and the use of gloves for contact with body fluids is therefore essential to prevent spread. Spills of vomit or faeces from affected patients should be treated with chlorine-based **disinfectants** to destroy any virus present (see p. 150).

Bloodborne viruses

Viruses transmitted by blood and body fluid are of particular importance to healthcare workers who may be at risk of acquiring infection through contact with body fluid. The most important bloodborne viruses are hepatitis B, hepatitis C and HIV. The hepatitis and HIV viruses are not related but will be considered together because the infection control implications are similar.

Viral hepatitis

Hepatitis, or inflammation of the liver, has infectious and non-infectious causes. Most primary viral infections of the liver are caused by hepatitis viruses. Hepatitis A and E are transmitted by the faecal–oral route, hepatitis B and C are bloodborne. The hepatitis D virus is not a true virus but can cause a severe, acute hepatitis if it infects an individual already infected with, or carrying, hepatitis B virus. Hepatitis can also be caused by other viruses, including Epstein–Barr virus and cytomegalovirus, leptospires and toxoplasma. Hepatitis causes malaise, nausea and, after a few days, jaundice.

Hepatitis B

Most infections caused by this virus are mild, but in a few cases result in extensive liver damage and liver failure that may be fatal. The incubation period is usually between 2 and 3 months, although it may be as long as 6 months. Between 2 and 10% of those infected do not completely eliminate the virus but continue to carry it in their blood. The risk of becoming a chronic carrier is greatest when the infection is acquired as a child. About 90% of those infected perinatally will become chronic carriers (Department of Health 1996). In some areas perinatal transmission is common and up to 20% of the population may be chronic carriers of hepatitis B virus (HBV) (e.g. South-East Asia, parts of Africa). Chronic HBV carriers are at increased risk of developing chronic progressive hepatitis, cirrhosis and primary carcinoma of the liver.

The prevalence of HBV varies in different parts of the world. In the UK and most other European countries it is less than 2%, although in some antenatal clinics in inner-city areas 1 in 100 women may carry the virus. Some groups are at increased risk of acquiring HBV (e.g. residents of institutions for people with learning difficulties whose behaviour may facilitate transmission, patients receiving renal dialysis, haemophiliacs, intravenous drug users who share needles and families of chronic carriers).

Tests to detect viral components and antibodies formed against them in the blood are used to determine previous infection and the carrier state. The surface antigen HBsAg is found on the outer protein coat of the virus and its presence in blood indicates an active infection or chronic carriage of hepatitis B. Anti-HBs are antibodies formed to the surface antigen and, if present in the blood, indicate that the individual has been infected in the past, the virus has been eliminated by the immune system and the patient is no longer infectious. HBeAg or the 'e' **antigen** is part of the virus's nuclear material and its presence in blood indicates a high level of viral replication and a highly infectious patient. Usually antibodies (anti-HBe) are formed against this antigen during the first few weeks of infection. The presence of anti-HBe in the blood indicates low infectivity. If anti-HBe is not formed, chronic carriage of the virus develops and the person remains highly infectious. Occasionally a mutation in the virus prevents the production of e antigen. Individuals infected with these mutant viruses appear to be e antigen negative but may in fact be highly infectious chronic carriers (Sundkvist et al 1998).

HBV is transmitted by sexual intercourse and perinatally from mother to baby. It is also transmitted when infected body fluids are inoculated through the skin, on instruments such as needles, via damaged or cut skin, or through contact with mucous membranes.

HBV has been isolated from virtually all body fluids but blood, semen and vaginal fluids are mostly implicated in transmission of the virus. Saliva has been found to contain the virus in much lower concentration than in blood and, although it does not appear to transmit infection through contact with mucous membranes, it has been associated with transmission through biting (Cancio-Bello et al 1982).

Healthcare workers are as much as five times more likely to become infected with HBV than other workers because of their regular and close contact with body fluids. The rate of transmission following needlestick injury with HBeAg-positive blood may be as high as 30% (Royal College of Pathologists 1992). Healthcare workers who are hepatitis B carriers may also transmit the virus to patients during invasive procedures such as surgery and obstetrical procedures and several outbreaks associated with HBV-infected surgeons have been reported (Communicable Disease Report 1996, Heptonstall 1991, Sundkvist et al 1998).

Hepatitis B immunization Vaccination is an effective method of protecting against infection. Healthcare workers who have direct contact with blood, bloodstained body fluids and tissues should be immunized against HBV. Immunization is particularly important for those who perform exposure-prone procedures (Box 6.1).

Box 6.1 Definition of exposure-prone procedures (EPPs)

'Exposure prone procedures are those where there is a risk that injury to the worker may result in the exposure of the patient's open tissues to the blood of the worker. These include procedures where the worker's gloved hands may be in contact with sharp instruments, needle tips and sharp tissues (spicules of bone or teeth) inside a patient's open body cavity, wound or confined anatomical space where the hands or fingertips may not be completely visible at all times.'

(UK Health Departments 1998)

Since 1993, healthcare workers who perform EPPs have been required to be immunized against HBV and have their antibody response tested. Those who are HBeAg positive are not able to perform EPPs. Healthcare workers who are HCV carriers may perform EPP provided they have not been associated with transmission of the virus to patients. Healthcare workers who are infected with HIV are not able to perform EPPs.

Examples of procedures considered to be exposure prone can be found in UK Health Departments (1994).

Current guidance recommends universal screening of women in antenatal clinics for HBV to identify carriers and to ensure that their infants are protected against infection by immunization at birth (NHS Executive 1998).

A course of three injections over a period of 6 months confers protection in about 80–90% of individuals, although those over the age of 40 years are less likely to develop immunity. A booster dose is recommended after 3–5 years. Specific immunoglobulin (HBIg) can be used to provide immediate, temporary, protection against infection with hepatitis B but it must be administered within 48 h of an exposure.

Hepatitis C

Before the introduction of a serological test for hepatitis C virus (HCV) in 1990, little was known about the epidemiology of a disease previously recognized only as non-A, non-B hepatitis. Although the primary infection with HCV is mild, often asymptomatic and rarely associated with jaundice, about 85% of those infected become chronic carriers of the virus. A significant proportion of those with chronic infection develop liver disease and cirrhosis. HCV infection is now a major indication for liver transplantation (Di Bisceglie 1998). The infection is generally transmitted by blood transfusion, although in developed countries this route has been eliminated by the introduction of blood donor screening. HCV is also prevalent amongst drug users and can spread rapidly where needle-sharing is practised. The virus may also transmit by sexual intercourse and from mother to baby (Di Bisceglie 1998). In the UK and other developed countries, the prevalence of HCV is low, with less than 1 in 1000 blood donors found to be carrying the virus (Neal et al 1997). However, the incidence amongst some populations of drug users may be as high as 90% (Goldberg et al 1998). Healthcare workers are at risk of acquiring HCV from needlestick injuries. The rate of transmission is lower than HBV, with between 5 and 10% of exposures to infected blood resulting in acquisition of the virus. HCV has also been acquired by blood splashing into the eyes (Rosen 1997). Transmission between patients in renal and haematology units has been reported (Allander et al 1994, 1995).

As with HBV, the virus may also be transmitted to the patient from an infected healthcare worker during exposure prone procedures (Box 6.1), although the risk of transmission is lower than that associated with HBV (Duckworth et al 1999, Esteban et al 1996).

Other hepatitis viruses

Hepatitis D is a defective virus that can only replicate with HBV. It is most prevalent in South America, parts of Russia and the Mediterranean, where coinfection with both viruses often causes serious, chronic illness. More recently hepatitis G virus has been identified. It is known to be transmitted by blood transfusions, and transmission to healthcare workers via needlestick injuries has also been reported (Shibuya et al 1998).

Human immunodeficiency virus (HIV)

HIV is a retrovirus. This means that the genetic information of the virus consists of RNA but it also has an enzyme, **reverse transcriptase**, that converts the RNA to DNA and then incorporates it into the DNA of the host cell.

The virus recognizes and infects cells in the body that carry a particular receptor protein on their surface, called CD4. The main target of the virus is the helper **T lymphocytes** of the immune system, but there are other cells that also carry CD4 and can be invaded by the virus (e.g. macrophages, dendritic cells of the mucous membranes). Two distinct forms of HIV have been identified so far: HIV-1 occurs throughout the world; HIV-2 has been found primarily in West Africa.

After the virus enters the body, the immune system mounts a response to the virus, but a few viruses survive inside the cells, and gradually replicate. As the T cells are gradually depleted, the immune response is impaired (Greene 1993). The virus has its greatest effect on the **cellular immune system**, whose main role is to destroy micro-organisms that invade host cells and cells that become malignant (see p. 66). Months or years may pass before the symptoms of infection, acquired immune deficiency syndrome (AIDS), become apparent. The underlying immunodeficiency enables a range of organisms normally held in check by the immune system to establish serious, often disseminated, infection; for example, *Pneumocystis carinii*, toxoplasmosis, cryptococcus, herpes simplex and atypical forms of mycobacteria. Early treatment with antiviral drugs does not cure the infection but will prolong survival and may reduce the risk of transplacental transmission in pregnant women (Rutter 1998).

HIV infection is diagnosed by detecting antibodies to the virus in the blood. These are not usually detectable until about 3 months after infection when the individual is said to have seroconverted. Tests to detect viral antigens and nucleic acid sequences are also available and play an important role in the management of the infection.

Infection with HIV will persist indefinitely. The infected person can transmit HIV to others soon after acquiring the infection, but becomes more infectious as immunodeficiency and the amount of virus in the blood increases. HIV is transmitted by sexual intercourse, by inoculation of infected body fluids through the skin or on to mucous membranes, transplantation of tissues or organs and by transfusion of contaminated blood. The virus is also transmitted from mother to baby, either through the placenta or during delivery: 15–20% of infants will acquire HIV infection by this route without antiretroviral treatment (European Collaborative Study 1996). Around one-third of the 8000 haemophiliacs in the UK acquired HIV from factor VIII derived from contaminated blood. Blood products are now screened and heat-treated to eliminate the risk of HIV infection.

The greatest concentration of virus is found in blood or body fluid containing visible blood. The virus has also been found in semen, vaginal secretions, tissues, cerebrospinal fluid, amniotic fluid and synovial fluid. HIV is probably transmitted by breast milk although the risk is likely to be greatest in the colostrum and early milk which contains more macrophages, and in mothers who have developed AIDS (Mok 1993). HIV has also been found in saliva and tears, although in much lower concentrations, and these fluids have not been associated with transmission of the infection unless they contain visible blood (Centers for Disease Control 1987, UK Health Departments 1998).

In the UK over 40 000 cases of HIV infection, and more than 16 000 cases of AIDS, have been reported since the epidemic was first recognized in the mid 1980s (Communicable Disease Report 2000a). Over 2000 new cases of AIDS are reported annually, mostly affecting young adults for whom it is a major cause of mortality (Mortimer et al 1997). Although the life expectancy associated with HIV infection has increased considerably since the adoption of highly active antiretroviral therapy (see p. 89), the disease remains ultimately fatal and the costs of treatment are high.

In the UK the major route of transmission is sexual intercourse between men, with 70% of patients with AIDS having been infected by this route. Although transmission had been declining, a recent increase in reported cases of HIV, as well as other sexually transmitted diseases, amongst homosexuals suggests a re-emergence of unsafe sexual practice (Mortimer et al 1997). Heterosexual intercourse is responsible for 15% of AIDS cases in the UK, although many of these are acquired abroad. Transmission of HIV by this route is facilitated by the presence of other sexually transmitted diseases (Cohen 1998). Some 6% of patients with

AIDS have acquired the infection through injecting drug use. This level of infection is lower than in many other European countries and the introduction of needle-exchange programmes has been successful in reducing the transmission of bloodborne viruses amongst injecting drug users (Madden et al 1997).

The prevalence of the infection varies considerably between regions. Over 70% of cases are reported from the Thames NHS regions (Molesworth 1998). The Unlinked Anonymous HIV Survey provides data on the prevalence of HIV in England and Wales by testing specimens obtained from genitourinary medicine clinics, injecting drug users, hospital patients and pregnant women (Table 6.2). The tests are taken from left-over blood that has been taken for other, routine clinical tests, and all patient-identifying information is removed before testing; the results cannot therefore be linked to the source patient. The data obtained from this testing programme are used to monitor the spread of the disease, to target health promotion programmes and to monitor their efficacy (Department of Health 1998b).

Occupational transmission of HIV to healthcare workers has been reported (Table 6.3). The first documented case of a healthcare worker who acquired HIV occupationally was reported in 1984 (Anonymous, 1984). By May 1999, 102 reports worldwide of healthcare workers who acquired HIV after a specific occupational exposure had been published in the literature, although this underestimates the actual number infected as only countries with well-developed surveillance systems are likely to report such infections (PHLS HIV & STD Centre 1999). Most occupational transmissions of HIV have followed inoculation of infected body fluid into the skin by a needle or other sharp instrument, although some have occurred after contamination of damaged skin or mucous membranes by infected body fluids (Table 6.3). Follow-up of healthcare workers exposed to HIV-infected body fluids indicates that the rate of transmission of HIV is much lower than that of hepatitis B. The risk of acquiring HIV from a needlestick injury with HIV-infected blood is estimated as 0.32%, although the volume of blood inoculated and the infectivity of the blood will influence whether transmission occurs. The risk of transmission associated with mucocutaneous exposure is lower, at around 0.03% (PHLS AIDS & STD Centre 1999). Although there is no vaccine available to protect against HIV infection, post-exposure prophylaxis with antiretroviral drugs is recommended should a healthcare worker have an injury involving HIV-infected material (see p. 146).

As with other bloodborne viruses, there is a risk of healthcare workers infected with HIV transmitting infection to others. Transmission of HIV from an infected dentist to five of his patients has been reported, although the exact route of transmission remains unclear (Centers for Disease Control 1991). More recently transmission of HIV from an infected orthopaedic surgeon to a patient was reported in France (Dorozynski 1997). Very few cases of HIV-2 have been identified in the UK and most have had some connec-

Table 6.2 Prevalence of HIV infection in the UK (Source: Department of Health 1998b)

Survey group	Prevalence (%)	
	London	England & Wales (excluding London)
GUM clinic attenders (men)		
Homosexual or bisexual	9.0	3.8
Heterosexual	0.8	0.12
GUM clinic attenders (women)	0.7	0.1
Injecting drug users		
Men	3.9	0.37
Women	1.5	0.41
Pregnant women at delivery	0.19	0.02
Pregnant women seeking terminations	0.55	–
Prisoners		
Men		0.3
Women		1.2

GUM, genitourinary medicine.

Table 6.3 Definite occupational transmission of human immunodeficiency virus. From PHLS AIDS & STD Centre, (1999)

Type of exposure	Healthcare workers infected
Percutaneous	85
Mucous membrane	2
Damaged skin	8
Source not reported	7
Total	102

tion with West Africa (Evans et al 1991). The incidence of infection in the UK is highest among homosexual men, intravenous drug users and sexual partners of these groups. However, in other parts of the world heterosexual intercourse is the major route of transmission. In some countries, particularly sub-Saharan Africa, HIV infection is endemic. In some cities in southern Africa over 40% of pregnant women are HIV positive. The prevalence of HIV is also increasing rapidly in other developing countries in South-East Asia (Davidson and Nicoll 1997, World Health Organization 1997). The World Health Organization (1998) has estimated that over 30 million people worldwide were infected with HIV at the end of 1997, with 16 000 new infections acquired every day.

Infection control precautions for bloodborne viruses The screening of blood donors for hepatitis B, treatment of blood products and the targeting of high-risk groups for immunization against hepatitis B, particularly infants born to infected mothers, has reduced the incidence of the infection in the UK (Department of Health 1996). The risk of acquiring HIV from blood products has been virtually eliminated by screening. However, the absence of a vaccine against HIV means that controlling the spread of infection depends on education to discourage behaviour that may transmit infection, such as unprotected sexual contact and the sharing of used needles to inject drugs.

Frequent contact with body fluids places many healthcare workers at particular risk of acquiring bloodborne viruses who may be infected in the following ways:

- inoculation of infected blood or body fluid through the skin on contaminated sharp instruments
- contamination of mucous membranes such as the eyes or mouth with infected blood or body fluid
- contamination of broken skin with infected blood or body fluid

In line with the Control of Substances Hazardous to Health Regulations (1994) the risk of exposure to hazardous biological agents such as bloodborne viruses should be assessed, and methods of minimizing the risk identified, for any activity involving contact with blood or body fluids. Healthcare workers can avoid exposure by using safety equipment, employing safe procedures and using protective clothing when exposure to body fluid is anticipated. The main risk is from contaminated sharp instruments. Healthcare workers are often unaware of patients who are infected with bloodborne viruses and any blood, and most body fluids, must therefore be considered potentially infectious and precautions used routinely in all situations. This approach, initially called universal precautions, was first recommended in 1987 by the Centers for Disease Control in the USA and has now been adopted widely (Centers for Disease Control 1987, 1988, UK Health Departments 1998). The main principles are listed in Box 6.2 and discussed in more detail in Chapter 7.

Patients known to be infected with bloodborne viruses do not require isolation unless contamination of the environment is likely (e.g. profuse bleeding). Infection cannot be transmitted by social contact with patients. Protective clothing is necessary only for

---

Box 6.2 Preventing the transmission of bloodborne viruses

Routine infection control precautions to be used in the care of all patients to prevent the transmission of bloodborne viruses from patient to healthcare worker and between patients. First recommended by the Centers for Disease Control in 1987, they have now been widely adopted and are also recognized as a means of minimizing the risk of transmission of other pathogens (Garner 1996, Wilson & Breedon 1990).

Sharps safety
- safety equipment
- safe handling procedures
- correct disposal
- managing and reporting injuries

Protective clothing
- use to protect against direct contact with body fluid
- assess risk of procedure and select appropriate protection

Cover cuts
- use waterproof dressing

Handwashing
- after gloves removed
- after contact with body fluid

Decontamination
- equipment contaminated with body fluid
- spills of body fluid

Waste disposal
- incinerate waste contaminated with body fluids

direct contact with blood or body fluids and not for the routine care of the patient. Patients with HIV infection may also be infected with other pathogens that present a risk to other patients, for example tuberculosis, salmonella. There is also evidence for the spread of opportunistic infections such as *Pneumocystis carinii* and cryptosporidium amongst patients with AIDS in hospital (Laing 1999). The use of long-term intravenous access to provide nutrition or therapy also places patients with AIDS at increased risk of bloodstream infection, and a high standard of care must be used to minimize the risk. Isolation may be indicated for such patients for the duration of their illness with these secondary pathogens. Transmission of hepatitis B amongst patients undergoing renal dialysis was a major problem in the 1970s but improved infection control, particularly the management of sharps and equipment, has reduced the incidence of infection. However, outbreaks of hepatitis C virus in haemodialysis and haematology units have been reported recently (Allander et al 1994, 1995).

Equipment that enters a sterile area of the body or has close contact with mucous membranes (e.g. fibreoptic endoscope) has the potential to transmit bloodborne viruses between patients. Chant et al (1993) reported an outbreak of HIV infection related to minor surgical procedures in private surgical consulting rooms, and Bronowicki et al (1997) reported HCV transmission on endoscopes used to perform colonoscopies. Such equipment must be decontaminated appropriately after each use to prevent cross-infection. Chapter 13 discusses methods of disinfection and sterilization in more detail

Injury with a contaminated sharp instrument is the most likely route of transmission to healthcare workers and every hospital should have a policy outlining the procedures to be followed in the event of a needlestick injury (see Fig. 7.6).

An active surveillance scheme for healthcare workers exposed to bloodborne viruses at work has been operated by the Public Health Laboratory Service since July 1997. So far, only one case of transmission of HCV has been reported (Communicable Disease Report 1999c). .

Transmission of bloodborne viruses from an infected healthcare worker to a patient may occur during procedures in which injury to the healthcare worker could result in blood contaminating the patient's open tissue, for example when hands are in contact with sharp instruments, bone or teeth. Healthcare workers infected with HIV or who are HBeAg positive should not perform exposure-prone procedures (EPPs) (Department of Health 1993, UK Health Departments 1994). Lookback investigations

where transmission of HCV from an infected healthcare worker has occurred have demonstrated a low risk of transmission, and current guidance is that HCV-positive healthcare workers may perform EPPs provided they have not transmitted HCV to a patient (Ramsay 1999). Healthcare workers who think that they may be infected with a bloodborne virus should seek medical advice and may need to modify their practice or avoid performing invasive procedures.

Virus-like agents: prions

These are abnormal proteins. They are not conventional infectious agents and have no nucleic acid. They appear to cause disease by replacing normal proteins on the surface of host cells, gradually compromising their function. They are associated with some rare diseases in humans and animals that cause progressive degeneration of the nervous system. Scrapie is a prion disease of sheep that has been recognized in the UK for many years, although with no evidence of transmission to humans. An epidemic of a prion disease in cattle, bovine spongiform encephalopathy (BSE) was first recognized in the UK in the mid 1980s and is thought to have affected a million cattle (Patterson & Painter 1999). The epidemic was probably related to changes in the methods used to render animal carcasses, which reduced heat and chemical decontamination and enabled the prion proteins to enter the meat and bone meal used as cattle feed supplements (Haywood 1997).

The main prion disease in humans is Creutzfeldt–Jakob disease (CJD). This is a spongiform encephalopathy associated with destruction of brain tissue and presenile dementia. The incidence of CJD in the UK, although very low (30–50 deaths per year), has increased in the last few decades. This increase is probably related to increased case ascertainment, especially amongst the elderly. Similar increases have been reported in other European countries and the USA (Cousins et al 1997). Since 1994, several cases of CJD with unusual neurological changes and symptoms have occurred amongst people aged under 30 years. It is likely that these cases of variant CJD (vCJD) are linked to exposure to BSE. At this stage, it is impossible to estimate how the epidemic may progress, as little is known about the risk of transmission, incubation period or susceptibility to the disease (Patterson & Painter 1999).

Unlike conventional CJD, there is evidence that vCJD affects the lymphoreticular systems. It can therefore be detected in lymph nodes, tonsils and spleen, and was detected in the appendix of an affected patient 8 months before the disease became clinically apparent (Hilton et al 1998). Prion proteins are highly resistant to conventional methods of decontamination, including cooking, irradiation, most chemical disinfectants and formaldehyde. The standard autoclave cycle of 134°C for 3 min does not reliably destroy the prion protein.

Infection control precautions   Currently there is no evidence that CJD is transmitted from person to person by close contact, and the routine precautions taken with blood and body fluids from all patients are sufficient for the care of patients known, or suspected to have, CJD (Box 6.2). There is no evidence that body secretions, excreta or saliva are infectious. Clinical waste (e.g. sharps, dressings) generated during the care of known or suspected patients, whether in hospital or the community, should be treated as clinical waste. Nervous tissue (e.g. cerebrospinal fluid) does present a risk and, although conventional CJD is not transmitted by blood, there is some experimental evidence to suggest that vCJD could be transmitted by blood transfusion (Advisory Committee on Dangerous Pathogens 1998). Blood from donors suspected to have CJD has been withdrawn (Department of Health 1998a) and methods of removing white blood cells from donated blood are being considered.

The main risk in healthcare settings is presented by invasive procedures, particularly those that involve the nervous system (e.g. lumbar puncture, neurosurgery) and the potential risk of transmission to other patients on contaminated instruments. Because the CJD agent is unusually resistant to conventional sterilization and disinfection processes, wherever possible single-use disposable instruments should be used on patients known or suspected to have CJD, these should then be destroyed by incineration, together with any protective clothing worn by those involved in the procedure. For any other invasive or surgical procedure, where disposable instruments are not available the instruments must not be sterilized or reused but disposed of by incineration.

When surgical procedures are performed on patients considered 'at risk' of CJD (i.e. asymptomatic but with family history of CJD, recipient of human growth hormone or dura mater grafts) the same precautions should be applied when the procedure involves the brain, spinal cord or eyes. For other procedures, protective clothing should be worn but can be reprocessed, single-use items should be used where possible and reusable instruments subjected to high-level decontamination before reuse (see p. 238). Instruments for incineration or high-level decontamination should be securely contained and clearly labelled.

Haemorrhagic fevers

A number of viral haemorrhagic fevers that do not occur in the UK are occasionally seen in patients recently returned from abroad, for example Lassa fever, Marburg and Ebola viruses. They are associated with a high rate of mortality. The viruses are transmitted to humans from animals such as rats and monkeys, but transmission to healthcare workers through handling of infected blood and body fluids has been reported. Acute hospitals should have a policy outlining the management of any patient admitted with unexplained fever. If viral haemorrhagic fever is strongly suspected, the patient should be transferred to a high security isolation unit. Otherwise, routine blood and body fluid precautions should be used until a diagnosis has been confirmed (see Box 6.2). Most patients returning from abroad with unexplained fever have malaria, and it is important to exclude this diagnosis (Advisory Committee on Dangerous Pathogens 1997).

REFERENCES

Advisory Committee on Dangerous Pathogens (1997) *Management and Control of Viral Haemorrhagic Fevers.* PL(97)1. The Stationery Office, London.
Advisory Committee on Dangerous Pathogens (1998) *Transmissible Spongiform Encephalopathy Agents; Safe Working and the Prevention of Infection.* PL/CO(98)2. The Stationery Office, London.
Allander T, Medin C, Jacobson SH et al (1994) Hepatitis C transmission in a haemodialysis unit: molecular evidence for spread of virus among patients not sharing equipment. *J. Med. Virol.,* **43**: 415–19.
Allander T, Gruber A, Naghavi M et al (1995) Frequent patient-to-patient transmission of hepatitis C in a haematology ward. *Lancet,* **345**: 603–7.

Anonymous (1984) Needlestick transmission of HTLV-III from a patient infected in Africa. *Lancet,* **ii**: 1376–7.
Ansari SA, Springthorpe S, Sattar SA et al (1991) Potential role of hands in spread of respiratory viral infections: studies with human parainfluenza virus 3 and rhinovirus 14. *J. Clin. Microbiol.,* **29**: 2115–19.
Barnes RA, Rogers TR (1989) Control of an outbreak of nosocomial aspergillosis by laminar air-flow isolation. *J. Hosp. Infect.,* **14**: 89–94.
Barrie DB, Wilson JA, Hoffman PN et al (1992) *Bacillus cereus* meningitis in two neurosurgical patients: an investigation into the source of the organism. *J. Infect.,* **25**: 291–7.

Benenson AS (ed.) (1995) *Control of Communicable Disease in Man*, 16th edn. American Public Health Association, Washington, DC.

Berlau J, Auken HM, Houang E et al (1999) Isolation of *Acinetobacter* spp including *A. baumannii* from vegetables: implications for hospital-acquired infections. *J. Hosp. Infect.*, **42**: 201–4.

Bhatti N, Law MR, Morris JK et al (1995) Increasing incidence of tuberculosis in England and Wales: a study of the likely causes. *BMJ*, **310**: 967–9.

Bignardi GE (1998) Risk factors for *Clostridium difficile* infection. *J. Hosp. Infect.*, **40**: 1–15.

Bignardi GE (1999) Surveillance of neonatal group B streptococcal infection in Sunderland. *Commun. Dis. Public Health*, **2**(1): 64–5.

Bodey GP (1988) The emergence of fungi as major pathogens. *J. Hosp. Infect.*, **11** (Suppl. A): 411–26.

Boyce JM (1996) Preventing staphylococcal infections by eradicating nasal carriage of *Staphylococcus aureus*: proceeding with caution. *Infect. Control Hosp. Epidemiol.*, **17**(12): 775–9.

Breathnach AS, de Ruiter A, Holdsworth GMC et al (1998) An outbreak of multidrug resistant tuberculosis in a London teaching hospital. *J. Hosp. Infect.*, **39**(2): 111–18.

Bronowicki JP, Vernard V, Botte C et al (1997) Patient-to-patient transmission of hepatitis C during colonoscopy. *N. Engl. J. Med.*, **337**(4): 237–40.

Burnett IA, Norman P (1990) *Streptococcus pyogenes*: an outbreak on a burns unit. *J. Hosp. Infect.*, **15**(2): 173–6.

Burnie JP, Odds FC, Lee W et al (1985) Outbreak of systemic *Candida albicans* in intensive care unit caused by cross infection. *BMJ*, **290**: 746–8.

Cancio-Bello TP, de Medina M, Shorey J et al (1982) An institutional outbreak of hepatitis B related to a human biting carrier. *J. Infect. Dis.*, **146**(5): 652–6.

Cartmill TDI, Panigrahi H, Worsley MA et al (1994) Management and control of a large outbreak of diarrhoea due to *Clostridium difficile*. *J. Hosp. Infect.*, **27**: 1–16.

Cartwright K, Logan M, McNulty C et al (1995) A cluster of cases of streptococcal necrotising fasciitis in Gloucestershire. *Epidemiol. Infect.*, **115**: 387–97.

Casewell MW, Desai N (1983) Survival of multiply-resistant *Klebsiella aerogenes* and other Gram-negative bacilli on finger-tips. *J. Hosp. Infect.*, **18** (Suppl. B): 23–8.

Casewell MW, Phillips I (1977) Hands as a route of transmission for Klebsiella species. *BMJ*, **2**: 1315–17.

Centers for Disease Control (1987) Recommendations for prevention of HIV transmission in healthcare settings. *MMWR*, **36**(2S): 3S–18S.

Centers for Disease Control (1988) Update: universal precautions for prevention of transmission of human immunodeficiency virus, hepatitis B virus and other blood-borne pathogens in healthcare settings. *MMWR*, **37**(24): 377–88.

Centers for Disease Control (1991) Update: transmission of HIV infection during invasive dental procedures – Florida. *MMWR*, **40**: 378–81.

Chadwick PR, McCann R (1994) Transmission of a small round structured virus by vomiting during a hospital outbreak of gastroenteritis. *J. Hosp. Infect.*, **26**: 251–60.

Chant K, Lowe D, Rubin G et al (1993) Patient to patient transmission of HIV in private surgical consulting rooms. *Lancet*, **342**: 1548–9.

Cohen MS (1998) Sexually transmitted diseases enhance HIV transmission: no longer a hypothesis. *Lancet*, **351**: 5–7.

Communicable Disease Report (1995) Scalp ringworm in London. *CDR*, **5**(38): 179.

Communicable Disease Report (1996) Transmission of hepatitis C virus from surgeon to patient prompts lookback. *CDR Weekly*, **9**(44): 387.

Communicable Disease Report (1997) Guidelines for the prevention of malaria in travellers from the United Kingdom. *CDR*, **7**(10): R138–51.

Communicable Disease Report (1998) An outbreak of influenza in four nursing homes in Sheffield. *CDR*, **8**(16): 139.

Communicable Disease Report (1999a) Seasonal rise in meningococcal disease: chief medical officer writes to all doctors. *CDR Weekly*, **9**(4): 29, 32.

Communicable Disease Report (1999b) Vaccination programme for group C meningococcal infection is launched. *CDR Weekly*, **30**(9): 261, 264.

Communicable Disease Report (1999c) Surveillance of healthcare workers exposed to bloodborne viruses at work, July 1997 to June 1999. *Commun. Dis. Rep. Weekly*, **9**(36): 319.

Communicable Disease Report (1999d) Cryptosporidiosis associated with swimming pools. *CDR Weekly*, **9**(48): 423.

Communicable Disease Report (1999e) Tuberculosis: incidence rising, resistance stable, surveillance enhanced, and communication improving. *CDR Weekly*, **9**(51): 453–6.

Communicable Disease Report (2000a) AIDS and HIV infection in the United Kingdom: monthly report. *CDR*, **10**(4): 37–40.

Communicable Disease Report (2000b) Legionella from guests of Welsh hotel indistinguishable from humidifier isolates. *CDR*, **10**(16): 141.

Cottrill MRB (1996) *Helicobacter pylori*. *Professional nurse*, **12**(1): 46–8.

Cousins SN, Zeidler M, Esmonde TF et al (1997) Sporadic Creutzfeldt–Jakob disease in the United Kingdom: analysis of epidemiological surveillance data for 1970–96. *BMJ*, **315**: 389–95.

Cradock-Watson JE (1990) Varicella-zoster virus infection during pregnancy. In *Current Topics in Clinical Virology*, pp. 1–28 (Morgan-Capner P, ed.) Public Health Laboratory Service, London.

Crowcroft NS, Cutts F, Zambon MC (1999) Respiratory syncitial virus: an underestimated cause of respiratory tract infections, with prospects of a vaccine. *Commun. Dis. Public Health*, **2**(4): 234–41.

Davidson K, Nicoll A (1997) The changing global epidemiology of HIV infections and AIDS. *Commun. Dis. Rep. Rev.*, **7**(9): R134–6.

Davies B, Blenkharn I (1987) On the right track. *Nursing Times* **83**(22): 64–8.

Dealler S (1998) Nosocomial outbreak of multi-resistant *Acinetobacter* spp. on an intensive care unit: possible association with ventilator equipment. *J. Hosp. Infect.*, **38**: 147.

De Louvois J (1993) Salmonella contamination of eggs. *Lancet*, **342**: 367–8.

Denton M, Hawkey PM, Hoy CM et al (1993) Co-existent cross-infection with *Streptococcus pneumoniae* and group B streptococci on an adult oncology unit. *J. Hosp. Infect.*, **23**: 271–8.

Department of Health (1993) *Protecting Health Care Workers and Patients from Hepatitis B: Recommendations of the Advisory Group on Hepatitis*. HSG(93)40. Addendum issued 1996. EL(96)77. HMSO, London.

Department of Health/Public Health Laboratory Service Joint Working Group (1994) *Clostridum difficile Infection. Prevention and Management*. Health Publications Unit, Heywood, UK.

Department of Health (1996) *Immunisation Against Infectious Disease*. HMSO, London.

Department of Health Interdepartmental Working Group on Tuberculosis (1996) *The Prevention and Control of Tuberculosis in the United Kingdom: Recommendations for the Prevention and Control of Tuberculosis at a Local Level*. Department of Health, London.

Department of Health (1998a) *New Variant CJD – Patients who have Received Implicated Blood Products*. PL(CO)(98) 1. DoH, London.

Department of Health (1998b) *Prevalence of HIV in England and Wales 1997*. Summary Report from the Unlinked Anonymous Surveys Screening Group. DoH, London.

Department of Health Interdepartmental Working Group on Tuberculosis (1998) *The Prevention and Control of Tuberculosis in the United Kingdom: UK Guidance on the Prevention and Control of Transmission of 1. HIV Related Tuberculosis and 2. Drug-resistant, Including Multiple Drug-resistant, Tuberculosis*. Department of Health, London.

Department of Health and Social Security (1989) *Listeriosis and Food*. Pl/CMO(89)3. HMSO, London.

Di Bisceglie AM (1998) Hepatitis C. *Lancet*, **351**: 351–5.

Djuretic T, Wall PG, Brazier JS (1999) *Clostridium difficile*: an update on its epidemiology and role in hospital outbreaks in England and Wales. *J. Hosp. Infect.*, **41**: 213–18.

Dorozynski A (1997) French patient contracts AIDS from surgeon. *BMJ*, **314**: 250.

Dowsett EG, Willson PA (1981) An outbreak of *Streptococcus pyogenes* infection in a maternity unit. *CDR*, **81**(17): 3.

Duckworth GJ, Heptonstall J, Aitkin C et al (1999) Transmission of hepatitis C virus from a surgeon to a patient. *CDR*, **2**: 188–92.

Edwards G, Hood J (1999) Vancomycin intermediate *Staphylococcus aureus* (VISA) update. *SCIEH Weekly Report*, **33**(99/24): 157.

Efstratiou A (1989) Outbreaks of human infections caused by the pyogenic streptococci of Lancefields group C and group G. *J. Med. Microbiol.*, **29**: 207–19.

Emori TG, Gaynes RP (1993) An overview of nosocomial infection, including the role of the microbiology laboratory. *Clin. Microbiol. Rev.*, **6**: 87–107.

Esteban JL, Gomez J, Martell M et al (1996) Transmission of hepatitis C virus by a cardiac surgeon. *N. Engl. J. Med.*, **334**: 555–60.

European Collaborative Study (1996) Vertical transmission of HIV-1; maternal immune status and obstetric factors. *AIDS*, **10**: 1675–81.

Evans BG, Gill ON, Gleave SR et al (1991) HIV-2 in the United Kingdom – a review. *CDR*, **1**(2): R19–23.

Evans HS, Madden P, Douglas C et al (1998) General outbreaks of infectious intestinal disease in England and Wales: 1995 and 1996. *Commun. Dis. Public Health*, **1**(3): 165–71.

Fekerty R, Kim KH, Brown D et al (1981) Epidemiology of antibiotic associated colitis. *Am. J. Med.*, **70**: 906–8.

Flanagan PG, Barnes RA (1998) Fungal infection in the intensive care unit. *J. Hosp. Infect.*, **38**(3): 163–77.

Fowler SL, Rhoton B, Springer SC et al (1998) Evidence for person-to-person transmission of *Candida lusitaniae* in a neonatal intensive care unit. *Infect. Control Hosp. Epidemiol.*, **19**(5): 343–5.

Fraise AP, Mitchell R, O'Brien SJ et al (1997) Methicillin-resistant *Staphylococcus aureus* (MRSA) in nursing homes in a major UK city: an anonymised point prevalence survey. *Epidemiol. Infect.*, **118**: 1–5.

French GL, Cheng AFB, Ling JML et al (1990) Hong Kong strains of methicillin-resistant and sensitive *Staphylococcus aureus* have similar virulence. *J. Hosp. Infect.*, **15**(2): 117–26.

Garner JS (1996) Hospital Infection Control Practices Advisory Committee Guideline for isolation precautions in hospitals. *Infect. Control Hosp. Epidemiol.*, **17**(1): 54–80.

George RH, Gully PR, Gill ON et al (1986) An outbreak of tuberculosis in a children's hospital. *J. Hosp. Infect.*, **8**: 129–142.

Glowacki LS, Hodsman AB, Hammerberg O et al (1994) Surveillance and prophylactic intervention of *Staphylococcus aureus* nasal colonisation in a haemodialysis unit. *Am. J. Nephrol.*, **14**: 9–13.

Goldberg D, Cameron S, McMenamin (1998) Hepatitis C virus antibody prevalence among injecting drug users in Glasgow has fallen but remains high. *Commun. Dis. Public Health*, **1**(2): 95–7.

Gorman LJ, Sanai L, Notman W et al (1993) Cross-infection in an intensive care unit by *Klebsiella pneumoniae* from ventilator condensate. *J. Hosp. Infect.*, **23**: 17–26.

Gray JW, George RH (2000) Experience of vancomycin-resistant enterococci in a children's hospital. *J. Hosp. Infect.*, **45**: 11–18.

Gray J, George RH, Durbin GM et al (1999) An outbreak of *Bacillus cereus* respiratory tract infections on a neonatal unit due to contaminated ventilator circuits. *J. Hosp. Infect.*, **41**: 19–22.

Greene WC (1993) AIDS and the immune system. *Sci. Am.*, **September**: 20–110.

Hannan MM, Bell A, Easterbrook P et al (1996) An outbreak of multi-drug resistant tuberculosis in a London teaching hospital HIV/GUM unit: outbreak investigations, infection control issues and molecular epidemiology. *Genitourin. Med.*, **72**: 307–8.

Hamory BH, Parisi JT (1987) *Staphylococcus epidermidis*: a significant nosocomial pathogen. *J. Infect. Control*, **15**: 59–74.

Haywood AM (1997) Transmissible spongiform encephalopathies. *N. Engl. J. Med.*, **337**: 1821–8.

Health and Safety Executive, Advisory Committee on Dangerous Pathogens (1990) *Statement on Cytomegalovirus and the Pregnant Woman*. HMSO, London.

Heptonstall J (1991) Outbreaks of hepatitis B virus infection associated with infected surgical staff. *CDR*, **1**: R81–5.

Hilton DA, Fathers E, Edwards P et al (1998) Prion immunoreactivity in appendix before clinical onset of Creutzfeldt–Jakob disease. *Lancet*, **352**: 703–4.

Hoffman PN (1993) *Clostridium difficile* and the hospital environment. *PHLS Microbiology Digest*, **10**(2): 91–2.

Hollyoaks V, Allison D, Summers J (1995) *Pseudomonas aeruginosa* wound infection associated with a nursing home's whirlpool bath. *CDR*, **5**(7): R100–2.

Howard AJ (1991) Nosocomial spread of *H. influenzae*. *J. Hosp. Infect.*, **19**(1): 1–4.

Humphries H, Johnson EM, Warnock DW et al (1991) An outbreak of aspergillosis in a general ITU. *J. Hosp. Infect.*, **18**(3): 167–78.

Hutchinson DN (1990) Nosocomial legionellosis. *Rev. Med. Microbiol.*, **1**: 108–15.

Johnson AP (1998) Antibiotic resistance among clinically important Gram positive bacteria in the UK. *J. Hosp. Infect.*, **40**: 17–26.

Joint Tuberculosis Committee of the British Thoracic Society (1990) An updated code of practice. *BMJ*, **30**: 995–1000.

Jones BL, Clark S, Curran ET et al (2000) Control of an outbreak of respiratory syncytial virus infection in immunocompromised adults. *J. Hosp. Infect.*, **44**: 53–7.

Jones D (1990) Foodborne listeriosis. *Lancet*, **336**: 1171–4.

Jones DM, Kaczmarski EB (1995) Meningococcal infections in England and Wales: 1994. *CDR Rev.*, **9**(5): R125–9.

Jones EM, Barnett J, Perry C et al (1997) Control of varicella-zoster infection on renal and other specialist units. *J. Hosp. Infect.*, **36**: 133–40.

Joseph CA, Palmer SR (1989) Outbreaks of Salmonella infection in hospitals in England and Wales 1978–87. *BMJ*, **298**: 1161–4.

Joseph CA, Harrison TG, Illjic-Car D et al (1999) Legionnaires' disease in residents of England and Wales: 1998. *Commun. Dis. Public Health*, **2**(4): 280–4.

Kelly CP, Lamont JP (1998) *Clostridium difficile* infection. *Ann. Rev. Med.*, **49**: 375–90.

Kleemola M, Jokinen C (1992) Outbreak of *Mycoplasma pneumoniae* infection amongst hospital personnel studied by a nucleic acid hybridisation test. *J. Hosp. Infect.*, **21**(3): 213–22.

Kluytmans JAJW, Mouton JW, Ijerman EPF et al (1995) Nasal carriage of *Staphylococcus aureus* as a major risk factor for wound infection after cardiac surgery. *J. Infect. Dis.*, **171**: 216–19.

Kluytmans JAJW, Mouton JW, Van den Bergh MFQ et al (1996) Reduction of surgical site infections in cardiothoracic surgery by elimination of nasal carriage of *Staphylococcus aureus. Inf. Control Hosp. Epidemiol.*, **17**: 780–5.

Kolmos HJ, Thuesen B, Nielsen SV et al (1993) Outbreak of infection in a burns unit due to *Pseudomonas aeruginosa* originating from contaminated tubing used for irrigation of patients. *J. Hosp. Infect.*, **24**: 11–21.

Korten V, Murray BE (1993) The nosocomial transmission of enterococci. *Curr. Opin. Infect. Dis.*, **6**: 498–505.

Krishnan PU, Pereira B, Macaden R (1991) Epidemiological study of an outbreak of *Serratia marcescens* in a haemodialysis unit. *J. Hosp. Infect.*, **18**: 57–61.

Laing RBS (1999) Nosocomial infections in patients with HIV disease. *J. Hosp. Infect.*, **43**: 179–85.

Laurichesse H, Grimand O, Wraight P et al (1998) Pneumococcal bacteraemia and meningitis in England and Wales: 1993 to 1995. *Commun. Dis. Public Health*, **1**(1): 22–7.

Levin MH, Olsen B, Nathan C et al (1984) Pseudomonas in the sinks of an intensive care unit: relation to patients. *J. Clin. Pathol.*, **37**: 424–7.

Lipman J, Saadia R (1997) Fungal infections in critically ill patents. *BMJ*, **315**: 266–7.

Livornese LL, Dias S, Samuel C et al (1992) Hospital-acquired infection with vancomycin-resistant *Enterococcus faecium* transmitted by electronic thermometers. *Ann. Intern. Med.*, **117**: 112–26.

Loomes S (1998) Is it safe to lie down in hospital? *Nursing Times*, **84**(49): 63–5.

Madden PB, Lamagni T, Hope V et al (1997) The HIV epidemic in injecting drug users. *CDR. Rev.*, **7**(9): R128–30.

Madge P, Payton JY, McColl JH et al (1992) Prospective controlled study of four infection control procedures to prevent nosocomial infection with respiratory syncytial virus. *Lancet*, **340**: 1079–83.

Maguire HC, Seng C, Onauters S et al (1998) Shigella outbreak in a school associated with eating canteen food and person to person spread. *Commun. Dis. Public Health*, **1**(4): 279–80.

Mangtani P, Jolley DJ, Watson JM et al (1995) Socio-economic deprivation and notification rates for tuberculosis in London during 1982–91. *BMJ*, **310**: 963–6.

Manuel RJ, Kibbler CC (1998) The epidemiology and prevention of invasive aspergillosis. *J. Hosp. Infect.*, **39**: 95–109.

Mitchell E, O'Mahoney M, McKeith I et al (1989) An outbreak of viral gastroenteritis in a psychiatric hospital. *J. Hosp. Infect.*, **14**(1): 1–8.

Mok J (1993) Breast milk and HIV-1 transmission. *Lancet*, **341**: 930–1.

Molesworth A (1998) Results of a survey of diagnosed HIV infections prevalent in 1996 in England and Wales. *Commun. Dis. Public Health*, **1**: 271–5.

Morgan M, Slamon R, Keppie N et al (1999) All Wales surveillance of methicillin-resistant *Staphylococcus aureus* (MRSA): the first year's results. *J. Hosp. Infect.*, **41**: 173–9.

Mortimer EA, Wolinsky E, Gonzaga AJ et al (1966) Role of airborne transmission in staphylococcal infections. *BMJ*, **1**: 319–22.

Mortimer JW, Evans BG, Goldberg DJ (1997) The surveillance of HIV infection and AIDS in the UK. *CDR Rev.*, **7**(9): R118–20.

Musa EK, Desai N, Casewell et al (1990) The survival of *Acinetobacter calcoaceticus* inoculated on fingertips and on formica. *J. Hosp. Infect.*, **15**(3): 219–28.

Mylotte JM (1994) Control of methicillin-resistant *Staphylococcus aureus*: the ambivalence persists. *Infect. Control Hosp. Epidemiol.*, **15**: 73–7.

Neal KR, Dornan J, Irving WL (1997) Prevalence of hepatitis C antibodies among healthcare workers of two teaching hospitals. Who is at risk? *BMJ*, **314**: 179–80.

Newton L, Hall SM, Pelevin M et al (1992) Listeriosis surveillance: 1991. *CDR Review*, **2**(12): R142–4.

NHS Estates (1993) *The Control of Legionella in Health Care Premises – A Code of Practice*. Health Technical Memorandum 2040. London.

NHS Executive (1998) *Screening of Pregnant Women for Hepatitis B and Immunisation of Babies at Risk*. HSC 1998/127. Online. Available: http://www.open.gov.uk/doh/coinh.htm

Olsen B, Weinstein RA, Nathan C et al (1984) Epidemiology of endemic *Pseudomonas aeruginosa*: why infection control efforts have failed. *J. Infect. Dis.*, **150**: 808–16.

Orsi GB, Aureli P, Cassonet et al (1999) Post surgical *Bacillus cereus* endophthalmitis outbreak. *J. Hosp. Infect.*, **42**(3): 250–1.

Pallett AP, Strangeways JEM (1988) Penicillin-resistant pneumococci. *Lancet*, **i**: 1452.

Patterson WJ, Painter MJ (1999) Bovine spongiform encephalopathy and new variant Creutzfeldt–Jakob disease: an overview. *Commun. Dis. Public Health*, **2**: 5–13.

Perez-Fontan M, Garcia-Falcon T, Rosales M et al (1993) Treatment of *Staphylococcus aureus* nasal carriers in continuous ambulatory peritoneal dialysis with mupirocin: long term results. *Am. J. Kidney Dis.*, **22**: 708–12.

Pfaller MA (1996) Nosocomial candidiasis: emerging species, reservoirs and modes of transmission. *Clin. Infect. Dis.*, **22** (Suppl.): S89–94.

Piedra PA, Kasel JA, Norton JH et al (1992) Description of an adenovirus type 8 outbreak in hospitalised neonates born prematurely. *Pediatr. Infect. Dis. J.*, **11**(8): 460–5.

Public Health Laboratory Service (1995a) Interim guidelines for the control of infections with verocytotoxin producing *Escherichia coli* (VTEC). *CDR Rev.*, **5**(6): R77–80.

Public Health Laboratory Service Meningococcal Infections Working Group and Public Health Medicine Environmental Group (1995b) Control of meningococcal disease: guidance for consultants in communicable disease control. *CDR Rev.*, **13**(5): R189–95.

Public Health Laboratory Service AIDS & STD Centre at the Communicable Disease Surveillance Centre (1999) Occupational transmission of HIV. Summary of published reports. Online. Available: http://www.phls.co.uk

Public Health Laboratory Service (2000a) *Surgical Site Infection. Analysis of Surveillance in English Hospitals, 1997–9*. Nosocomial Infection National Surveillance Scheme, London.

Public Health Laboratory Service (2000b) *Hospital-acquired Bacteraemia. Analysis of Surveillance in English Hospitals, 1997–9*. Nosocomial Infection National Surveillance Scheme, London.

Ramage L, Green K, Pyskir D et al (1996) An outbreak of fatal nosocomial infections due to group A streptococcus on a medical ward. *Infect. Control. Hosp. Epidemiol.*, **17**: 429–31.

Ramsay ME (1999) Guidance on the investigation and management of occupational exposure to hepatitis C. *Commun. Dis. Public Health*, **2**(4): 258–62.

Reid JA, Breckon D, Hunter PR (1990) Infection of staff during an outbreak of viral gastroenteritis in an elderly persons' home. *J. Hosp. Infect.*, **16**: 81–5.

Reybrouck G (1983) Role of hands in the spread of nosocomial infection: 1. *J. Hosp. Infect.*, **4**: 103–10.

Ridgeway EJ, Allen KD, Galloway A et al (1991) Penicillin-resistant pneumococci in a Merseyside hospital. *J. Hosp. Infect.* **17**: 15–23.

Rosen HR (1997) Acquisition of hepatitis C by a conjunctival splash. *Am. J. Infect. Control*, **25**: 242–7.

Rowan NJ, Anderson JG (1998) Growth and enterotoxin production by diarrhoegenic *Bacillus cereus* in dietary supplements prepared for hospitalized HIV patients. *J. Hosp. Infect.*, **38**: 139–46.

Royal College of Pathologists (1992) *HIV Infection: Hazards of Transmission to Patients and Health Care Workers During Invasive Procedures*. Royal College of Pathologists, London.

Rutter T (1998) Short course of zidovudine cuts transmission of HIV. *BMJ*, **316**: 645.

Sanderson PJ, Weissler S (1992) Recovery of coliforms from the hands of nurses and patients: activities leading to contamination. *J. Hosp. Infect.*, **21**: 85–94.

Schlech WF (1991) Listeriosis: epidemiology, virulence and the significance of contaminated foodstuffs. *J. Hosp. Infect.*, **19**(4): 211–24.

Shibuya A, Takeuchi A, Sakurai K, Saigenji K (1998) Hepatitis G virus infection from needle-stick injuries in hospital employees. *J. Hosp. Infect.*, **40**: 287–90.

Skaliy P, Sciple GV, Savannah GA (1964) Survival of staphylococci on hospital surfaces. *Arch. Environ. Health*, **8**: 636–41.

Stansfield R, Caudle S (1997) *Bacillus cereus* and orthopaedic surgical wound infection associated with incontinence pads manufactured from virgin wood pulp. *J. Hosp. Infect.*, **37**(4): 336–7.

Strausburgh LJ, Sewell DL, Ward TT et al (1994) High frequency of yeast carriage on hands of hospital personnel. *J. Clin. Microbiol.*, **32**: 299–300.

Stover BH, Bratcher DF (1998) Varicella-zoster virus: infection control and prevention. *Am. J. Infect. Control*, **26**: 369–84.

Sundkvist T, Hamilton GR, Rimmer D et al (1998) Fatal outcome of transmission of hepatitis B from an e antigen negative surgeon. *Commun. Dis. Public Health*, **1**(1): 48–50.

Takahashi A, Yomoda S, Tarimoto K et al (1998) *Streptococcus pyogenes* hospital acquired infection within a dermatological ward. *J. Hosp. Infect.*, **40**(2): 135–40.

Tassios PT, Gennimata V, Spaliara-kalogeropoulou L et al (1997) Multi-resistant *Pseudomonas aeruginosa* serogroup O:11 outbreak in an intensive care unit. *Clin. Microbiol. Infect.*, **3**(6): 621–8.

Thomas CGA (1988) *Medical Microbiology*, 6th edn. Baillière Tindall, London.

Tookey P, Peckham CS (1991) Does cytomegalovirus present an occupational risk? *Arch. Dis. Child.*, **66**: 1009–10.

UK Health Departments (1993) *Protecting Health Care Workers and Patients from Hepatitis B. Recommendations of the Advisory Group on Hepatitis*. HMSO, London.

UK Health Departments (1994) *AIDS/HIV Infected Health Care Workers: Guidance on the Management of Infected Health Care Workers*. DoH, Wetherby, UK.

UK Health Departments (1997) *Guidance on Post-exposure Prophylaxis for Health Care Workers Occupationally Exposed to HIV*. DoH, London.

UK Health Departments (1998) *Guidance for Clinical Health Care Workers: Protection Against Infection with Blood-borne Viruses. Recommendations of the Expert Advisory Group on AIDS and the Advisory Group on Hepatitis*. DoH, Wetherby, UK.

Valenti WM, Wehrle PF (1986) In *Hospital Infections*, 2nd edn, pp. 531–60 (Bennett JV, Brachman PS, eds). Little, Brown, Boston.

Vincent JL, Bihari DJ, Suter PM et al (1995) The prevalence of nosocomial infection in intensive care units in Europe. Results of the European prevalence of infection in intensive care units in Europe study. *JAMA*, **274**: 639–44.

Voss A, Doebbeling BN (1995) The world-wide prevalence of methicillin-resistant *Staphylococcus aureus*. *Int. J. Antimicrob. Agents*, **5**: 101–6.

Wade JJ, Desai N, Casewell MW (1991) Hygienic hand disinfection for the removal of epidemic vancomycin-resistant *Enterococcus faecium* and gentamicin-resistant *Enterobacter cloacae*. *J. Hosp. Infect.*, **18**(3): 211–18.

Watson JM (1991) Tuberculosis in perspective. *CDR Review*, **1**(12): R129–31.

Weber DJ, Rutala WA (1997) Role of environmental contamination in the transmission of vancomycin-resistant enterococci. *Infect. Control Hosp. Epidemiol.*, **18**: 306–9.

Weems JJ (1993) Nosocomial outbreak of *Pseudomonas cepacia* associated with contamination of reusable electronic ventilator temperature probes. *Infect. Control Hosp. Epidemiol.*, **14**(10): 583–6.

Wenzel RP, Perl TM (1995) The significance of nasal carriage of *Staphylococcus aureus* and the incidence of post-operative wound infection. *J. Hosp. Infect.*, **31**(1): 13–24.

Willcocks L, Crampin A, Milne L et al (1998) A large outbreak of cryptosporidiosis associated with a public water supply from a deep chalk borehole. *Commun. Dis. Public Health*, **1**: 239–43.

Williams CL (1999) *Helicobacter pylori* and endoscopy. *J. Hosp. Infect.*, **41**: 263–8.

Williams REO (1963) Healthy carriage of *Staphylococcus aureus*: its prevalence and importance. *Bacteriol. Rev.*, **27**: 56–71.

Wilson J, Breedon P (1990) Universal precautions. *Nursing Times*, **86**(37): 67–70.

World Health Organization (1997) *The World Health Report 1997*. WHO, Geneva.

World Health Organization (1998) *Report on the Global HIV/AIDS Epidemic*. Joint United Nations Programme on HIV/AIDS and WHO, Geneva.

Worsley MA (1993) A major outbreak of antibiotic-associated diarrhoea. *PHLS Microbiology Digest*, **10**(2): 97–9.

FURTHER READING

Cameron S, Blakely A (1993) A protocol for the detection of *Chlamydia*. *Nursing Standard*, **8**(5): 25–7.

Communicable Disease Report (1996) The incidence and prevalence of AIDS and prevalence of severe HIV disease in England and Wales for 1995 to 1999: projection using data to the end of 1994. Report of an Expert Group. *CDR Rev.*, **6**(10): R1–24.

Donal M, Hughes N (1997) Hepatitis C: a bloody business. *Nursing Times*, **93**(45): 71–4.

Greer P (1998) Vaginal thrush: diagnosis and treatment options. *Nursing Times*, **94**(4): 50–2.

Handysides S (1999) All the history that you can remember. *Commun. Dis. Public Health*, **2**(4): 229–32.

Handyside S (2000) All the history you can remember from the twentieth century. *Commun. Dis. Public Health*, **3**(1): 3–6.

Hannan MM, Azadian BS, Gazzard BG et al (2000) Hospital infection control in an era of HIV infection and multidrug resistant tuberculosis. *J. Hosp. Infect.*, **44**: 5–11.

Hughes G (1997) An overview of the HIV and AIDS epidemic in the UK. *CDR Rev.*, **7**(9): R121–2.

Mims C, Playfair J, Roitt I, Wakelin D, Williams R (1998) *Medical Microbiology*, 2nd edn. Mosby, London.

Omerod Pl, Shaw RJ, Mitchell DM (1994) Tuberculosis in the UK, 1994: current issues and future trends. *Thorax*, **49**: 1085–9.

Pratt R (1995) *AIDS: A Strategy for Nursing Care*, 4th edn. Edward Arnold, London.

Public Health Laboratory Service website: http://www.phls.co.uk.

Purcell RH (1994) Hepatitis C virus: historical perspective and current topics. *FEMS Microbiol. Rev.*, **14**: 181–92.

Terence Higgins Trust (1992) *HIV: How to Protect Yourself and Others*. Terence Higgins Trust, London.

7

The central principles of infection control

INTRODUCTION

Infection is a common, but largely avoidable, complication of healthcare which has a major impact on the patient and the health service (see Ch. 3)

A small proportion of patients admitted to hospital will have an **infectious** disease and precautions are necessary to prevent transmission to other patients or staff. Patients may be infectious before the clinical illness. For example, individuals with chickenpox are infectious for two or three days before the rash appears. This is particularly the case with bloodborne viruses such as human immunodeficiency virus (HIV), hepatitis B and C, which are associated with prolonged asymptomatic carriage of which even the patient may be unaware. The implementation of special precautions on diagnosis of infection may therefore not prevent cross-infection before the diagnosis is made. In addition, approximately 6% of patients admitted to hospital will acquire an infection during their stay (Glenister et al 1992), often as a consequence of an invasive procedure or device. It has been estimated that up to one-third of these infections could be prevented by improved infection control practice (Haley et al 1985, National Audit Office 2000).

Infection control procedures are also important to protect staff from infection. Healthcare workers are healthy and are generally less susceptible to infection than their patients. However, healthcare workers may acquire skin infections caused by streptococci, staphylococci, herpes simplex, fungi and scabies (Greaves et al 1980, Ross et al 1998); respiratory infections such as chickenpox, respiratory syncytial virus and *Mycobacterium tuberculosis* (George et al 1986, Hall 1981); and enteric infections, particularly viral gastroenteritis (Reid et al 1990). Healthcare workers are also at risk from the bloodborne viruses hepatitis B and C (West 1984). At least 102 healthcare workers worldwide have acquired HIV occupationally since it was first recognized as the cause of acquired immune deficiency syndrome (AIDS) in the 1980s (Public Health Laboratory Service 1998, AIDS & STD Centre 1998, 1999).

Healthcare workers infected with bloodborne viruses may transmit infection to their patients, although the main risk of transmission is associated with invasive procedures in which injury to the healthcare worker could result in blood entering the patient's open tissues (UK Health Departments 1994, 1998).

PRINCIPLES OF INFECTION CONTROL

This chapter reviews the key procedures that should be used as part of the everyday care of all patients to minimize the transmission of infection to staff and between patients. They are applicable to all healthcare environments in hospitals, clinics, surgeries or the patient's home (Box 7.1). Chapters 8, 9, 10 and 11 examine the more specific precautions required to prevent infection associated with invasive devices such as urinary catheters, intravenous devices, and respiratory therapy and wounds. Chapter 12 describes the principles of sterilization and disinfection of equipment.

Isolation precautions were originally developed to prevent the spread of infectious disease amongst vul-

nerable hospital patients and are used to prevent or control outbreaks or **epidemics** of infection in hospital, for example of antibiotic-resistant bacteria. They are initiated when an infectious disease is diagnosed in a particular patient and are discussed in more detail in Chapter 14.

Universal blood and body fluid precautions

Background to routine precautions

In the past, infection control precautions have tended to be focused on special measures intended to prevent the transmission of infection from patients known to have infectious disease. The concept of using a range of infection control precautions routinely in the care of all patients, regardless of whether they are known to have an infection, was first recommended in the late 1980s (Centers for Disease Control 1987). This approach, called universal precautions, was developed in response to the emerging HIV epidemic which was highlighting the problem of identifying patients with infection (see Box 7.2). Universal precautions were originally applied to all body fluids but when it became clear that bloodborne viruses were not transmitted by all fluids (e.g. faeces, urine, sputum), a recommendation to exclude those fluids from universal precautions, unless they contained visible blood, was made (CDC, 1988).

Box 7.1 Routine infection control precautions

Handwashing
- before and after contact with patients
- after gloves removed
- after contact with body fluid

Maintain integrity of skin
- cover cuts to skin with waterproof dressing
- dry skin properly and use handcream

Protective clothing
- use to protect against direct contact with body fluid
- assess risk of procedure and select appropriate protection

Sharps safety
- use equipment with safety devices
- use safe handling and disposal procedures
- provide hepatitis B vaccination for staff at risk
- report exposures to blood or body fluid

Safe handling of clinical waste
- use safe handling and disposal procedures
- discard excreta directly into drainage system
- incinerate contaminated disposable material

Decontamination of equipment
- clean and decontaminate equipment after use
- disinfect used linen by laundering
- use protective clothing whilst handling and cleaning

Decontamination of environment
- keep environment clean and free from dust
- disinfect spills of body fluid

Box 7.2 Universal precautions

Universal precautions were first recommended by the Centers for Disease Control in Atlanta, USA, in 1985 in response to growing concerns about the risk to healthcare workers from the human immunodeficiency virus (HIV) (CDC 1987). Until then, special precautions had been taken only with body fluids from patients known or suspected to be infected with bloodborne viruses. HIV had highlighted the difficulty of identifying people who were incubating a disease and were infectious, but who had no outward signs of the infection. Universal precautions recognized that there were a few simple practices that could be used in the care of all patients that would minimize the risk of bloodborne viruses being transmitted to healthcare workers. These included the safe management of sharps, the use of protective clothing in situations where open skin lesions or mucous membrane may have contact with blood or body fluid, the use of waterproof dressings to cover cuts, and handwashing after any contact with body fluids.

Since universal precautions were first proposed, other workers have recognized their benefit as a means of protecting staff and patients from other pathogens that have a propensity to spread in clinical settings (Lynch et al 1990, Wilson & Breedon 1990).

In the UK the Department of Health advised similar measures to protect clinical healthcare workers against infection with bloodborne viruses (UK Health Departments 1990) and endorsed the use of the same level of precaution with all patients. The concept was initially controversial. It was suggested that where the prevalence of bloodborne viruses was low the precautions were unnecessary and should be used only with individuals known or suspected to be infected (Speller et al 1990). As body fluids are involved in the transmission of a wide range of other pathogens, the introduction of universal precautions stimulated interest in the use of routine precautions to prevent other hospital-acquired infection (Wilson & Breedon 1990). However, if universal precautions were to be effective in preventing cross-infection between patients, as well as protecting staff from bloodborne viruses, then it was important to ensure that protective clothing was both used and changed appropriately. Thus, by changing protective clothing after each procedure, microorganisms acquired during contact with body fluid would not be introduced to a susceptible site on the same or another patient.

In 1987, Lynch et al addressed this issue by proposing a new system called body substance isolation. This recommended the use of universal precautions with all moist body substances as a means of preventing the transmission of hospital pathogens. Healthcare workers were required to use clean gloves where contact with moist body substances was anticipated, for contact with mucous membranes and non-intact skin, and to change them after each procedure. By ensuring that these basic precautions were taken to prevent transmission from patients who are unknowingly incubating infection or colonized with pathogens, isolation procedures for patients known to have infectious disease could be simplified and focused on a smaller number of pathogens (Jackson & Lynch 1985).

There has been some concern about the cost of these precautions and whether they can be maintained as a routine (Garner & Hierholzer 1993). However, a number of studies have demonstrated a reduction in infection rates associated with the routine use of gloves and other protective clothing (Klein et al 1989, Leclair et al 1987, Weinstein & Kabins 1981).

The value of routine infection control precautions both to protect healthcare workers from bloodborne viruses and to minimize the risk of transmission of other pathogens is now generally accepted. In the recent guideline on isolation precautions (Garner 1996), the principles of universal precautions and body substance isolation have been synthesized with a level of 'standard precautions' recommended for use with the care of all patients. UK guidelines contain similar advice (Pratt et al 2001, Ward et al 1997).

Risk assessment

As well as protecting the patient, infection control precautions are important for the protection of staff. Employers are responsible for ensuring that hazards in the workplace are identified, the risks they pose are assessed and appropriate precautions are taken to protect against them (Health & Safety Executive 1992a) (Box 7.3). This general risk assessment will determine whether the provisions contained within other more specific regulations are relevant to the work area, for example the Personal Protective Equipment at Work (PPE) Regulations or the Control of Substances Hazardous to Health (COSHH) Regulations. The latter regulations cover exposure to hazardous micro-organisms present in body fluids or tissues as well as chemicals and carcinogens.

Risk assessment requires a structured approach, termed risk analysis, and should take into account both workers and other people affected by the work (Advisory Committee on Dangerous Pathogens 1996, Health & Safety Executive 1992a) (Box 7.4). Where a hazard is identified, a hierarchy of controls to prevent or minimize the risk associated with it should be devised. These should begin by considering whether the hazard can be eliminated completely, for example whether a hazardous chemical can be replaced by a

---

Box 7.3   Hazards and risks

Hazard   an intrinsic danger associated with an object, substance or activity
Risk   the probability of the hazard resulting in harm

Box 7.4   Risk analysis: a structured approach to the reduction of risk

1. Risk assessment
Identify hazards and conditions under which they occur. Quantify the risk related to each hazard and make a formal record

2. Risk management
Decide on and implement the actions required to eliminate or minimize the risk

3. Risk communication
Inform and train staff about risks and risk management and control measures

4. Risk monitoring
Assess the effectiveness of control measures

safer one. If this is not possible, other controls such as those listed in Box 7.5 should be implemented. The use of protective clothing to minimize risk should be considered only where adequate protection cannot be achieved by engineering or work practice controls.

The COSHH Regulations were first introduced in 1989 and have undergone several amendments since then. They include a general Approved Code of Practice (ACOP) for hazardous substances, and separate ACOPs for carcinogenic substances and biological agents. The ACOP for biological agents applies where people are liable to be exposed to any micro-organism that can cause infection or other risk to health. They apply to situations where micro-organisms are being used or worked on, for example in laboratories, as well as activities that may result in incidental exposure such as refuse disposal, food production and healthcare. Assessments should take into account the type of biological agent that may be present (Box 7.6).

Risk assessments should be made in all areas of work to identify those procedures likely to involve exposure to body fluids or tissue and the options available to minimize the risk of exposure. The identification of

---

Box 7.6	Biological agents: hazard groups
Group 1	Unlikely to cause human disease
Group 2	Can cause human disease and may be a hazard; is unlikely to spread to the community, there is usually effective prophylaxis or treatment available
Group 3	Can cause severe human disease and may be a serious hazard; may spread to the community but there is usually effective prophylaxis or treatment available
Group 4	Causes severe human disease and is a serious hazard; likely to spread to the community and there is usually no effective prophylaxis or treatment available

Source: Control of Substances Hazardous to Health Regulations 1999

---

hazards and the development of associated control measures should involve a multidisciplinary group of staff familiar with the clinical area under consideration. This will help to ensure that control measures are practical and relevant. Changing work practices may enable the risk to be minimized or avoided, for example using disposable instruments or sending reusable ones to a central sterile supply department for automatic decontamination, rather than cleaning them by hand. There may also be equipment available with safety features that can prevent injury, such as blunt suture needles or needles with automatic resheathing devices. Only if exposure to the hazard cannot be prevented should the use of protective clothing be recommended (Health and Safety Executive, 1992b) (see Box 7.5).

First aid equipment should be available to enable prompt treatment if inadvertent exposure to a hazardous substance occurs (e.g. eye wash solutions). In addition, administrative controls should be in place. These should include systems for ensuring that staff know about the risks, are trained to comply with controls, and are aware of the actions to take should exposure to the hazard occur, for example following a needlestick injury. Mechanisms for monitoring adherence to health and safety policies and for recording accidents should be in place and the information used to evaluate and review practice (Gerberding 1993).

ROUTINE INFECTION CONTROL PRECAUTIONS

The infection control precautions outlined below represent the standard of care that should be used routinely

---

Box 7.5 Hierarchy of controls to prevent or minimize risks in the workplace

1. Eliminate or substitute hazard
Avoid activity or substance or replace with a safer one
Example: use peracetic acid in place of glutaraldehyde to disinfect endoscopes

2. Engineering controls
Use of equipment that may prevent injury
Example: shielding devices, blunt-tipped needles

3. Work practice controls
Adopt systems of work that prevent or minimize risk
Example: discard used sharps directly into sharps container

4. Protective clothing
Select appropriate clothing for activities likely to result in exposure to a hazard
Example: use gloves to clean instruments, wear eye protection during surgical procedures

5. Administrative controls
Ensure relevant personnel know about hazards and recommended controls
Example: policies, training programmes

6. Monitoring and evaluation
Record and analyse accident data, provide health surveillance where indicated
Example: monitor sharps injuries, adverse health effects in glutaraldehyde users

Source: Control of Substances Hazardous to Health Regulations 1999; Gerberding (1993)

with all patients to minimize the spread of pathogens between patients and staff.

Handwashing

The hands of staff are the most common vehicle by which micro-organisms are transmitted between patients, and hands are frequently implicated as the route of transmission in outbreaks of infection (Box 7.7). Although there is little direct evidence that hands are involved in passing micro-organisms from one person to another, it is generally accepted that pathogens are frequently acquired on the hands in clinical settings and that handwashing is essential to remove them. There are two categories of micro-organisms present on the skin; the transient and the resident flora. Ansari et al 1991a, Bryan et al 1995, Simmons et al 1990).

Transient skin flora

Microbes acquired on the surface of the skin through contact with other people, objects or the environment are known as transient skin flora. They are particularly easily acquired on the hands when the object touched is moist (Marples & Towers 1979). The composition of this transient flora varies but reflects the extent of contact with patients or their environment and the prevalent micro-organisms. For example, **methicillin-resistant** *Staphylococcus aureus* **(MRSA)** is frequently found on the skin of nurses who are caring for patients infected with the organism (Cookson et al 1989). The antibacterial properties of skin prevent the survival of these transient micro-organisms for more than a few hours (Reybrouck 1983) but within this time the organisms are readily transferred to other people or objects (Mackintosh & Hoffman 1984).

The potential for transmission has been demonstrated by experiments using a fluorescent powder, visible only under ultraviolet light, to represent micro-organisms. This study demonstrated that 2 h after the powder was applied to a baby, traces of it were found on the hands of all the nurses responsible for the care of the baby, the hands of at least one other nurse and in the environment (Scanlon & Leikkanen 1973).

Pathogens are likely to be acquired on the hands in greatest number when handling moist, heavily contaminated substances such as body fluids. However, Casewell & Phillips (1977) showed that, even during routine procedures such as touching, lifting or washing a patient, transient bacteria are easily acquired on the hands. They are also acquired simply by touching the buttocks of a baby, even if the nappy is not soiled (Sprunt et al 1973) and have been recovered from hands after bedmaking, handling curtains or using the sluice (Sanderson & Weissler 1992). Pathogens present on the skin surrounding an infected wound are readily transferred to the hands even if forceps are used to dress the wound (Tomlinson 1987). Viruses are also easily acquired, for example during nappy changing (Samadi et al 1983), and hands are commonly contaminated by respiratory viruses (Ansari et al 1991a) (Fig. 7.1).

Pittet et al (1999) demonstrated that contamination of the hands cumulated during time in contact with skin or secretions. They also found that respiratory care was associated with particularly high levels of hand contamination.

Resident skin flora

The skin is an inhospitable environment for most micro-organisms: it is dry, acidic and poor in nutrients (Hoffman & Wilson 1994). However, some micro-organisms have adapted to these conditions and exist in stable populations known as the resident or normal flora. These organisms live in deep crevices in the skin, in hair follicles and sebaceous glands. The type and distribution of organisms varies according to humidity, temperature, body site and the person's general health. The micro-organisms present in largest numbers are Gram-positive bacteria, mainly coagulase-negative staphylococci, micrococci and coryneforms. Although not conventionally considered part of the resident flora, some Gram-negative bacilli appear able to survive in some areas, notably moist areas beneath rings (Hoffman et al 1985).

Box 7.7 Hands and the spread of infection

Over a period of 1 month the same type of *Klebsiella pneumoniae* was isolated from the respiratory secretions of six patients on an intensive care unit. Four patients developed infections caused by the organism. During the investigation to identify the source of the organism it was noticed that the water traps collecting condensate from ventilator tubing were emptied into foil dishes. These remained by the beside until full when they were emptied into the sink. Although hands were washed after contact with tracheal secretions, hands were not washed after handling the condensate.

Klebsiella was found in samples of the condensate and in the foil bowls and was also recovered from the hands of staff. No further cases of infection occurred once staff had been alerted to the hazard of the condensate and handwashing after contact with ventilator tubing and traps had been instituted.
Gorman et al (1993)

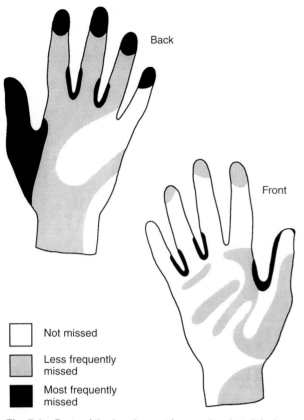

Back

Front

□ Not missed

▨ Less frequently missed

■ Most frequently missed

Fig. 7.1 Parts of the hands most frequently missed during handwashing.

Removing micro-organisms from the hands

In clinical situations, transient micro-organisms acquired on the hands through contact with patients, their body fluids or environment need to be removed if cross-infection is to be avoided. Fortunately, the majority of transient micro-organisms are easily removed mechanically by washing with soap and water, even by a brief, 10 s wash (Sprunt et al 1973) (Plate 7.1). Ideally, hands should be washed to remove these transient organisms before and after any episode of patient care that involves any direct contact with their skin, dressings or devices (Pratt et al 2001). However, as a minimum, they should always be washed *before* an activity that could introduce infection to a susceptible site on the patient (e.g. handling an invasive device or wound) and *after* an activity that could result in the hands becoming contaminated by micro-organisms (e.g. contact with urine or faeces) (Box 7.8).

The removal of resident skin flora during routine clinical care is not necessary in many situations as

Box 7.8 Indications for handwashing

Hands should be washed with soap and water before any direct contact with patients and especially:

● before and after handling invasive devices
● before and after dressing wounds
● before and after contact with immunocompromised patients
● before and after handling food/drink
● after handling equipment contaminated with body fluid
● after contact with blood or body fluid
● after handling clinical waste and used laundry
● after removing gloves
● after using the toilet
● before leaving the clinical area

these micro-organisms are not readily transferred to other people or surfaces and most are of low pathogenicity. However, some resident bacteria could cause infection if introduced during invasive procedures into normally sterile body sites or on to particularly vulnerable individuals (e.g. neonates, patients in intensive care). The resident microbial flora are not easily removed by the mechanical action of washing with soap, but their numbers can be reduced by the combination of a detergent and a microbiocide, such as chlorhexidine or povidone–iodine. Both these antiseptic soap solutions have a cumulative effect on the resident flora if used repeatedly (Lowbury & Lilley 1973).

Antiseptic soap solutions are only slightly more effective at removing transient skin flora than soap and water (Ayliffe et al 1988). Originally designed for use by surgeons only a few times a day, when used frequently for handwashing in ward situations they have been associated with damage to skin and increased levels of bacteria on the hands (Ojajärvi et al 1977). Their use is therefore best restricted to situations where the removal of resident flora is indicated, such as in operating theatres and before invasive procedures. They are of dubious value as a means of routine handwashing in most clinical areas. Occasionally their use is recommended to assist in the control of outbreaks of infection. Gram-negative bacilli, especially antibiotic-resistant strains, are often difficult to remove by the mechanical action of soap and water and antiseptic detergents may be helpful in preventing their spread (Wade et al 1991) (Box 7.9).

One of the prime considerations in ensuring that handwashing takes place is selecting a handwash preparation that is acceptable to the users (Hoffman & Wilson 1994). Irritation and drying effects of handwash preparations have been reported to affect compliance with handwashing guidelines (Zimakoff et al

Box 7.9   Guide to selecting hand-cleaning preparations

	Handwashing preparation		
	Soap	**Alcohol rub or gel**	**Antiseptic soap**
Removes transient micro-organisms	✓	✓	✓
Removes resident micro-organisms		✓	✓
Effective on physically soiled hands	✓		✓
Routine use in clinical areas	✓	✓	
Preoperative hand preparation		✓	✓
Hand preparation before invasive procedures		✓	✓

General principles
- Use liquid soap for routine use to wash physically soiled hands
- Use alcohol hand rub or gel for routine use to decontaminate physically clean hands and as a preoperative hand preparation
- Use antiseptic soap solution to remove resident flora before surgical or invasive procedures

1992). Preparations should therefore contain emollients and moisturizers to minimize skin damage that may be caused by frequent use.

Gram-negative micro-organisms may grow on soap bars and in solutions, even in the presence of disinfectants (Archibald et al 1997a). Soap should therefore be supplied in liquid form in a dispenser fitted with disposable cartridges. Recently Sartor et al (2000) reported an outbreak of *Serratia marcescens* associated with contaminated soap pumps. The micro-organisms were transferred from one soap bottle to another on the contaminated pump, and then multiplied in the soap. The authors recommended the use of disposable sealed pumps and small-volume soap cartridges to address the problem.

Handwashing technique

Hands should be washed properly to ensure micro-organisms are removed. Taylor (1978) observed that nurses washed their hands for an average time of 20 s and that large areas of the skin were frequently left unwashed. Micro-organisms may remain on parts of the hands not exposed to soap and water, and would still be available for transfer to other patients. The greatest concentration of micro-organisms is found beneath fingernails (McGinley et al 1988). There is evidence that nurses with long fingernails are more likely to become colonized with Gram-negative pathogens and to transmit infection to vulnerable patients (Moolenaar et al 2000). Long fingernails may also interfere with the handwashing process.

Hands should be washed by systematically rubbing all parts of the hands and wrists with soap and water, being particularly careful to include the areas that are most frequently missed (Fig. 7.1). Similarly, the efficacy

of antiseptic soap solutions depends on the adequacy of the handwash; micro-organisms will be removed by these solutions only if all parts of the hands are reached. Some infection control teams recommend a six-stage technique for ensuring that all parts of the hands are covered (Ayliffe et al 1978). However, because even a brief handwash appears to remove transient micro-organisms effectively (Sprunt et al 1973), the relevance of such a detailed technique is debatable, particularly if it acts to discourage handwashing.

Thorough drying afterwards is also an important part of the procedure. More bacteria are probably removed by the towel or hot-air drier (Ansari et al 1991b) and moisture remaining on the skin may cause it to become dry and cracked.

Unfortunately, research has shown that healthcare staff frequently do not wash their hands at all after contact with patients, even after dirty procedures (Glynn et al 1997, Gould 1993). Medical staff have been found to be especially unlikely to wash their hands (Albert & Condie 1981, Glynn et al 1997). Handwashing activity may not reflect the risk of contamination or cross-infection. Pittet et al (1999) found that staff were more likely to decontaminate their hands after an activity associated with a low risk of acquiring micro-organisms than before an activity associated with a high risk of introducing infection. Hands were washed between a dirty and clean body site on only 11% of occasions. This suggests that the risk to the patient of transferring micro-organisms into a susceptible site was not appreciated or was being overlooked.

A number of factors influence handwashing frequency, notably staff workload, shortage of sinks, lack of soap, hand towels or water temperature controls (Archibald et al 1997b, Pittet et al 1999). Williams &

Buckles (1988) demonstrated that, even though handwashing frequency increased significantly after an extensive promotional campaign, six months later the rate of handwashing had decreased to the previous level. This finding has been confirmed by Larson et al (1997), who found that focus groups, automated sinks and feedback on handwashing frequency had a minimal long-term effect on handwashing frequency. Raising the profile of handwashing as a key infection control measure and finding novel ways of encouraging staff to wash their hands (Fig. 7.2) remains an important challenge (Handwashing Liaison Group 1999).

Alcohol handrubs or gels

Although a single handwash and dry takes about 1 min to perform properly, a considerable amount of time is spent on repeated handwashing – more if there is some distance between the patient and the nearest sink. An inadequate supply of handwashing facilities may adversely affect the frequency of handwashing (Kaplan & McGuckin 1986).

One means of encouraging effective and frequent handwashing is by using alcohol handrubs. These can be applied more quickly (15–20 s) without the need for a handwash basin and will remove both transient organisms and resident bacteria. A recent study found that alcohol preparations were more effective than both soap and water and antiseptic soap solutions, at removing rotavirus from the hands (Bellamy et al 1993). In most situations alcohol handrubs can be used as an alternative to routine handwashing with soap and water, but should not be used if hands are visibly soiled (Mackintosh & Hoffman 1984, Pratt et al 2001). Handrubs are particularly useful during aseptic techniques, outside isolation rooms, in intensive care settings where hands may need to be washed frequently, and in the patient's home where access to handwashing facilities may be difficult. They are associated with less skin damage than antiseptic soap solutions and have a better suppressive effect on the regrowth of resident micro-organisms (Rotter et al 1980). They are therefore also an ideal surgical scrub which can be applied quickly (Hoffman & Wilson 1994).

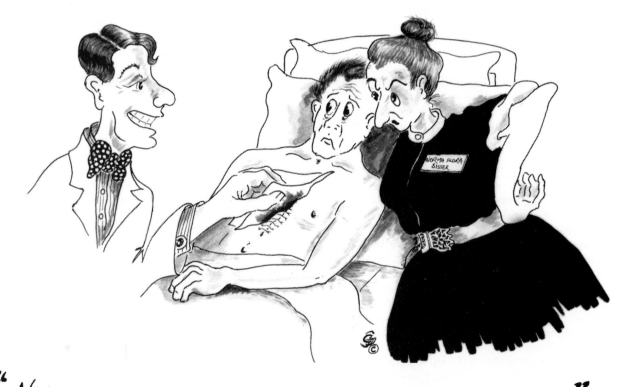

"NOW WASH YOUR HANDS – OR, DON'T PEEK!"

Fig. 7.2

Handcreams

Frequent handwashing, especially with antiseptic soap solutions or if hands are not properly dried, can cause damage to skin. Cracked skin may harbour more bacteria and increase the risk of cross-infection (Larson et al 1986). Soap should always be applied to wet hands to minimize irritation to the skin. Regular use of handcreams may help to prevent skin damage but communally used creams can become a potential source of infection (Morse & Schonbek 1968).

Covering cuts

Intact skin protects tissue from invasion by micro-organisms. Damaged skin may become infected superficially by bacteria or fungi, and bloodborne viruses may enter the body through damaged skin. Whilst at work, healthcare workers should therefore always protect any damaged skin, particularly on the hands and forearms, with a waterproof dressing. Healthcare workers with dermatitis are at particular risk of acquiring infection and should seek advice from the occupational health department.

Protective clothing

Many excretions and secretions of the body are a major source of **pathogenic micro-organisms** associated with hospital-acquired infection (Box 7.10). Protective clothing should therefore be worn for any direct contact with these body fluids, to protect the skin of staff from contamination with body fluid and micro-organisms, and to reduce the risk of transmission of micro-organisms between patients and staff.

The protective clothing selected depends on the anticipated risk of exposure to body fluid during the particular activity. This assessment should consider the risk both to the patient and to the healthcare worker. Many clinical activities involve no direct contact with body fluid and do not require the use of protective clothing, for example washing a patient or taking a pulse, blood pressure or temperature. Other procedures may result in contamination of the hands or clothing and require the use of gloves and a plastic apron, for example assisting a patient with a commode or handling specimens. Procedures in which there is a risk that splashing of blood or body fluid may occur require the use of a mask and eye protection to protect these mucous membranes, and a water-resistant gown will be necessary. In the operating theatre, waterproof boots or shoes may also be required in some situations. Fig. 7.3 illustrates the principles of risk assessment in the selection of protective clothing. They should be applied in all situations, with all patients and in all areas of clinical practice, and clothing should be changed after each procedure or activity to prevent the transmission of infection to other patients.

Gloves

The contribution that the hands of staff make to the transmission of infection in healthcare settings has already been demonstrated (see p. 34). Disposable gloves for direct contact with body fluids and moist body sites provide a reliable method of reducing the acquisition on hands of micro-organisms from these sources. Some studies have demonstrated a reduction in the incidence of infection where gloves are used routinely for handling body fluids, although they must be used appropriately (Gerding et al 1988, Leclair et al 1987, Lynch et al 1990). Gloves will also protect the healthcare worker from infection if cuts and abrasions are present on the hands.

Gloves should be worn for any activity where body fluid may contaminate the hands, but to prevent transmission of infection gloves must be discarded after each procedure (Patterson et al 1991). This principle even applies for procedures on the same patient, where, for example, gloves worn for tracheal suction must be changed before dressing a wound otherwise micro-organisms colonizing the respiratory tract may be transferred into the wound and establish infection. Gloves must always be changed between patients, even if being used for routine procedures such as emptying urine drainage bags. Latex gloves should also be changed regularly during prolonged procedures as hydration of the latex may cause the gloves to become porous (UK Health Departments 1998). Washing gloves between patients is not recommended; the

---

Box 7.10 Potentially infectious body fluids
Body fluids that may contain bloodborne viruses
Blood
Blood-stained body fluids
Semen
Vaginal secretions
Tissues
Cerebrospinal fluid
Amniotic fluid, synovial fluid, pleural fluid, etc.
Body fluids that may contain other pathogens
Faeces
Urine
Vomit
Sputum
Saliva

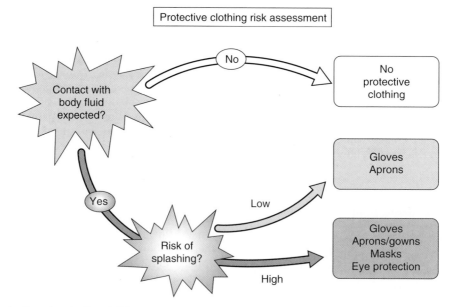

Fig. 7.3 The selection of protective clothing.

gloves may be damaged by the soap solution and, if punctured unknowingly, may cause body fluid to remain in direct contact with skin for prolonged periods (Adams et al 1992, Centers for Disease Control 1993). Hands should be washed after removal because gloves may be punctured and hands are easily contaminated as the gloves are taken off (Olsen et al 1993).

Gloves should also be worn for procedures involving direct contact with mucous membranes, for example mouth care and vaginal examination. Micro-organisms colonizing or infecting mucous membranes may easily be transmitted on hands and infect another person, for example papilloma virus or candida in the vagina, herpes simplex virus or candida in the mouth (Burnie et al 1985).

Type of glove material Disposable gloves must be readily available in all clinical areas. Medical gloves are made from rubber latex, synthetic latex or vinyl. Each type has slightly different properties and may be suited to a different range of activities. Latex gloves conform to the hands and are most suitable for procedures requiring a degree of dexterity, although sensitization to latex is increasingly recognized as a problem amongst health-care workers (Booth 1996) (Box 7.11). Synthetic formulations of latex, with similar conforming properties, are becoming more widely available. Vinyl gloves are looser fitting but not associated with adverse skin reactions. Korniewicz et al (1990) have suggested that vinyl gloves are more likely to develop holes during use than

latex gloves, although their study demonstrated a significant difference only where gloves were being used in prolonged simulated tests. Latex does have some resistance to puncture and resealing properties, so that these gloves are probably more appropriate for procedures involving the handling of sharp instruments. De Groot-Kosolcharoen & Jones (1989) demonstrated that a proportion of both latex and vinyl medical gloves have small holes in them before use, and point to the importance of ensuring that good-quality gloves are purchased. Medical gloves should comply with British Standard EN455 (British Standards Institution 1994), should be free from pinholes and not split or tear easily. None the less, they should be regarded as a means of minimizing the risk of acquiring pathogens on the hands rather than as an impermeable barrier. Handwashing after glove removal is still necessary. Gloves do not need to be sterile unless used in a sterile body site (e.g. surgical or other invasive procedures).

Gloves with very long cuffs are available for procedures where blood contamination of the arms is likely (e.g. obstetrics).

Gloves and the prevention of percutaneous injury Whilst disposable gloves cannot prevent percutaneous injury, there is evidence that they can be used to reduce the risk of injury (Palmer & Rickett 1992, UK Health Departments 1998). A number of studies in operating theatres have demonstrated that wearing two pairs of latex gloves (double-gloving) significantly reduces the risk of exposure to blood.

Box 7.11   Latex allergy

Latex gloves are made from natural rubber latex. The latex is treated with chemicals called accelerators to increase its strength and flexibility and to enable it to retain its moulded shape. When dry, the gloves are washed to remove residual traces of chemicals and latex proteins. Cornstarch powder is commonly added to latex gloves to improve the ease with which they can be put on and removed. Since the introduction of universal precautions in the 1980s, the use of gloves has increased considerably and there has been a corresponding increase in reports of allergy to latex (Yessin et al 1994). Users may react to latex proteins, chemical accelerators or the cornstarch powder. Allergy to the latex proteins is mediated by immunoglobulin (Ig) E and causes an itchy rash on exposed skin, itching eyes and nose, wheezing or asthma (Johnson 1998, Medical Devices Agency 1996). Allergy to accelerators causes contact dermatitis with red, cracked and thickened skin developing a few hours after contact with the gloves. Cornstarch powder can absorb latex proteins and enable them to become airborne when gloves are put on or removed; this can expose other sensitized people to the allergens in areas where gloves are being used. Cornstarch powder in gloves has also been linked with adhesions in surgical wounds and poor healing (Medical Devices Agency 1998). People who are 'atopic', that is they are predisposed to producing IgE on exposure to an allergen (e.g. hayfever, asthma, eczema) may be more easily sensitized to latex. There is also a link between latex sensitization and some foods (Medical Devices Agency 1996).

In recognition of these problems, reputable glove manufacturers produce powder-free latex gloves, coated with hydrogel polymer for donning and removal. They will also use thorough washing processes to ensure that the levels of accelerators and extractable latex proteins in the gloves are low.

Local supplies departments should convene a multidisciplinary group to consider these issues in relation to the purchase of gloves for clinical use, and ensure that gloves comply with the relevant British Standard (British Standards Institution 1994, Medical Devices Agency 1996). The Medical Devices Agency recommends that only powder-free gloves should be purchased (Medical Devices Agency 1998).

Gerberding et al (1990) found that where two pairs of gloves were worn 17% of outer gloves were punctured during the procedure but only 5% of the inner gloves, and Tokars et al (1992) recorded a 70% reduction in exposure to blood in surgeons who double-gloved. Wearing two pairs of gloves does not appear to have a significant effect on comfort, but the recommended combination is an outer glove of the usual size and inner glove half a size larger (Telford & Quebberman 1993). Double-gloving is recommended for procedures associated with a high risk of glove tear or percutaneous injury (e.g. gynaecology and orthopaedic surgery, obstetric procedures). Indicator glove systems are available that use a coloured inner glove to alert the user to punctures of the outer glove (Zimmerman & Junghans 1996).

Gloves should also be worn for venepuncture, especially by inexperienced personnel. Several healthcare workers have acquired bloodborne viruses as a result of blood exposure during venepuncture (PHLS AIDS & STD Centre 1999, UK Health Departments 1998).

MASKS AND EYE PROTECTION

Masks were introduced at the turn of the twentieth century to protect patients from micro-organisms expelled from the respiratory tract of staff during surgical procedures, and to provide protection for staff caring for patients with infectious disease. Evidence of their ineffectiveness followed much later. It is now recognized that, unless the mask fits closely around the mouth and nose, air is inhaled and exhaled around its edge and is therefore not filtered. If worn for prolonged periods moisture, which collects in the fabric, interrupts the passage of air through the mask and increases the flow around the outside (Belkin 1997).

Close-fitting masks are recommended for some aspects of care of patients with open tuberculosis, but are not generally necessary for patients with other infectious diseases (see p. 250). They are also of limited value in protecting sites on the patient that are susceptible to infection as healthy staff expel few micro-organisms from the respiratory tract (Ayliffe 1991). Although still used in operating theatres for this purpose, there is little evidence that they reduce the risk of surgical wound infection (Hubble et al 1996). However, staff are vulnerable to infection by blood-borne viruses and other pathogens if infected body fluid is splashed on to the mucous membranes of the eyes and mouth (PHLS AIDS & STD Centre 1999).

Eye protection and a mask should be worn for any activity where there is a risk of body fluid splashing into the face (Fig. 7.4). Such activities are not commonly encountered in ward settings, where the main risks are associated with respiratory suction if excessive secretions are present, or cleaning of instruments and equipment. Staff at greatest risk from splashing of blood or other body fluids are those involved in surgical or obstetrical procedures. Tokars et al (1995) found that contact between blood or other infective fluids and the eyes or mouth of surgical staff occurred in 2% of surgical procedures, particularly

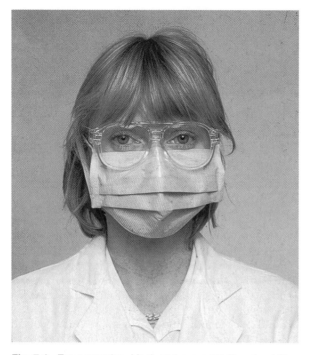

Fig. 7.4 Eye protection. Mask and eye protection should be worn for procedures where there is risk of splashing of blood or body fluids.

orthopaedic and gynaecological. Short & Bell (1993) reported a high risk of splashing into the face associated with obstetrical procedures.

In common with people in other occupations whose work involves a risk of damage to the eyes, healthcare workers are often reluctant to protect their eyes properly. Masks and eye protection must be readily available in any clinical area where such procedures are performed. In the past, eye protection has been cumbersome to wear, but now a variety of types is available and some look similar to conventional spectacles. Information on different types of eyewear can be found in British Standard BS7028 (British Standards Institution 1999).

Water-repellent aprons or gowns

Water-repellent protection should be worn for procedures anticipated to cause significant contamination of skin or clothing with blood or body fluid. This will protect the skin of the healthcare worker from contamination by potentially infected body fluid and reduce the risk of **cross-infection** of micro-organisms to other patients on the clothing. Cotton gowns are not water-repellent and, when wet, micro-organisms pass through them easily (Callaghan 1998, Holborn 1990).

Because the front of the body is the part most frequently contaminated by body fluid, plastic disposable aprons provide adequate protection in most circumstances (e.g. dealing with body fluid spills, handling bedpans, dressing wounds). Plastic aprons should be readily available in all clinical areas and must be replaced after each procedure to prevent the transfer of micro-organisms to other patients.

Exposure to body fluid during surgical procedures varies; minor surgery such as biopsy, lump removal or laparoscopy involves little exposure to body fluid. Some orthopaedic, abdominal and cardiac procedures may result in considerable contamination with blood or body fluid and then a water-repellant gown should be worn (Tokars et al 1995, UK Health Departments 1998). Gowns with water-repellant sleeves, together with a plastic apron underneath, may also provide adequate protection.

Water-repellant gowns may be disposable or reusable and made from specially woven or treated cotton. The most impervious have a plastic layer, but are expensive. For procedures where the legs and feet may be contaminated (e.g. obstetrics), the gown must be long enough to cover the legs, and calf-length over-boots should be worn rather than clogs.

All contaminated clothing must be removed before leaving the area, and any blood that has inadvertently contaminated the skin washed off immediately.

Safe handling of sharp instruments

'Sharps' include needles, scalpels, broken glass or other items that may cause a laceration or puncture.

Sharp instruments frequently cause injury to healthcare workers and are a major cause of transmission of bloodborne viruses (PHLS AIDS & STD Centre 1999) (see p. 123). They are reported to account for 16% of occupational injuries in hospitals, but since many go unreported this figure is likely to be a considerable underestimate (National Audit Office 1999).

The risk of transmission following a single sharps (percutaneous) injury depends on the type of bloodborne virus involved. The risk is one in three when the instrument is contaminated with hepatitis B virus from a patient who is e antigen positive (see p. 119); approximately one in 30 when the instrument is contaminated by hepatitis C; and one in 300 when contaminated by HIV. In the UK, four healthcare workers have acquired HIV following a percutaneous injury, and a further eight probably acquired the virus by this route, since the epidemic was first recognized in the early 1980s (PHLS AIDS & STD Centre 1999). The risk of acquiring HIV depends on the infectivity of the source patient;

this is highest at the time of seroconversion and during the later stages of HIV disease when the level of virus is high (Department of Health 1997).

Hollow 'sharps', such as hypodermic needles or cannulas, are more likely to transmit infection than solid items such as suture needles and scalpels (PHLS AIDS & STD Centre 1999, Royal College of Pathologists 1992).

Causes of sharps injuries

A number of studies have investigated the causes of percutaneous injuries in healthcare workers. Injuries are commonly associated with the disassembly of devices such as vacuum blood-taking systems or intravenous cannulas; recapping of needles; transfer of used sharps to point of disposal; sharps not discarded after use or overfilled sharps containers (Eisenstein & Smith 1992, Jagger et al 1988, Weltman et al 1995). Resheathing of needles is particularly dangerous because if the needle misses the sheath it will puncture the hand holding it. In one study resheathing was responsible for 33% of injuries (Becker et al 1990, Jagger et al 1988).

Preventing needlestick injuries

Used sharps must be handled as little as possible to avoid injury. Needles should not be disconnected from syringes but discarded as one unit. In situations where resheathing is essential, a device should be used (Fig. 7.5). If such a device is unavailable, the sheath should be placed on a flat surface and the needles inserted without holding the sheath by hand.

Immediate disposal of used sharps diminishes the risk that they will cause injuries. Disposal of used sharps in inappropriate places may present a considerable risk to other people, for example used needles left on trolleys or blood glucose lancets left on lockertops. Every healthcare worker has a responsibility to ensure proper disposal of the sharps that they have used. Sharps should always be discarded into appropriate containers, and these should be readily accessible at the point where sharps are used. Containers used for sharps should conform to the British Standard for sharps containers, which is summarized in Box 7.12. Small, portable sharps bins are available for use in community settings. Containers must be assembled properly and sealed securely for disposal before discarded sharps protrude from the aperture (Medical Devices Agency 1993, Saghafi et al 1992). In areas where children may be present, containers must be kept out of their reach. Box 7.13 outlines the principles of good practice for the safe management of

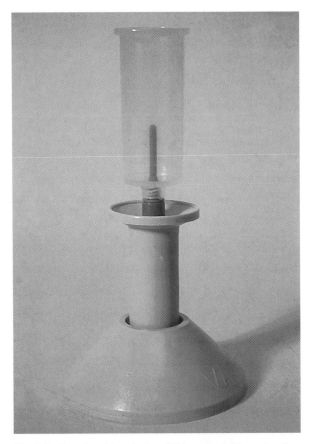

Fig. 7.5   A resheathing device. If it is essential to resheathe a needle, a resheathing device should be used.

Box 7.12   Summary of contents of the British Standard for sharps containers (BSI 1990)

Containers intended to hold sharps should:

- have a handle
- have a closure device that remains closed when the container is carried or dropped
- be resistant to penetration
- not leak or break open when dropped
- be yellow
- be marked with the words:
  Danger
  Contaminated sharps only
  Destroy by incineration
- be marked to indicate when 70–80% full

---

sharp instruments. Many devices for preventing needlestick injuries are available but not all are effective and they may have limited application or be associated with adverse consequences (Do et al 1999, Pratt et al 2001).

> **Box 7.13** Safe handling of used sharp instruments
>
> - Do not disassemble needles from syringes or other devices, discard as a single unit
> - Do not resheathe needles (if essential use a resheathing device)
> - Do not carry used sharps by hand or pass to another person
> - Discard sharps immediately after use into a sharps container
> - Ensure sharps containers are placed at points of use
> - Use sharps containers that conform to BS7320
> - Ensure containers are securely closed when three-quarters full

Each clinical area should take a systematic approach to minimizing percutaneous injuries by undertaking a risk assessment of local practices and instituting appropriate controls (see Box 7.5). Data collected from injury reports can help to pinpoint the important hazards in a particular area. If sharp instruments cannot be replaced, for instance by blunt needles, then engineering controls such as safety devices or retractable needles and changes to work practices, such as arrangements for sealing and closing bins when three-quarters full, should be considered. A clear, written policy outlining recommended practices and control measures should be available to all staff, together with information on the management of injuries (see Fig. 7.6).

Handling sharps in operating departments

The risk of percutaneous injury is particularly high during surgical procedures. A comprehensive study undertaken by Tokars et al in 1992 found that a percutaneous injury occurred during 7% of surgical procedures. In vaginal hysterectomies the rate was as high as 21%, probably because of the poor visibility associated with this procedure. Suture needles caused 77% of injuries; commonly these were inflicted on the index finger of the non-dominant hand as it was used to guide the needle. One-quarter of injuries were inflicted on a co-worker. This type of study provides an important insight into factors associated with injury and where preventive measures should be directed. Blunt suture needles are now available and can be used to suture most tissues, apart from skin. Needle-holders with needle-tip guards, blade removal devices and safety containers for storage of used sharps should be used routinely (Davies 1994, Stafford et al 1995). Double-gloving can also be employed to reduce the risk of sharps penetrating the skin (see p. 141). Systems of work should be established to ensure that sharp instruments are not handed directly to co-workers, but passed on a tray or via a neutral zone. Magnets should be used to pick up blades or needles that have fallen on to the floor (Box 7.14).

Vacuum blood collection systems These systems are now widely used for venepuncture and are generally considered safer than taking blood with a needle and syringe, as blood is drawn directly into the specimen bottle and not injected in after collection.

Some vacuum collection systems incorporate a reusable barrel from which the needle has to be unscrewed. This can be done safely only if the needle is resheathed in a resheathing device (Fig. 7.5) and it is better if the barrel and needle are discarded together.

Treatment of sharps injuries

Exposure to blood or body fluid, from a sharps injury, bite or from splashing into the eyes, mouth or broken skin, must always be followed up properly because of the risk of infection from bloodborne viruses (Fig. 7.6).

The occupational health department will assess whether any action is necessary to prevent infection with hepatitis B or HIV. The recipient of the injury may need a blood test to establish whether he or she has immunity to hepatitis B virus. If the source of the blood or body fluid is known, the patient can be tested, with informed consent, for bloodborne viruses. If the injured person is not immune to hepatitis B, specific immunoglobulin can be given. This will prevent or moderate the infection by hepatitis B virus, provided that it is administered quickly, preferably within 48 h of the injury. A full course of hepatitis B **vaccination** should also be given.

At present, there is no vaccination or specific immunoglobulin available for hepatitis C or HIV. The occupational health department can offer counselling and arrange, with his/her consent, for the healthcare

> **Box 7.14** Prevention of percutaneous injuries in operating departments
>
> - Use blunt suture needles where possible and remove sharp needles before tying the suture
> - Use a device to handle needles and remove blades
> - Store used needles and blades in a safety container
> - Do not pass sharps from hand to hand
> - Use instruments, not fingers, to retract tissue
> - Use double gloves for procedures where there is a risk of sharps injury
> - Ensure sharps containers of an appropriate size are available

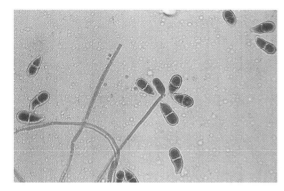

Plate 1.1   A filamentous fungus. Tubular hyphae with groups of spores.

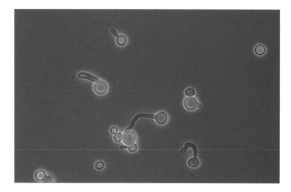

Plate 1.2   *Candida albicans*. When incubated in serum the cells produce characteristic outgrowths called germ tubes.

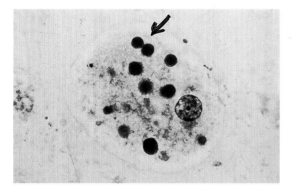

Plate 1.3   *Entamoeba histolytica*. These protozoa cause amoebic dysentery. The black dots are red blood cells that have been engulfed. The nucleus can be seen in the lower right of the cell.

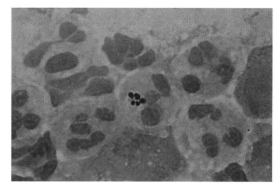

Plate 2.1   A clump of Gram positive staphylococci in or on a neutrophil ('pus cell') and surrounded by other neutrophils.

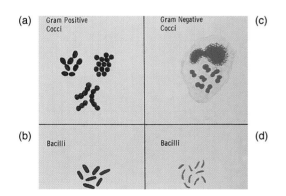

Plate 2.2   There are four main groups of bacteria: (a) Gram-positive cocci, (b) Gram-positive bacilli (rods), (c) Gram-negative cocci, and (d) Gram-negative bacilli (rods).

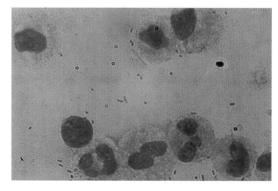

Plate 2.3   Cerebrospinal fluid from two patients with meningitis. Large mononuclear cells and neutrophils can be seen with a number of small Gram-negative rods. Provisional diagnosis: *Haemophilus influenzae* meningitis.

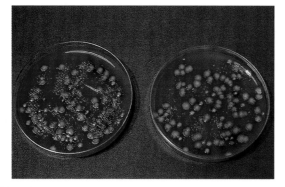

Plate 2.4 Large colonies of *Bacillus cereus*.

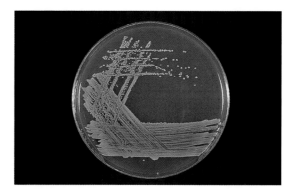

Plate 2.5 *Staphylococcus aureus*.

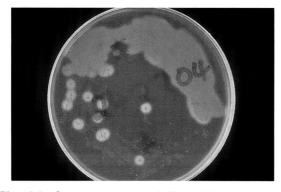

Plate 2.6 Streptococcus group A. Haemolysins produced by streptococcus lyse the red blood cells in blood agar, producing a clear area around the colonies.

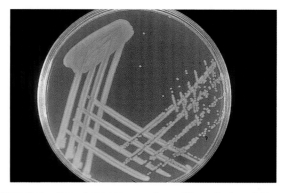

Plate 2.7 *Pseudomonas aeruginosa*. The colonies of *P. aeruginosa* appear green when grown on nutrient agar.

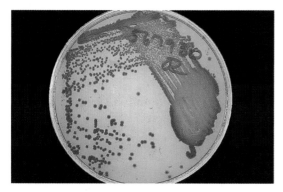

Plate 2.8 *Serratia marcescens*. The colonies of *S. marcescens* have a characteristic red coloration.

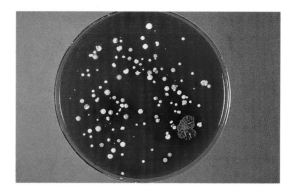

Plate 2.9 Mixed growth of organisms. Specimens often contain more than one type of bacterium, illustrated by the different forms of colony on this plate.

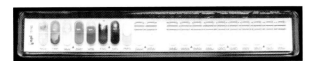

Plate 2.10 Each chamber contains a different biochemical test. Positive tests are indicated by a colour change and the set of results are used to identify the species of bacteria present.

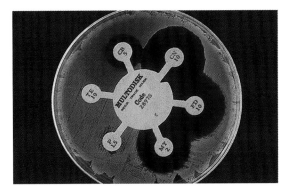

Plate 2.11 Antibiotic sensitivity testing. Antibiotics in each disc diffuse into the agar. Bacteria cannot grow around the discs unless they are resistant to the antibiotic in the disc.

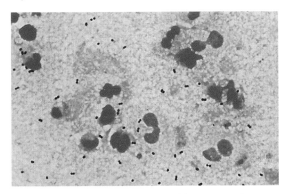

Plate 2.12 Sputum from a patient with suspected pneumonia. Gram-positive cocci, mostly in pairs, can be seen amongst the numerous large pus cells. Provisional diagnosis: pneumococcal pneumonia.

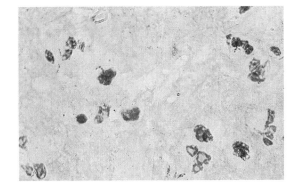

Plate 2.13 Tubercle bacilli appear as clumps of fine rods.

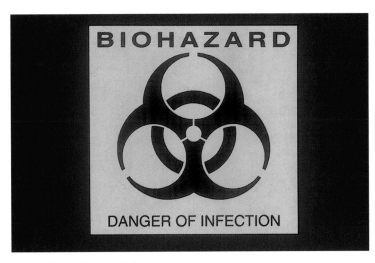

Plate 2.14 Biohazard label.

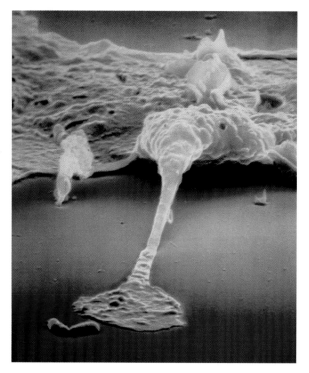

Plate 4.1 A macrophage extends a pseudopod to ingest a bacterium.

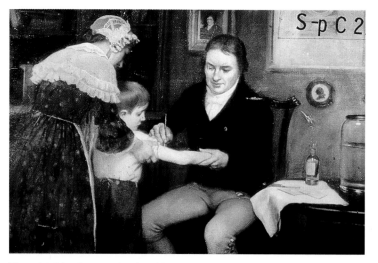

Plate 4.2 The first vaccination (Edward Jenner).

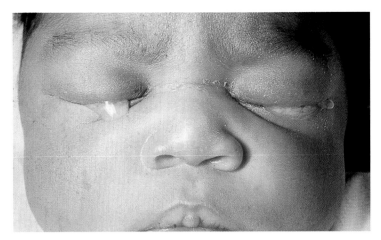

Plate 6.1 Staphylococcal infection of the eyes.

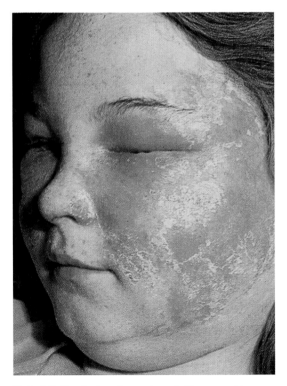

Plate 6.2 Erysipelas. An acute cellulitis caused by streptococcus.

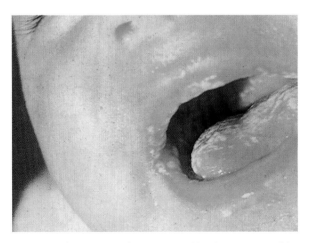

Plate 6.3 Oral thrush infection caused by the yeast candida.

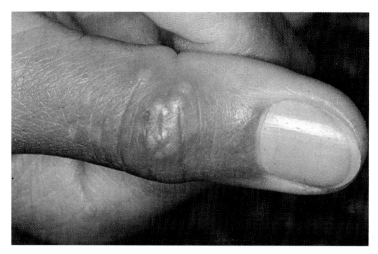

Plate 6.4 Herpetic whitlow caused by the herpes simplex virus.

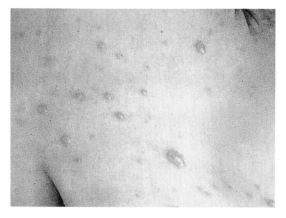

Plate 6.5 Chickenpox infection.

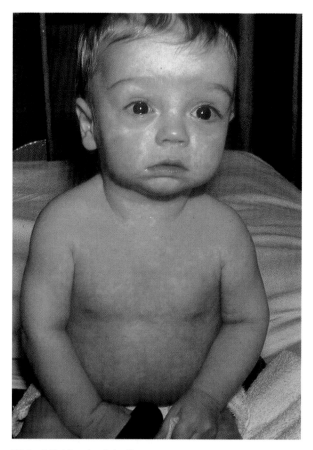

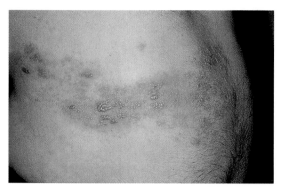

Plate 6.6 Herpes zoster (shingles).

Plate 6.7 Measles infection.

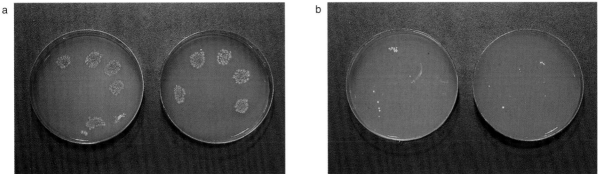

Plate 7.1 The effect of handwashing. (a) Fingertips pressed on to blood agar before washing. (b) Fingertips pressed on to blood agar after washing with soap and water.

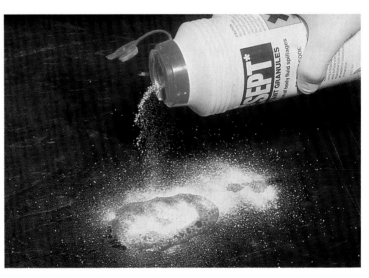

Plate 7.2 Chlorine-based granules can be used to soak up spills of blood.

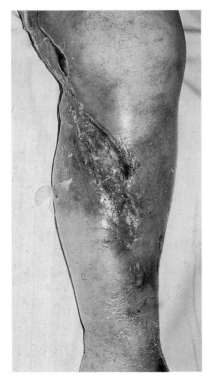

Plate 8.1 Infection in a surgical wound.

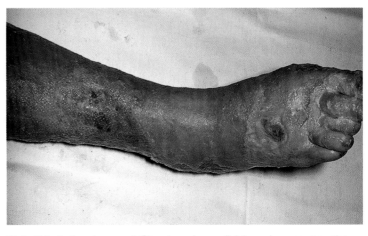

Plate 8.2 A chronic wound. Slough and superficial pus is present on the surface of the wound but with no signs of infection.

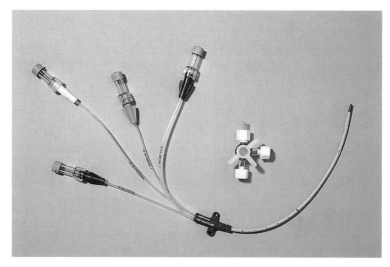

Plate 9.1 A set of access points and a three-way tap used with intravascular devices.

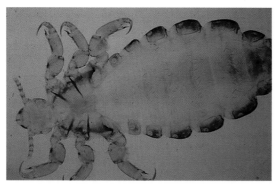

Plate 15.1 The female head louse (*Pediculus humanus capitis*).

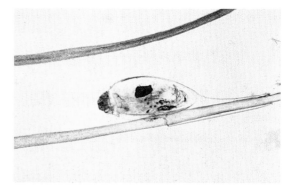

Plate 15.2 A louse egg (nit) attached to a hair.

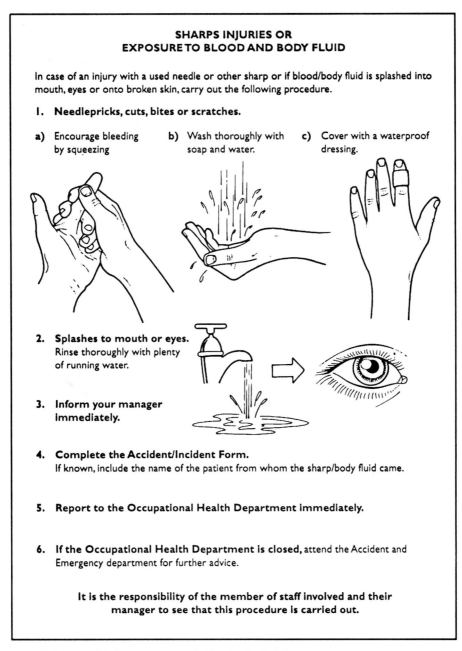

SHARPS INJURIES OR
EXPOSURE TO BLOOD AND BODY FLUID

In case of an injury with a used needle or other sharp or if blood/body fluid is splashed into mouth, eyes or onto broken skin, carry out the following procedure.

1.   Needlepricks, cuts, bites or scratches.

a) Encourage bleeding by squeezing

b) Wash thoroughly with soap and water.

c) Cover with a waterproof dressing.

2.   Splashes to mouth or eyes. Rinse thoroughly with plenty of running water.

3.   Inform your manager immediately.

4.   Complete the Accident/Incident Form. If known, include the name of the patient from whom the sharp/body fluid came.

5.   Report to the Occupational Health Department immediately.

6.   If the Occupational Health Department is closed, attend the Accident and Emergency department for further advice.

It is the responsibility of the member of staff involved and their manager to see that this procedure is carried out.

Fig. 7.6   Management of sharps injuries or exposure to blood or body fluid.

worker to be tested for HIV infection (including repeat testing 3, 6 and 12 months after the exposure). Storage of a baseline sample of the healthcare worker's blood is recommended for subsequent testing if the worker acquires HIV, to demonstrate that **seroconversion** occurred as a result of the incident.

Unfortunately, a significant proportion of needlestick injuries are not reported. Reasons commonly cited for non-reporting are lack of knowledge about the risk or standard procedures (Leliopoulou et al 1999, Waterman et al 1994). This illustrates the importance of clear, accessible policies and regular training for all groups of staff on sharps injuries, their significance, prevention and management.

Exposure-prone procedures

Healthcare workers who perform exposure-prone procedures (EPPs) (see Box 6.1) are not only at increased risk of acquiring bloodborne viruses from patients, but if infected themselves may transmit the virus to the patient during the procedure. Healthcare workers who perform EPPs should be immunized against hepatitis B virus (HBV) and their response to the vaccine checked (Department of Health 1993 – addendum 1996). A small proportion of people do not respond to HBV vaccine and can only perform EPPs provided they have been investigated to exclude HBV infection. Healthcare workers infected with HIV or who are HBV e antigen positive may not perform EPPs.

There is a legal requirement for employers to keep records of accidents to staff, and the records provide an important method of identifying hazardous procedures or inadequate equipment. Healthcare workers who acquire HIV or hepatitis B at work are considered eligible for industrial injury compensation. Accurate records of the time of the injury are essential if compensation is to be awarded.

Hepatitis B vaccination

A safe and effective **vaccine** against hepatitis B is available and recommended for immunization of healthcare workers who have direct contact with blood, blood-stained body fluids or tissues; for staff and clients in residential homes; for people with learning difficulties, where there is known to be a high prevalence of hepatitis B carriage and where behavioural problems increase the risk to staff. **Immunization** should also be considered for other staff who may not directly handle blood but who are at risk from injury by blood-contaminated sharps (Department of Health 1993).

Management of percutaneous or mucocutaneous exposure to material known, or strongly suspected, to be infected with HIV

Although the risk of acquiring HIV following a needlestick injury with infected blood is small, and even smaller for mucocutaneous exposures, there is evidence that the risk can be reduced by commencing prophylactic antiretroviral therapy as soon as possible after the exposure.

Currently, it is recommended that 4 weeks of post-exposure prophylaxis (PEP) should be given to healthcare workers exposed to high-risk body fluids or tissues percutaneously or mucocutaneously. The decision about whether to recommned PEP should take into account factors in the source patient that may increase the risk of transmission, such as the viral load if known, and the type of injury or exposure, for example whether the injury was deep or involved a hollow-bore needle. This type of risk assessment requires expert advice which is usually provided by the occupational health department. However, because PEP should be commenced within 1 h of the injury, starter packs containing the relevant drugs should be available in designated places (e.g. occupational health, accident and emergency, pharmacy departments) and specific staff given appropriate training to administer the drugs. The decision about whether treatment should be continued can then be made once expert advice is available.

Every healthcare organization should have a policy describing how to obtain immediate advice and treatment and who is responsible for long-term follow-up.

Healthcare workers who choose to take PEP will need regular monitoring during the period of therapy for side-effects to the drugs, and may also need psychological support (Department of Health 1997).

The safe disposal of waste

Waste from hospitals, clinics, surgeries, veterinary practices or pharmacies which may be toxic, hazardous or infectious is described as **clinical waste** (Box 7.15). Clinical waste needs to be properly segregated, handled, transported and disposed of to ensure it does not harm staff, patients, the public or the environment. The responsibilities of those who produce waste are described in the Environmental Protection Act 1990 and the Environmental Protection (Duty of Care) Regulations 1991.

Box 7.15   Definition of clinical waste

- human or animal tissue
- blood, other body fluids and excretions
- drugs, other pharmaceutical products
- soiled surgical dressings, swabs and instruments
- discarded syringes, needles, cartridges, broken glass and other sharp surgical instruments in contact with the above
- other waste arising from medical, nursing, dental, veterinary, pharmaceutical or other similar practice that may cause infection to persons coming into contact with it.

Source: Controlled Waste Regulations 1992

These Regulations require the producers of waste to manage it safely and to transfer it only to an authorised person. They also include duties to control polluting emissions and discharges to sewers, and producers must be satisfied that arrangements for treatment and disposal are appropriate. Most clinical waste is classified as controlled waste, requiring those who keep, treat or dispose of it to be licensed by an Environment Agency. Some is classified as 'special waste' (e.g. untreated waste from patients with viral haemorrhagic fever, pharmaceutical waste) and requires more stringent controls. Clinical waste must be incinerated and usually this requires designated incinerators that are able to meet the conditions for handling the waste and controlling emissions. Waste from human hygiene only (e.g. nappies, sanitary towels, incontinence pads) is considered as clinical waste only if it is generated from a population that cannot be assumed to be healthy, such as in a nursing home. Otherwise this waste can be treated as household waste.

Most hospitals employ external contractors to handle the disposal of waste, as on-site incinerators are usually unable to meet the stringent controls on emissions (Department of Health 1991).

Segregation of waste

Disposing of waste safely and cost-effectively depends on the proper segregation of different types of waste. This can be achieved by ensuring that waste is discarded into an appropriate colour-coded bag (Table 7.1). Information about where different waste items should be discarded should be clearly displayed and all staff should receive training. A considerable proportion of waste generated in clinical areas is not hazardous and can be safely disposed of as household waste. It is important to ensure that this waste is not sent for incineration to minimize both disposal costs and damage to the environment (Audit Commission 1997).

Waste bags must meet the appropriate regulations, and from January 2002 waste transported off-site will have to be enclosed in approved rigid containers (Health Services Advisory Committee 1999).

Handling and storage

Waste containers should be closed and sealed when three-quarters full to prevent spillage of the contents. Clinical waste should be labelled with the point of origin so that any problems that arise during disposal can be investigated. Sharps bins should be clearly visible and not enclosed inside plastic bags. If leakage

Table 7.1 Colour coding for the disposal of clinical waste

Colour of bag	Type of waste	Method of disposal
Black	Household waste, treated clinical waste (e.g. paper, food, flowers, etc.)	Landfill
Yellow	Clinical waste (e.g. material contaminated with blood or body fluid, human or animal tissue)	Incineration
Yellow sharps containers	Needles, syringes, broken glass and any other contaminated sharp item	Incineration
Blue or transparent with blue inscription	Waste for autoclaving (e.g. pathology specimens)	Landfill (once autoclaved)
Yellow, black stripes	Non-infectious human waste (e.g. sanitary towels, incontinence pads)	Landfill

Source: Health Services Advisory Committee (1999).

of body fluids is likely, a second bag or a special impervious container should be used. This particularly applies to the disposal of human tissue, which should not be mixed with other waste. The safest method of waste handling uses containers to transport waste bags and automatically discharges them into collection containers at the disposal point.

Training

Training is of key importance in ensuring safe and effective waste management, and should include all grades of staff involved in the process. It should cover the procedures specific to their work and the actions to take in an emergency, such as how to deal with and report accidents or spills. First aid kits and protective clothing must be readily available.

Waste policy

A local policy, accessible to all staff and taking account of different levels of knowledge, must be available. This should form part of the overall risk management strategy for the organization and should clearly define the responsibilities of line managers (e.g. for staff training). A waste manager should be designated to monitor, evaluate and review the policy regularly (Health Service Advisory Committee 1999, NHS Executive 1999).

Efforts to minimize the volume of clinical waste produced are essential, as incineration is both costly and damaging to the environment. Alternatives to incineration are being developed, such as sterilization and gasification, and increasing the use of reusable and recyclable materials has been proposed (Daschner & Dettenkofer 1997, Phillips 1999). Others advocate a reclassification of clinical waste as there is little evidence that it is more hazardous than household waste (Collins & Kennedy 1992).

Disposal of clinical waste in the home

The situation in the home is different as the amounts of clinical waste generated are much smaller and householders are exempt from the 'duty of care' for their own household waste. Waste produced and handled only by the patient or his or her family can usually be discarded with the normal household waste where, because it is mixed with large amounts of ordinary waste, it does not present a hazard. Used needles, such as those used by insulin-dependent diabetics, must not be discarded into household waste even if a device is used to destroy them. Arrangements for disposal should be made with local hospitals, clinics, pharmacies or local authorities (Health Services Advisory Committee 1999).

Healthcare workers who produce clinical waste in the home, for example community nurses or dialysis technicians, are obliged under the Health and Safety at Work Act to transport and dispose of the clinical waste safely but are exempted from being registered carriers. Small amounts of waste can be discarded into sharps bins and discarded via the employer's clinical waste disposal system. Employers may need to make arrangements for the collection and disposal of larger amounts (Environmental Protection Act 1990; Department of the Environment 1991). In Scotland, the importance of risk assessment in choosing a safe method of disposal for clinical waste is emphasized (NHS in Scotland 1998). This approach is particularly helpful for staff working in the community where a large proportion of clinical waste generated in the patient's home is of low risk and small volume.

Local authorities have a legal obligation to provide a collection service for infectious waste if requested, but this usually applies only to waste from dialysis patients or those known to be infected with blood-borne viruses. This in itself presents difficulties to the client who may fear possible loss of anonymity if an infected waste collection service is arranged for them. They may prefer to make their own arrangements to take waste to a health centre or GP surgery.

Linen

Used hospital linen may become contaminated with micro-organisms from patients with infection or when soiled by blood, excreta or other body fluids. It is decontaminated in the laundry process by a combination of detergent, dilution and mechanical action to remove particles, and temperatures that destroy micro-organisms. The process must include sufficient time for all parts of the load to reach an adequate temperature, for example 71°C for 3 min or 65°C for 10 min. Failure in the process has been associated with outbreaks of infection, notably with spore-forming bacteria such as *Bacillus cereus* (Barrie et al 1992).

Laundries that process hospital linen have to comply with Department of Health guidance on disinfection, staff protection and effluent control (NHS Executive 1995). Most linen will be washed in large tunnel washers that carry several batches at one time in a continuous process (Barrie 1994). Laundry staff sort linen by hand into batches of sheets, pillow cases, towels, etc. before washing and may be exposed to potential pathogens on soiled linen, particularly where instruments or 'sharps' are carelessly discarded with linen (Fig. 7.7). The risks may be minimized by the use of protective clothing and the segregation of particularly hazardous linen for disinfection by washing prior to sorting, for example linen from patients infected with enteric pathogens or heavily blood-stained linen (Table 7.2). This infected linen should be sealed in a water-soluble or soluble stitched bag and distinguished from other linen by placing it in a red outer bag. The water-soluble bag can then be removed from the outer bag and placed directly into a designated washing machine without opening (NHS Executive 1995).

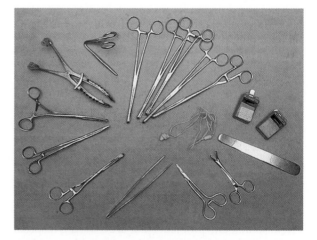

Fig. 7.7 Sharps found in laundry bags. These sharps present a considerable hazard to laundry staff.

Table 7.2 Categories of hospital linen

Category	Bag colour	Description	Recommended process
Used	White linen or clear plastic	Used, soiled and foul linen	Thermal disinfection by washing at 65°C for 10 min or 71°C for 3 min
Infected	Water-soluble bag, with red outer bag	Linen used by patients with certain infectious diseases or as advised by Infection Control Team	Not sorted prior to washing, thermal disinfection as used linen
Heat-labile	Orange stripe	Fabrics likely to be damaged by thermal disinfection (e.g. wool)	Wash at 40°C and add hypochlorite to penultimate rinse

Source: NHS Executive (1995).

Micro-organisms that remain after washing may also be destroyed by tumble drying and ironing. Some fabrics are damaged by high wash temperatures and must be decontaminated by the addition of a chemical disinfectant to the rinse cycle instead. Bedlinen made from these types of fabrics should be avoided because these chemicals damage the fire-retardancy of the fabric.

Contaminated linen may release pathogens on lint and should be handled carefully on the ward prior to disposal (Overton 1988). See Guidelines for practice.

Some wards use domestic washing machines to wash patients' clothing. Whilst satisfactory for this purpose, they should not be used to wash bedlinen or other items that will be used by different patients. The normal wash temperatures of 40°C or 60°C may not achieve satisfactory heat disinfection and the items can be difficult to dry quickly and thoroughly.

Increasingly, duvets are used in clinical areas. Fabric duvets must withstand a wash temperature of 71°C and comply with Department of Health standards of fire retardancy. The duvet cover should be washed between patients and when soiled. The duvet should be washed when soiled and at least once every three months (Ayton 1983, Croton 1990). PVC-coated duvets should be cleaned with detergent and water between patients in the same way as mattresses.

In the home, contaminated linen can be decontaminated in a hot wash of a domestic washing machine (UK Health Departments 1998).

Uniforms

Uniforms worn by staff in clinical areas may become contaminated by a range of pathogens, although such contamination is unlikely to be heavy unless there has been direct contact with body fluids, infected wounds or burns (Hambreaus 1973, Speers et al 1969). The appropriate use of plastic aprons will protect the uniform from contamination in most circumstances (Babb et al 1983). Uniforms should be decontaminated in the same way as other hospital linen, by washing in hot water (or water as hot as the fabric will tolerate) either in hospital or domestic washing machines.

Excreta

Excreta and other body fluids may contain considerable numbers of pathogens and must be discarded safely to minimize the risk of transmission of infection to others. Excreta should be discarded directly into the bedpan washer, macerator or toilet. There is no advantage in adding disinfectant to excreta prior to disposal as it is unlikely to penetrate the organic material. Pathogens are constantly introduced to the drainage system from infected people in the community and there is therefore no value in attempting to remove them from the relatively small amounts entering the system from hospitals.

To prevent the transmission of micro-organisms between patients on bedpans these should be decontaminated in a bedpan washer with a heat-disinfection cycle. The bedpan is disinfected during the cycle by flushing with water at a temperature of 80°C for a few minutes after washing. Faults in these machines must be reported promptly.

Guidelines for practice: safe handling of linen

- Wear a plastic apron during bed-making and discard afterwards
- Wash hands after contact with soiled linen
- Place linen carefully into an appropriate linen bag
- Use linen bags that comply with Health Service guidance (HSG(95)18; NHS Executive 1995)
- Place linen that is heavily soaked in body fluid in a plastic bag to prevent leakage
- Securely fasten the linen bag when full

Disposable bedpans should be discarded into bedpan macerators. These should have an effective seal around the door to prevent the escape of aerosols that may contain pathogenic micro-organisms.

Decontamination of equipment

There are numerous examples of infection transmitted between patients on inadequately decontaminated equipment, and concerns about the transmission of HIV have highlighted the need to ensure that equipment used for invasive procedures is properly decontaminated after every patient, not only those known to be infected.

The method selected should be sufficient to prevent transmission of any pathogens and usually it should not be necessary to use a higher level of decontamination after equipment has been used on patients known to have an infection.

In some instances it is possible to reduce exposure to equipment contaminated by body fluid by changing practice. For example, swabs used during operations present a considerable hazard to staff who handle and count them on to a swab rack. This risk can be reduced if such swabs are counted directly into clear plastic bags so that contamination of the swab rack can be avoided.

Departments such as intensive care and theatres, which use suction frequently, may choose a disposable suction system to avoid the need to decontaminate suction jars.

Any equipment contaminated by body fluid that requires servicing or repair must be decontaminated before it is given to the engineer or returned to the manufacturer (NHS Management Executive 1993). The principles of decontamination are discussed in more detail in Chapter 13.

Treatment of spills of blood or body fluid

Dealing with spills of blood or body fluid may expose the healthcare worker to bloodborne viruses or other pathogens. The task can be carried out more safely if any pathogens in the spillage are first destroyed by a disinfectant (Coates & Wilson 1989).

High concentration chlorine-releasing compounds provide the most economical and effective method of treating many spills, especially large spills of blood (Box 7.16). Chlorine-releasing granules have the advantage of containing the spill rather than adding to it; they have a longer shelf-life than hypochlorite solutions and are more portable (Plate 7.2). In the home, good quality thick bleaches, such as Domestos or Parazone, contain a high concentration of available chlorine (see p. 234) and

---

Box 7.16 Methods of treating body fluid spills

Chlorine-releasing granules*
- put on disposable gloves and apron
- cover fluid completely with chlorine granules
- leave for 2 min
- remove granules and discard into yellow waste bag
- wash the area with detergent and water

Hypochlorite solution*
- put on disposable gloves and apron
- cover spill with disposable paper towels
- pour hypochlorite (10 000 ppm available chlorine) over the towels
- leave for 2 min
- remove towels and discard into a yellow waste bag
- wash area with detergent and water

Detergent and water
- put on disposable gloves and apron
- soak up spill with disposable paper towels
- discard into a yellow waste bag
- wash area with detergent and water

*Do not use for large spillages of urine

---

can be diluted and used to treat spills. However, chlorine compounds are corrosive to many materials and will bleach the colour from fabrics. They should not be used on carpets or furnishings and residual disinfectant should be removed from surfaces with detergent and water. If chlorine disinfectants cannot be used, spills should be removed using detergent and hot water.

Unfortunately, acidic solutions such as urine may react with the hypochlorite and cause the release of chlorine vapour. Hypochlorite solutions should therefore not be used on large urine spills (Department of Health 1990).

It may be impractical to treat large spills of blood or body fluid such as may occur in labour wards or operating theatres with hypochlorite. The spill should be soaked up with disposable paper towels or wipes and discarded into a yellow waste bag. The area should then be cleaned with detergent and water.

EDUCATION AND TRAINING

The adoption of a routine standard of infection control is essential for the safety of both patients and staff (Fig. 7.8). Employers have an obligation to protect workers from hazards encountered during their work, including microbiological hazards (COSHH Regulations 1999, Health and Safety at Work Act 1974, HSE 1992a).

The health and safety legislation acknowledges the importance of training and the provision of suitable equipment in establishing safe working practices. The

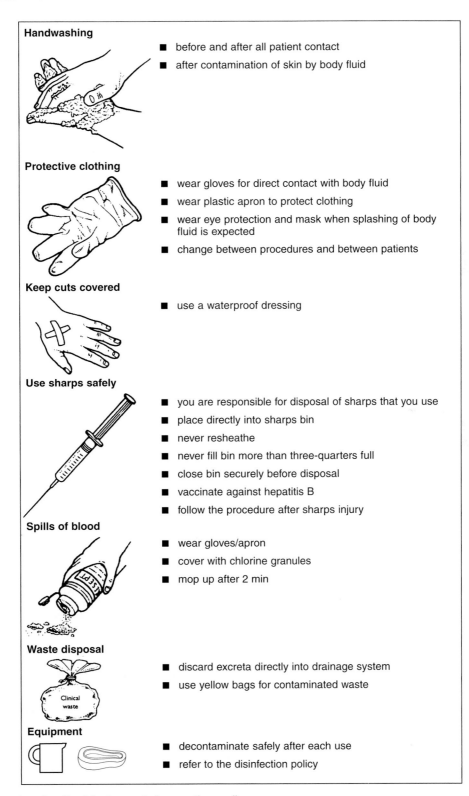

Handwashing

- before and after all patient contact
- after contamination of skin by body fluid

Protective clothing

- wear gloves for direct contact with body fluid
- wear plastic apron to protect clothing
- wear eye protection and mask when splashing of body fluid is expected
- change between procedures and between patients

Keep cuts covered

- use a waterproof dressing

Use sharps safely

- you are responsible for disposal of sharps that you use
- place directly into sharps bin
- never resheathe
- never fill bin more than three-quarters full
- close bin securely before disposal
- vaccinate against hepatitis B
- follow the procedure after sharps injury

Spills of blood

- wear gloves/apron
- cover with chlorine granules
- mop up after 2 min

Waste disposal

- discard excreta directly into drainage system
- use yellow bags for contaminated waste

Equipment

- decontaminate safely after each use
- refer to the disinfection policy

Fig. 7.8   Examples of routine infection control precautions policy.

adoption of a routine standard of infection control depends on regular and appropriate education and training to ensure that all healthcare workers understand the procedures and know what standards are expected (Fahey et al 1991). Gershon et al (1995), in their assessment of compliance with universal precautions amongst hospital staff, identified organizational commitment to safety as a key factor in increasing compliance.

Written policies or standards should be developed to clarify the local arrangements for minimizing the risks from hazards identified by the risk assessment process (see p. 133), for example situations where the use of protective clothing is indicated, local arrangements for the disposal of sharps, and recommended methods of passing used instruments in theatre. Gerberding (1993) emphasizes the importance of involving all groups of staff in the process of identifying hazards and risk management solutions. These policies can form the basis for informing and training all staff who work in the area, and then need to be the subject of regular monitoring and review. Seto et al (1989) suggest that education programmes should also actively involve staff if they are to be effective in altering behaviour and maintaining change over a prolonged period. Essential equipment such as protective clothing and sharps containers must also be readily available in all clinical areas.

REFERENCES

Adams D, Bagg J, Limaye M et al (1992) A clinical evaluation of glove washing and re-use in dental practice. *J. Hosp. Infect.*, **20**: 153–62.

Advisory Committee on Dangerous Pathogens (1996) *Microbiological Risk Assessment: An Interim Report.* HMSO, London.

Albert RK, Condie F (1981) Handwashing patterns in medical intensive care units. *N. Engl. J. Med.*, **304**: 1465–6.

Ansari SA, Springthorpe VS, Sattar SA et al (1991a) Potential role of hands in the spread of respiratory viral infections: studies with human parainfluenza virus 3 and rhinovirus 14. *J. Clin. Microbiol.*, **29**: 2115–19.

Ansari SA, Springthorpe VS, Sattar SA et al (1991b) Comparison of cloth, paper and warm air drying in eliminating viruses and bacteria from washed hands. *Am. J. Infect. Control*, **9**: 243–9.

Archibald L, Corl A, Shah B et al (1997a) *Serratia marcescens* outbreak associated with extrinsic contamination of 1% chloroxylenol soap. *Infect. Control Hosp. Epidemiol.*, **18**: 704–9.

Archibald LK, Manning ML, Bell LM et al (1997b) Patient density, nurse-to-nurse patient ratio and nosocomial infection risk in a pediatric cardiac intensive care unit. *Pediatr. Infect. Dis. J.*, **16**: 1045–8.

Audit Commission (1997) *Getting Sorted – The Safe and Economic Management of Hospital Waste.* Bookpoint, Oxon.

Ayliffe GAJ (1991) Masks in surgery? *J. Hosp. Infect.*, **18**: 165–6.

Ayliffe GAJ, Babb JR, Quoraishi AH et al (1978) A test for hygienic hand disinfection. *J. Clin. Pathol.*, **31**: 923.

Ayliffe GAJ, Babb JR, Davies JG et al (1988) Hand disinfection: a comparison of various agents in laboratory and ward studies. *J. Hosp. Infect.*, **11**: 226–43.

Ayton M (1983) Continental quilts – their use in hospitals. *Nursing Times*, **79**(30): 64–5.

Babb JR, Davies JG, Ayliffe GAJ (1983) Contamination of protective clothing and nurses' uniforms in an isolation ward. *J. Hosp. Infect.*, **4**: 49–57.

Barrie D (1994) How hospital linen and laundry services are provided. *J. Hosp. Infect.*, **27**(3): 219–36.

Barrie D, Wilson J, Hoffman PN, Kramer J (1992) *Bacillus cereus* meningitis in two neurosurgical patients: an investigation into the source of the organism. *J. Infect.*, **25**: 291–7.

Becker MH, Janz NK, Band J et al (1990) Non-compliance with universal precautions policy: why do physicians and nurses recap needles? *Am. J. Infect. Control*, **18**: 232–9.

Belkin NL (1997) The evolution of the surgical mask: filtering efficiency versus effectiveness. *Infect. Control Hosp. Epidemic.*, **18**(1): 49–56.

Bellamy K, Alcock R, Babbb JR et al (1993) A test for the assessment of 'hygienic' hand disinfection using rotavirus. *J. Hosp. Infect.*, **24**: 201–10.

Booth (1996) Latex allergy: a growing problem in healthcare. *Prof. Nurse*, **11**: 316–19.

British Standards Institution (1990) *Specification for Sharps Containers. BS 7320.* BSI, London.

British Standards Institution (1994) *Medical Gloves for Surgical Use. BS EN455.* BSI, London.

British Standards Institution (1999) *Eye Protection for Industrial and Other Uses. Guidance on Selection, Use and Maintenance. BS 7028.* BSI, London.

Bryan JL, Cohran J, Larson EL (1995) Handwashing: a ritual revisited. *Crit. Care Nurs. Clin. North Am.*, **4**: 617–25.

Burnie JP, Odd FC, Lee W et al (1985) Outbreak of systemic *Candida albicans* in intensive care unit caused by cross-infection. *BMJ*, **290**: 746–8.

Callaghan I (1998) Bacterial contamination of nurses' uniforms: a study. *Nursing Standard*, **13**(1): 37–42.

Casewell M, Phillips I (1977) Hands as a route of transmission for *Klebsiella* species. *BMJ*, **ii**: 1315–17.

Centers for Disease Control (1987) Recommendations for the prevention of HIV transmission in healthcare settings. *MMWR*, **36**: 2S.

Centers for Disease Control (1988) Update: Universal precautions for prevention of transmission of human immunodeficiency virus, hepatitis B virus and other bloodborne pathogens in healthcare settings. *MMWR*, **37**: 24.

Centers for Disease Control (1993) Recommended infection control practices in dentistry. *MMWR*, **42**: RR1–8.

Collins CH, Kennedy DA (1992) The microbiological hazards of municipal and clinical wastes. *J. Appl. Bacteriol.*, **73**: 1–6.

Coates D, Wilson M (1989) Use of dichloroisocyanurate granules for spills of body fluids. *J. Hosp. Infect.*, **13**: 241–52.

Cookson B, Peters B, Webster M et al (1989) Staff carriage of epidemic methicillin-resistant *Staphylococcus aureus*. *J. Clin. Microbiol.*, **27**: 1471–6.

Croton CM (1990) Duvets on trial. *Nursing Times*, **86**(26): 63–7.

Daschner FD, Dettenkofer M (1997) Protecting the patient and the environment – new aspects and challenges in hospital infection control. *J. Hosp. Infect.*, **36**: 7–16.

Davies MS (1994) Blunt-tipped suture needles. *Inf. Control. Hosp. Epidemiol.*, **15**(4): 191.

De Groot-Kosolcharoen J, Jones JM (1989) Permeability of latex and vinyl gloves to water and blood. *Am. J. Infect. Control*, **17**: 196–201.

Department of the Environment (1991) Environmental Protection Act 1990. *Waste Management: The Duty of Care. A Code of Practice*. HMSO, London.

Department of Health (1990) Spills of urine: potential risk of misuse of chlorine-releasing disinfecting agents. *Safety Advice Bulletin*, **59**(90): 41.

Department of Health (1991) *Strategic Guide to Waste Management*. Circular EL(90)M/I. DoH, London.

Department of Health (1993) *Protecting Health Care Workers and Patients from Hepatitis B: Recommendations of the Advisory Group on Hepatitis*. HSG(93)40. Addendum (1996) EL(96)77. DoH, London.

Department of Health (1997) *Guidance on Post-exposure Prophylaxis for Health Care Workers Occupationally Exposed to HIV*. PL/CO(97)1. DoH, London.

Do AN, Ray BJ, Bannerjee SN et al (1999) Bloodstream infection associated with needle-less device use and the importance of infection control practice in the home healthcare setting. *J. Infect. Dis.*, **179**: 442–8.

Eisenstein HC, Smith DA (1992) Epidemiology of reported sharps injuries in tertiary care hospital. *J. Hosp. Infect.*, **20**: 271–80.

Fahey BJ, Koziol DE, Banks SM et al (1991) Frequency of nonparenteral occupational exposures to blood and body fluids before and after universal precautions training. *Am. J. Med.*, **90**: 145–53.

Garner JS (1996) Hospital Infection Control Practices Advisory Committee. Guideline for isolation precautions in hospitals. *Infect. Control Hosp. Epidemiol.*, **17**(1): 54–80.

Garner JS, Hierholzer WJ (1993) Controversies in isolation policies and practice. In *Prevention and Control of Nosocomial Infections*, 2nd edn, pp. 70–81 (RP Wenzel, ed.). Williams & Wilkins, Baltimore, MD.

George RH, Gully PR, Gill ON et al (1986) An outbreak of tuberculosis in a children's hospital. *J. Hosp. Infect.*, **8**: 129–42.

Gerberding JL (1993) Procedure-specific infection control for preventing intra-operative blood exposures. *Am. J. Infect. Control.*, **21**: 364–7.

Gerberding JL, Littell C, Tarkington A et al (1990) Risk exposure of surgical personnel to patients' blood during surgery at San Francisco general hospital. *New. Engl. J. Med.*, **322**: 1788–93.

Gerding DN, Johnson S, Olson M et al (1988) Prospective controlled study of vinyl glove use to interrupt *Clostridium difficile* nosocomial transmission. *Abstracts of the 88th Annual Meeting American Society for Microbiology*, **416**: L32.

Gershon RM, Vlahor D, Felknor SA et al (1995) Compliance with universal precautions among healthcare workers at three regional hospitals. *Am. J. Infect. Control*, **23**: 225–36.

Glenister HM, Taylor LJ, Bartlett CLR et al (1992) An 11 month incidence study of infections in ward of a district general hospital. *J. Hosp. Infect.*, **21**(4): 261–73.

Glynn A, Ward V, Wilson J (1997) *Hospital Acquired Infection: Surveillance, Policies and Practice*. PHLS, London.

Gorman LJ, Sanai L, Notman W et al (1993) Cross-infection in an intensive care unit by *Klebsiella pneumoniae* from ventilator condensate. *J. Hosp. Infect.*, **23**(1): 27–34.

Gould D (1993) Assessing nurses' hand decontamination performance. *Nursing Times*, **89**(25): 47–50.

Greaves WL, Kraiser AB, Alford RH et al (1980) The problem of herpatic whitlow among hospital personnel. *Infect. Control.*, **1**: 181–5.

Haley RW, Culver DH, White JW et al (1985) The efficacy of surveillance and control programs in preventing nosocomial infections in US hospitals. *Am. J. Epidemiol.*, **121**: 182–205.

Hall CB (1981) Nosocomial viral respiratory infections: perennial weeds on paediatric wards. *Am. J. Med.*, **70**: 670–6.

Hambreaus A (1973) Transfer of *Staphylococcus aureus* via nurses' uniforms. *J. Hyg. Camb.*, **71**: 799–14.

Handwashing Liaison Group (1999) Handwashing. *BMJ*, **318**: 686.

Health and Safety Executive (1992a) *The Management of Health and Safety at Work Regulations* (The Management Regulations). HSE Books, Sudbury.

Health and Safety Executive (1992b) *Personal Protective Equipment at Work. Regulations* (EEC Directive). HMSO, London.

Health Services Advisory Committee (1999) *Safe Disposal of Clinical Waste*. HSE Books, Sudbury.

Hoffman PN, Wilson JA (1994) Hands, hygiene and hospitals. *PHLS Micro. Dig.*, **11**(4): 211–16.

Hoffman PN, Cooke EM, McCarville MR et al (1985) Micro-organisms isolated from skin under wedding rings worn by hospital staff. *BMJ*, **290**: 206–7.

Holborn J (1990) Wet strike through and the transfer of bacteria through operating barrier fabrics. *Hygiene Med.*, **15**: 15–20.

Hubble MJ, Weale AE, Perez JV et al (1996) Clothing in laminar flow operating theatres. *J. Hosp. Infect.*, **32**: 1–7.

Jackson MJ, Lynch P (1985) Isolation practices: a historical perspective. *Am. J. Infect. Control*, **13**: 21–31.

Jagger J, Hunt EH, Brand-Elnaggar J et al (1988) Rates of needlestick injury caused by various devices in a university hospital. *N. Engl. J. Med.*, **318**: 284–8.

Jagger I, Hunt EH, Pearson RD (1990) Sharp object injuries in the hospital: causes and strategies for prevention. *Am. J. Infect. Control*, **18**: 227–31.

Johnson G (1998) Latex allergy: reducing the risks. *Nursing Times*, **94**(44): 69–73.

Kaplan LM, McGuckin M (1986) Increasing handwashing compliance with more accessible sinks. *Infect. Control*, **7**: 408–9.

Klein BS, Perloff WH, Maki DG (1989) Reduction of nosocomial infection during pediatric intensive care by protective isolation. *N. Engl. J. Med.*, **320**: 1714–21.

Korniewicz DM, Laughton BE, Howard CYR et al (1990) Leakage of virus through used vinyl and latex examination gloves. *J. Clin. Microbiol.*, **28**(4): 787–8.

Larson E, Leyden JJ, McGinley KJ et al (1986) Physiologic and microbiologic changes in skin related to frequent handwashing. *Infect. Control*, **7**: 59–63.

Larson EL, Bryan JL, Adler LM et al (1997) A multifaceted approach to changing handwashing behaviour. *Infect. Control Hosp. Epidemiol.*, **25**: 3–10.

Leclair JM, Freeman J, Sullivan BF et al (1987) Prevention of nosocomial respiratory syncitial virus infections through compliance with glove and gown isolation precautions. *N. Engl. J. Med.*, **6**: 317–34.

Leliopoulou C, Waterman H, Chakrabarty S (1999) Nurses failure to appreciate the risk of infection due to needle stick accidents: a hospital based survey. *J. Hosp. Infect.*, **42**: 53–9.

Lowbury EJL, Lilley HA (1973) Use of 4% chlorhexidine detergent solution (Hibiscrub) and other methods of skin disinfection in wards. *J. Hyg. (Camb.)*, **76**: 75.

Lynch P, Jackson MM, Cummings MJ et al (1987) Rethinking the role of isolation practices in the prevention of nosocomial infections. *Ann. Intern. Med.*, **107**: 243–6.

Lynch P, Cummings MJ, Roberts PL et al (1990) Implementing and evaluating a system of generic infection control precautions: body substance isolation. *Am. J. Infect. Control*, **18**: 1–13.

McGinley KL, Larson EL, Leyden JJ (1988) Composition and density of microflora in the subungual space of the hand. *J. Clin. Microbiol.*, **26**: 950–3.

Mackintosh CA, Hoffman PN (1984) An extended model for the transfer of micro-organisms and the effect of alcohol disinfection. *J. Hyg.*, **92**: 345–55.

Marples RR, Towers AG (1979) A laboratory model for the investigation of contact transfer of micro-organisms. *J. Hyg.*, **82**: 237–48.

Medical Devices Agency (1993) *Use and Management of Sharps Containers*. Action Bulletin No. 102. DoH, Wetherby, UK.

Medical Devices Agency (1996) *Latex Sensitisation in the Healthcare Setting (Use of Latex Gloves)*. DB9601. DoH, Wetherby, UK.

Medical Devices Agency (1998) *Powdered Latex Medical Gloves (Surgeons and Examination)*. Safety Notice SN9825. HMSO, London.

Moolenaar RL, Crutcher JM, San Joaquin VN et al (2000) A prolonged outbreak of *Pseudomonas aeruginosa* in a neonatal intensive care unit: did staff fingernails play a role in disease transmission? *Infect. Control Hosp. Epidemiol.*, **21**: 80–5.

Morse LJ, Schonbek LE (1968) Hand lotions and potential nosocomial hazard. *N. Engl. J. Med.*, **278**: 376–8.

National Audit Office (1999) *The Management of Medical Equipment in Acute NHS Trusts in England*. The Stationery Office, London.

National Audit Office (2000) *The Management and Control of Hospital Acquired Infection in Acute NHS Trusts in England. Report by the Comptroller and Auditor General*. The Stationery Office, London.

National Health Service in Scotland (1998) *Management and Disposal of Clinical Waste*. Scottish Hospital Technical Note No. 3. Estates Environment Forum, April 1998.

NHS Executive (1995) *Hospital Laundry Arrangements for Used and Infected Linen*. HSG(95)18. HMSO, London.

NHS Executive (1999) *Controls Assurance Standard. Waste Management*. DoH, Wetherby, UK.

NHS Management Executive (1993) *Decontamination of Equipment Prior to Inspection, Service or Repair*. HSG(93)26. HMSO, London.

Ojajärvi J, Mäkelä P, Rautasalo I (1977) Failure of hand disinfection with frequent handwashing: a need for prolonged field studies. *J. Hyg. (Camb.)*, **79**: 107–12.

Olsen RJ, Lynch P, Coyle MB et al (1993) Examination gloves as barriers to hand contamination in clinical practice. *JAMA*, **270**(3): 350–3.

Overton E (1988) Bed-making and bacteria. *Nursing Times*, **85**(9): 69–71.

Palmer JD, Rickett JWS (1992) The mechanisms and risks of surgical glove perforation *J. Hosp. Infect.*, **22**: 279–86.

Patterson JE, Vecchio J, Pantelick EL (1991) Association of contaminated gloves with transmission of *Acinetobacter calcoaceticus* var. *anitratus* in an intensive care unit. *Am. J. Med.*, **91**: 479–83.

Phillips G (1999) Microbiological aspects of clinical waste. *J. Hosp. Infect.*, **41**: 1–6.

Pittet D, Dharan S, Touveneau S et al (1999) Bacterial contamination of the hands of hospital staff during routine patients care. *Arch. Intern. Med.*, **159**: 821–6.

Pratt RA, Pellowe CM, Loveday HP et al (2001) The Epic project: developing national evidence-based guidelines for preventing healthcare associated infections. *J. Hosp. Infect.*, **47**: Supp. A.

Public Health Laboratory Service AIDS & STD Centre (1998) Occupational transmission of HIV infection. *CDR Weekly*, **8**(22): 193.

Public Health Laboratory Service AIDS & STD Centre (1999) Occupational transmission of HIV. Summary of published reports. Online. Available: http://www.phls.co.uk

Reid JA, Breckon D, Hunter PR (1990) Infection of staff during an outbreak of viral gastro-enteritis in an elderly persons' home. *J. Hosp. Infect.*, **16**: 81–6.

Reybrouck G (1983) Role of the hands in the spread of nosocomial infections. 1. *J. Hosp. Infect.*, **4**: 103–10.

Ross DJ, Cherry NM, McDonald JC (1998) Occupationally acquired infectious disease in the United Kingdom: 1996 to 1997. *Commun. Dis. Public Health*, **1**(2): 98–102.

Rotter M, Koeller W, Wewalka G (1980) Povidone–iodine and chlorhexidine gluconate containing detergents for disinfection of hands. *J. Hosp. Infect.*, **1**: 49–58.

Royal College of Pathologists (1992) *HIV Infection: Hazards of Transmission to Patients and Health Care Workers During Invasive Procedures*. Royal College of Pathologists, London.

Saghafi L, Raselli P, Francillon C et al (1992) Exposure to blood during various procedures: results of two surveys before and after implementation of universal precautions. *Am. J. Infect. Control*, **20**(2): 53–7.

Samadi AR, Huq MI, Ahmed QS (1983) Detection of rotavirus in handwashings of attendants of children with diarrhoea. *BMJ*, **286**: 188.

Sanderson PJ, Weissler S (1992) Recovery of coliforms from the hands of nurses and patients: activities leading to contamination. *J. Hosp. Infect.*, **21**: 85–93.

Sartor C, Jacomo V, Duvivier C et al (2000) Nosocomial *Serratia marcescens* infections associated with extrinsic contamination of liquid non-medicated soap. *Infect. Control Hosp. Epidemiol.*, **21**: 196–9.

Scanlon JW, Leikkanen M (1973) The use of fluorescein powder for evaluating contamination in a newborn nursery. *J. Pediatr.*, **82**: 966–71.

Seto WH, Ching PTY, Fung JPM et al (1989) The role of communication in the alteration of patient-care practices in hospital – a prospective study. *J. Hosp. Infect.*, **14**: 29–37.

Short LJ, Bell DM (1993) Risk of occupational infection with bloodborne pathogens in operating and delivery room settings. *Am J. Infect. Control*, **21**: 343–50.

Simmons B, Bryant J, Neiman K et al (1990) The role of handwashing in prevention of endemic intensive care unit infections. *Infect. Control Hosp. Epidemiol.*, **11**(11): 589–94.

Speers R, Shooter RA, Gaya H et al (1969) Contamination of nurses' uniforms with *Staphylococcus aureus*. *Lancet*, **ii**: 233–5.

Speller DCE, Shanson DC, Ayliffe GAJ et al (1990) Acquired immune deficiency syndrome. Recommendations of a Working Party of the Hospital Infection Society. *J. Hosp. Infect.*, **15**: 17–34.

Sprunt K, Redman W, Leidy G (1973) Antibacterial effectiveness of routine handwashing. *Pediatrics*, **52**: 264–71.

Stafford K, Kitchen VS, Smith JR et al (1995) Reducing the risk of bloodborne infection in surgical practice. *Br. J. Obstet. Gynaecol.*, **102**(6): 439–41.

Taylor L (1978) An evaluation of handwashing techniques. *Nursing Times*, **74**: 108–10.

Telford GL, Quebberman EJ (1993) Assessing the risk of blood exposure in the operating theatre. *Am. J. Infect. Control*, **21**: 351–6.

Tokars JI, Bell DM, Culver DH et al (1992) Percutaneous injuries during surgical procedures. *JAMA*, **267**: 2899–904.

Tokars JI, Culver DH, Mendelson MH et al (1995) Skin and mucous membrane contacts with blood during surgical procedures: risk and prevention. *Infect. Control Hosp. Epidemiol.*, **16**: 703–11.

Tomlinson D (1987) To clean or not to clean? *Nursing Times*, **83**: 71–5.

UK Health Departments (1990) *Guidance for Clinical Health Care Workers: Protection Against Infection with HIV and Hepatitis Viruses*. Recommendations of the Expert Advisory Group on AIDS. HMSO, London.

UK Health Departments (1994) *AIDS/HIV Infected Health Care Workers: Guidance on the Management of Infected Health Care Workers and Patient Notification*. Expert Advisory Group on AIDS. HMSO, London.

UK Health Departments (1998) *Guidance for Clinical Health Care Workers: Protection Against Infection with Blood Borne Viruses. Recommendation of the Expert Advisory Group on AIDS and Advisory Group on Hepatitis*. Department of Health, Wetherby, UK.

Wade JJ, Desai N, Casewell MW (1991) Hygienic hand disinfection for the removal of epidemic vancomycin-resistant *Enterococcus faecium* and gentamicin-resistant *Enterobacter cloacae*. *J. Hosp. Infect.*, **18**(3): 211–18.

Ward V, Wilson J, Glynn A et al (1997) *Preventing Hospital-acquired Infection: Clinical Guidelines*. PHLS, London.

Waterman J, Jankowski R, Madan I (1994) Under-reporting of needlestick injuries by medical students. *J. Hosp. Infect.*, **26**: 149–53.

Weinstein RA, Kabins SA (1981) Strategies for prevention and control of multiple drug-resistant nosocomial infection. *Am. J. Med.*, **70**: 449–54.

Weltman AC, Short LJ, Mendelson MH et al (1995) Disposal – related sharps injuries at a New York City teaching hospital. *Infect. Control Hosp. Epidemiol.*, **16**: 268–74.

West DJ (1984) The risk of hepatitis B infection among health professionals in the United States: a review. *Am. J. Med. Sci.*, **287**: 26–33.

Williams E, Buckles A (1988) A lack of motivation. *Nursing Times*, **84**: 60–4.

Wilson J, Breedon P (1990) Universal precautions. *Nursing Times*, **86**: 67–70.

Yessin MS, Lieri MB, Fischer TJ et al (1994) Latex allergy in hospital employees. *Ann. Allergy*, **72**(3): 245–9.

Zimakoff J, Kjelsberg AB, Larse SO et al (1992) A multicenter questionnaire investigation of the attitudes toward hand hygiene, assessed by staff in fifteen hospitals in Denmark and Norway. *Am. J. Infect. Control*, **23**: 251–69.

Zimmermann C, Junghams K (1996) Use of a new peroration indicator system. *Hyg. Med.*, **21**: 9.

FURTHER READING

Ayton M (1983) Continental quilts – their use in hospitals. *Nursing Times*, **July 27**: 64–5.

British Dental Association (1996) *Infection Control in Dentistry*. Advice Sheet 12. BDA Advisory Service, London.

British Medical Association (1990) *A Code of Practice for the Safe Use and Disposal of Sharps*. BMA, London.

Health & Safety Executive (1992) *Personal Protective Equipment at Work Regulations: Guidance on Regulations*. The Stationery Office, London.

Health & Safety Executive (1999) A guide to risk assessment requirements. *Common Provisions in Health and Safety Law*. HSE Books, Sudbury.

Infection Control Nurses Association (1999) *Guidelines for Hand Hygiene*. ICNA, Bathgate, West Lothian.

Infection Control Nurses Association (1999) *Glove Usage Guidelines*, ICNA, Bathgate, West Lothian.

Jackson MM, Lynch P (1986) Education of the adult learner: a practical approach for the infection control practitioner. *Am. J. Infect. Control*, **14**: 257–71.

Larson E (1988) A causal link between handwashing and risk of infection? Examination of the evidence. *Infect. Control Hosp. Epidemiol.*, **9**(1): 28–36.

Larson EL (1995) APIC guideline for handwashing and hand antisepsis in healthcare settings. *Am. J. Infect. Control*, **23**: 251–69.

Sherwoood E (1995) Motivation: the key factor. *Nursing Times*, **91**(20): 65–6.

Simmons BP (1983) CDC guidelines for the prevention and control of nosocomial infection. Guideline for hospital environmental control. *Am. J. Infect. Control*, **11**(3): 97–115.

8

Preventing wound infection

INTRODUCTION

A wound has been defined as a loss of continuity of skin or tissue (Ayton 1985) and may result from accidental trauma, an underlying disease process (e.g. venous ulceration) or a surgical procedure. When considering the prevention of infection in wounds it is important to distinguish between wounds healing by **secondary intention** in which there is loss of tissue and the remaining tissues are exposed for many days or weeks, and the surgical wound where exposure of the underlying tissue occurs for only a few minutes or hours and healing is by **primary intention** (Fig. 8.1). In healing by secondary intention the gap must be gradually filled from the base by new tissue. This process is accelerated by contraction; contractile cells in the wound gradually move the edges of the wound into the centre and decrease its size.

Epithelial cells are constantly shed and replaced from the surface of the skin. When skin is damaged these cells migrate across the living tissue, towards areas where cells are lost or depleted. This process is called **epithelialization** and is particularly important for healing by secondary intention.

The processes that take place in a wound as it heals are summarized in Box 8.1.

THE SURGICAL WOUND

Surgical wound infections account for between 10% and 20% of infections acquired by patients in hospital (Emmerson et al 1996, Haley et al 1985). Infections may affect the superficial cutaneous layer, the deep fascial layers or nearby organs, and other sites such as joints or abdomen manipulated during the procedure. Most infections are acquired at the time of operation (Kluytmans 1997). The bacteria may be introduced from a variety of sources but the most common is the patient's own microbial flora (Box 8.2). Intra-abdominal wound infection caused by Gram-negative bacteria can

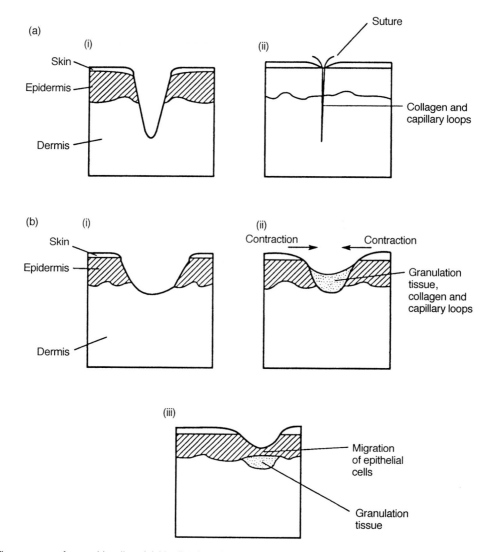

Fig. 8.1   The process of wound healing. (a) Healing by primary intention. (b) Healing by secondary intention.

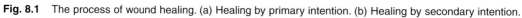

Box 8.1 Stages in wound healing	
Stage 1 (0–3 days) *Inflammation phase*	Injured blood vessels thrombose; clot forms. Damaged tissue releases histamine causing vasodilation. Increased blood supply brings macrophages and polymorphonucleocytes. Epithelialization begins
Stage 2 (2–5 days) *Destructive phase*	Polymorphs and macrophages remove dead tissue and stimulate multiplication of fibroblasts
Stage 3 (3–24 days) *Proliferation phase*	Fibroblasts begin to produce fibres of collagen (a protein that is the main constituent of structural tissue, e.g. skin, bone, ligaments). New capillary loops grow into the collagen to form granulation tissue
Stage 4 (24 days to 1 year) *Maturation phase*	More collagen fibres are made and reorganized to increase the strength of the scar

---

Box 8.2 Surgical wound infections: potential sources of bacteria

Patient	Theatre	Ward
Skin	Staff	Staff
Colonized hollow organs	Instruments	Dressings
	Airborne particles	Airborne particles
Other infection, abscesses		

Box 8.3 Factors that increase the risk of surgical wound infection

In the wound	**In the patient**
Number of bacteria	Malnourishment
Dead tissue	Obesity
Haematoma	Underlying illness (e.g. diabetes)
Tissue damage during procedure	Immune deficiency
Foreign material	Infection at a remote site

---

be particularly serious because the endotoxins released may trigger a systemic inflammatory response and subsequent multiorgan failure (Henderson et al 1996). The risk of infection developing in a surgical wound depends on a delicate balance between the host immune defences and the number of bacteria present in the wound at the end of the operation. This balance is influenced by the condition of the wound and the susceptibility of the patient to infection (Box 8.3).

Factors influencing the risk of wound infection

Bacterial contamination of the wound

Wounds are able to heal despite the presence of quite large numbers of bacteria. Kriezek & Robson (1975) found that wound infection occurred only if more than 100 000 bacteria per gram of tissue were present when the wound was closed.

As the bacteria that cause surgical wound infections are frequently derived from the patient's own **normal flora**, the number of bacteria in the wound at the end of the procedure depends on the site of the body involved. Some parts of the body, for example the intestines, are **colonized** by large numbers of bacteria which readily enter the wound when surgery is performed on the bowel. Before operating on the colon various methods are used to reduce the number of bacteria in the bowel (e.g. elemental diets, purgatives, antibiotics). Surgery involving a site with pre-existing infection, or where necrosed tissue is present, is significantly more likely to result in wound infection. Other types of surgery, for example orthopaedic surgery, are less likely to encounter colonizing bacteria and the risk of surgical wound infection developing is correspondingly smaller (Fig. 8.2; Table 8.1).

Some types of procedure are more likely to result in wound infection than others. For example, when internal mammary arteries rather than saphenous veins are used for coronary artery bypass grafts, the rate of surgical wound infection is much higher. This is probably because the mammary arteries are important for providing a blood supply to the sternum and, if this is reduced, the site becomes more susceptible to infection (Sethi et al 1991).

Surgical technique

A considerable proportion of surgical wound infection has been attributed to the technique of the surgeon (Cruse 1986, Holzheimer et al 1997, Kluytmans 1997). Minimizing the amount of trauma to the tissue improves

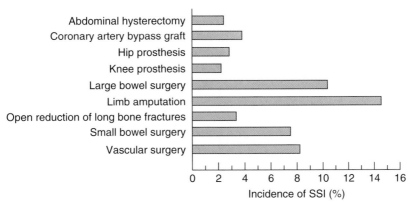

Fig. 8.2 Incidence of surgical site infection (SSI) by category of surgical procedure. Source: Public Health Laboratory Service (2000).

Table 8.1 Classification of wound contamination

Category	Description	Type of surgery	Approximate no. of wound infections per 100 operations
Clean	GI, GU or respiratory tract not entered; no evidence of inflammation or infection; no break in technique	Orthopaedic; neurosurgery; cardiac surgery	2–5
Clean-contaminated	GI, GU or respiratory tract entered but no spillage of contents	Abdominal hysterectomy; resection of prostate	8
Contaminated	Open traumatic wounds; major break in technique; spillage from GI tract; inflamed tissue encountered	Reduction of open fracture; some large bowel surgery	15
Dirty	Delayed treatment of traumatic wounds; pre-existing clinical infection, perforated viscera at site of operation	Drainage of abscess	40

GI, gastrointestinal; GU, genitourinary.

wound healing and reduces the risk of infection (Holzheimer et al 1997). Important factors include maintaining a good blood supply, removing devitalized tissue, minimizing bleeding and preventing tissues from drying out by using saline irrigation. Control of haemorrhage is also important because of the increased surgical wound infection rate associated with blood transfusion. This is thought to be due to an adverse effect on cell-mediated immunity: the risk increases for each unit administered but is significantly lower when autologous blood is used (Heiss et al 1993). In a study on major vascular surgery the rate of surgical site infection increased to over 50% if five or more units of blood were given (Verwaal et al 1992). The presence of haematomas and dead tissue in the wound encourages the multiplication of bacteria which may then be able to establish infection. Inadvertent breaks in surgical technique, for example spillage of bowel contents, may also increase the risk of subsequent wound infection.

Foreign bodies

The presence in tissue of even a small amount of foreign material has a dramatic effect on the immune defences. This was first demonstrated by Elek & Conen (1957), who inoculated the forearms of medical students with *Staphylococcus aureus*. They found that only 100 bacteria were necessary to produce infection in the presence of a silk suture, compared with the 6.5 million bacteria required without a suture. Small areas of **inflammation** around skin sutures on surgical wounds are frequently observed, although they rarely develop into infection.

Some bacteria, e.g. *S. epidermis*, are able to adhere to implanted material such as joint replacements and prosthetic heart valves where they multiply to produce infection, with devastating consequences for the patient (Sanderson, 1991).

Duration of operation

The longer that tissues are exposed, the greater the chance that bacteria carried by airborne particles will settle on to the tissues or be carried into the wound on hands or instruments (Whyte et al 1982). Longer procedures also provide more opportunity for tissue damage or a break in surgical technique to occur. The duration of operation is therefore an important risk factor for wound infection (Cruse & Foord 1973, Culver et al 1991).

Susceptibility of the patient to infection

The risk of patients acquiring a wound infection is influenced by their susceptibility to infection and the ability of the wound to heal.

Underlying disease may depress the response of the immune system and patients with serious underlying illness are more susceptible to infection. Diabetes mellitus interferes with **phagocytosis** by **white blood cells** and causes a general increase in susceptibility to infection, as well as an increased risk of surgical wound infection (Slaughter et al 1993). **Immunosuppressive** therapy or steroid treatment also depresses the immune response and enables bacteria to multiply in the wound.

There is a significant correlation between increasing age and the risk of developing wound infection, probably related to diminished immune defences (Cruse 1986). Poor nutrition and nicotine use have been associated with delayed wound healing. Obesity has been shown to be an important risk factor for surgical wound infection (Cruse & Foord 1973, Nicholson et al 1994). Deep layers of adipose tissue can increase the complexity of the procedure and reduce the blood flow to the wound during healing (Mangram et al 1999). In breast surgery, larger breast size also increases the risk of surgical wound infection (Rotstein et al 1992).

Patients who already have an infection, for example pneumonia or urinary tract infection, at the time of operation are more prone to develop a wound infection, and infections should be treated before surgery is performed (Valentine et al 1986).

An awareness of the underlying factors that predispose patients to infection can help to identify patients at greatest risk, enhance their resistance to infection as much as possible before operation and observe them closely after operation for early signs of infection.

Nasal colonization with Staphylococcus aureus

Although *S. aureus* is an important pathogen, it is also commonly present as part of the normal flora of the skin and nose. About 20% of people carry *S. aureus* in their nose all the time, and a further 60% some of the time (Williams 1963). *S. aureus* is an important cause of surgical wound infection, accounting for approximately 50% of infections (Public Health Laboratory Service 2000). An association between nasal carriage of *S. aureus* and the development of surgical wound infection has been recognized for many years, but a number of recent studies have emphasized its importance as a major risk factor (Kluytmans et al 1995). The use of topical mupirocin to remove nasal carriage before operation has been used successfully to reduce surgical site infections following major surgery

(Kluytmans 1998). However further studies are required to demonstrate its efficacy (Casewell 1998).

Reducing the risk of surgical wound infection

Preoperative hospitalization

From the time of admission to hospital, the normal harmless flora of the patient's skin is gradually replaced by hospital **pathogens**, which may then be introduced into the surgical wound (Noone et al 1983). Cruse & Foord (1980) demonstrated that the longer a patient stayed in hospital before operation, the greater the probability that the wound would become infected. When the preoperative stay was 1 day, 1.2% of wounds became infected, whilst 3.4% of wounds became infected if the patient had been in hospital for more than 2 weeks. However, some of this increase in risk is probably linked to the patient's underlying illness. More seriously ill patients are more likely to require preparation and treatment in hospital before surgery (Mangram et al 1999).

For most patients hospital stay can be reduced to a minimum by performing essential preoperative investigations in assessment clinics and admitting them on the day before or the day of surgery.

Preoperative bathing

Bacteria present on the patient's skin can be introduced into the wound during operation. Reducing bacterial colonization of the skin before incision has therefore been advocated as a means of minimizing the risk of infection. A bath or shower using an antiseptic such as chlorhexidine or povidone–iodine before operation reduces the number of bacteria on the skin, but a clear association with reduction in wound infection rate has not been demonstrated (Ayliffe et al 1983, Lynch et al 1992).

Alcoholic solutions of iodine or chlorhexidine should be used to cleanse around the site of the incision to reduce the number of skin bacteria present when the incision is made and to minimize the risk of introducing them into the wound (Mangram et al 1999). Sterile occlusive drapes can then be used to reduce the transfer of bacteria from the patient's skin into the wound.

Shaving the skin

A number of studies have shown that shaving the skin before operation increases the risk of wound infection

(Alexander et al 1983, Cruse 1986). Bacteria multiply in microabrasions caused by the razor on the surface of the skin, particularly if the skin is shaved some hours before surgery. Removal of hair with an electric shaver is associated with a lower infection rate, but shavers present their own cross-infection problems if used between patients (Millward 1992). Hair clippers may provide a suitable alternative and cause less damage (Pettersson 1986). The use of depilatory creams instead of razors reduces the risk of wound infection but they can cause an allergic reaction and may not remove hair of male patients (Seropian & Reynolds 1971). Some studies have suggested that any form of hair removal increases the risk of infection (Winston 1992).

Hair is no more heavily colonized with microbial flora than the skin, and the criteria for hair removal should be based on the need to view or access the operative site rather than to remove bacteria. If hair removal is essential, the best approach is to remove the minimum amount of hair as near to the time of operation as possible.

Antibiotic prophylaxis

The use of antibiotics to prevent infection is recommended for surgery associated with a high risk of infection or when a prosthesis is inserted and an infection at the site, although unusual, would be disastrous. The aim is to inhibit bacterial growth in the wound and other areas prone to postoperative infection. For example, an appendicectomy for an inflamed appendix may be complicated by an infected wound and peritonitis, and antibiotic prophylaxis is intended to prevent both. Prophylactic antibiotics have undoubtedly had a major effect in reducing the risk of surgical wound infection but their efficacy depends on selecting an appropriate agent and time of administration. The choice of antibiotic should be based on the species of bacteria most likely to contaminate the wound. In some circumstances more than one agent may be required to prevent infection by bacteria resistant to common antibiotics, such as enterococci (Korten & Murray 1993). The administration of the antibiotics should be timed to achieve the right levels in blood and tissue before bacterial contamination occurs and to maintain them during operation. The first dose should therefore be given before the incision is made. Further doses should not be continued for more than a few hours after operation as this will encourage the selection of resistant bacteria (Holzheimer et al 1997).

Procedures in the operating department

Ventilation and air filtration Air contains micro-organisms on airborne particles such as skin squames, dust, lint or respiratory droplets. In theatre, the main source of airborne bacteria is the staff.

The number of airborne microbial particles in an operating room is proportional to the number of humans present and their level of activity. Each person has been estimated to emit approximately 10 000 organisms per minute at rest, increasing to 50 000 per minute during activity as friction of clothing against the skin releases more squames (Howarth 1985). These particles may settle on to instruments, gloved hands or into the wound itself and subsequently result in wound infection (Hambreus 1988, Whyte et al 1982). Barrie et al (1992) reported an unusual outbreak of surgical wound infection caused by linen contaminated with *Bacillus cereus*. Lint from the contaminated linen was thought to have entered the wound directly or after settling on instruments, but infection occurred during two neurosurgical operations which lasted for many hours and provided ample opportunity for bacteria to enter the wound and establish infection.

Special ventilation systems are used to filter out airborne micro-organisms and to prevent micro-organisms from entering the theatre in the air supply from corridors or other parts of the hospital. Air is forced into the theatre through filters in the ceiling which remove particles and bacteria; the volume of air in the room will be changed approximately 20 times an hour (less frequently in scrub-up and anaesthetic rooms). Theatres are plenum ventilated; that is, a higher pressure is maintained in the room to prevent unfiltered air from outside flowing in through the doors (Fig. 8.3).

The number of airborne particles can be reduced by keeping the number and activity of people present during operation to a minimum and ensuring that the ventilation system is not disrupted by opening operating room doors during the procedure. Dust should not be allowed to collect on surfaces where it may be disturbed and become airborne. Ultra-clean air systems have been recommended to reduce the incidence of infection in orthopaedic surgery, particularly prosthetic hip and knee replacements. Such procedures are susceptible to infection even if only small numbers of bacteria are introduced into the wound (Gosden et al 1998). These systems direct a laminar flow of filtered air over the operating table and use over 600 air changes per hour (Lidwell et al 1982). Early studies demonstrated a significant reduction in wound infection rates, although similar results may be achieved by using only prophylactic antibiotics (Mangram et al 1999).

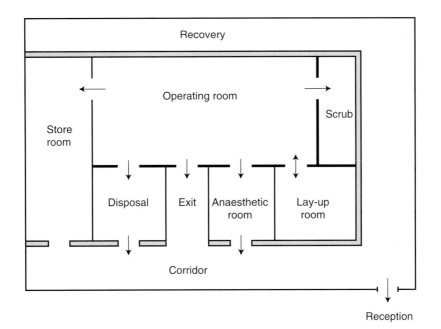

Fig. 8.3 Ventilation of an operating theatre. Air moves from the cleanest areas to the least clean areas. Arrows indicate direction of air flow.

Handwashing The transfer of micro-organisms from the surgeon's hands to the wound may be reduced by handwashing. Whilst soap removes the transient flora of the skin, microbicidal detergents (surgical scrubs) are used to reduce the resident microbial flora of the skin (see Ch. 7). To achieve maximum reduction, the hands and arms should be washed thoroughly, ensuring that all parts are covered with the detergent. Chlorhexidine and povidone–iodine have a persistent effect on skin micro-organisms; therefore repeated washes through the day gradually reduce the number of bacteria on the skin (Ojajärvi 1976, O'Shaughnessy et al 1991). Alcohol handrub solutions containing a microbicide such as chlorhexidine are equally effective and could be used in place of surgical scrubs (Lilley et al 1979). Artificial nails can increase bacterial colonization of the hands and outbreaks of wound infections associated with artificial nails have been reported (Passaro et al 1997).

Operating room clothing Micro-organisms are constantly shed from skin; therefore, personnel directly involved in the operation wear sterile gowns to limit the transmission of their microbial skin flora into the open wound. Although gowns provide some protection against contamination by body fluid, they do not completely prevent bacteria shed from the skin escaping from the openings at the neck, ankles and wrists as

well as through pores in the fabric (Whyte et al 1976). The passage of bacteria is enhanced if the material becomes wet (Hoborn 1990). Gowns made of nonwoven materials or close-woven polyester fabrics can reduce the dispersal of bacteria (Matthews et al 1985, Whyte et al 1990) and are often recommended for orthopaedic surgery.

Masks are conventionally worn to prevent bacteria from the upper respiratory tract entering the wound. There is little evidence to suggest a significant risk of transmission by this route (Ayliffe 1991a). The mask rubbing against the skin may actually increase the shedding of skin squames and, unless they fit very well, exhaled air will escape from the sides. Air flow around the sides will increase as the material becomes wet with moist exhaled air (Belkin 1997, Schweizer 1976). Masks are, of course, necessary to protect those close to the operating site from blood or body fluid splashing on to mucous membranes, but the value of masks to other personnel in the theatre is questionable (Hubble et al 1996, Mitchell & Hunt 1991) (see p. 141).

Whilst head covers may prevent bacteria on hairs from entering the operative sites, they probably have limited impact on counts of bacteria in the air (Humphries et al 1991a). They are therefore probably of little value for non-scrubbed staff assisting most types of surgery. Overshoes also appear to have no effect on bacterial counts on the floor (Humphries et al 1991b) and, because the open wound has no contact with the floor, there seems to be no logical reason for their use.

Sterile gloves are worn to prevent the transmission of the operator's skin flora into the wound. Evidence from operations performed with punctured gloves suggests that there is no increase in the rate of wound infection as a result of bacteria leaking out of the glove from the skin (Cruse 1986, Whyte et al 1991). Gloves are essential to protect the operator from exposure to blood and may provide some protection against needlestick injury (see Ch. 7). The use of two pairs of gloves (double-gloving) can significantly reduce the risk of puncturing the inner glove and is recommended for procedures associated with a high risk of injury (e.g. gynaecology) (Tokars et al 1995, UK Health Departments 1998).

Instruments and equipment   Items used for invasive procedures should be sterile when used (see Ch. 13). The sterility of packs can be maintained indefinitely, provided they remain intact and are not exposed to moisture, direct sunlight or heat. Those who are working close to the operation field must adhere to the principles of asepsis to minimize the risk of surgical wound infection.

Cleaning   In a modern well-managed theatre, the risk of infection from the environment is low (Ayliffe 1991b). Smears of blood and body fluid on surfaces should be removed with detergent and water after each operation and large spills removed using chlorine-releasing granules (see Ch. 7). Horizontal surfaces, which readily collect dust, should be cleaned daily and the minimum amount of equipment should be kept in the operating room to prevent the collection of dust and avoid unnecessary cleaning. Tacky mats outside the entrance to the theatre do not reduce the risk of wound infection (Ayliffe 1991b).

There is usually no need to allocate infected patients to the end of an operating list provided that spills of blood or body fluid are removed at the end of the operation, dust is removed from surfaces and ventilator tubing is changed. There is no evidence to support special cleaning procedures (Mangram et al 1999). Suspended particles will be rapidly removed by the air filtration system and the next patient can be brought into the room as soon as it has been cleaned.

Wound drains   A wound is more likely to become infected if a drain leading from the tissues out through the skin is inserted as it will provide a route through which bacteria can enter the wound (Cruse 1986). However, drains can facilitate wound healing by preventing the formation of haematomas. When required, a closed drainage system, for example emptying directly into a bag or bottle, is recommended because this reduces the risk of bacteria entering the wound. Making a separate incision for the drain has also been advocated so that the incision is not affected when the drain is shortened or if it becomes infected (Mangram et al 1999). Drains should not be left in place for too long as this may enable bacteria to colonize the site (Drinkwater & Neil 1995).

Postoperative care

Although the first signs of infection in a surgical wound become apparent during postoperative care, usually 4–10 days after operation, most of these infections will probably have been introduced during surgery. As soon as the wound has been sutured, a loose mesh of fibrin is formed and is gradually infiltrated by fibroblasts and collagen. Within a few hours this structure has become impervious to the entry of bacteria and, provided the dressing applied in theatre remains undisturbed for the first 48 hours, pathogens are unlikely to gain access to the wound.

Surveillance of wound infection

Surgical wound infections are an important problem: they delay the recovery of the patient, increase the length of hospital stay and may result in readmission to hospital for treatment. These have obvious economic consequences. A recent study by Plowman et al (1999) found that patients with a surgical wound infection had an additional hospital stay of 6.5 days and their hospital costs were doubled.

Surveillance of the incidence of surgical site infections in England has demonstrated marked differences in infection rate between hospitals even when the rates are adjusted by the most important risk factors for infection (Public Health Laboratory Service 2000). Although some of these differences may reflect variations in patient mix or case-finding, the standard of clinical practice in the operating theatre and ward and skills of the operating surgeon have a major effect.

A major study of the efficacy of infection control measures in the USA in the 1980s demonstrated the value of surveillance of surgical wound infection and reporting the rates of infection to individual surgeons (Haley et al 1985) (Table 8.2). The feedback of these data to surgeons focuses attention on the importance of good surgical technique in preventing wound infection and can be used to motivate change in practice where high rates are identified (Cruse & Foord 1980, Haley 1986). Major reductions in wound infection rates have

Table 8.2 Efficacy of infection control programmes in preventing surgical site infection. Source: Haley et al (1985), by permission of Oxford University Press

Components of programme	Percentage of SSIs prevented
Organized infection control programme with:	
intensive surveillance and control activity SSI rates reported to surgeons	20
plus	
physician or surgeon with expertise in infection control	38

SSI, surgical site infection.

been reported when such **surveillance** and feedback programmes are used (Cruse 1986, Olsen et al 1990).

In 1996, the Department of Health in England with the Public Health Laboratory Service established an English scheme (Nosocomial Infection National Surveillance Scheme; NINSS) for the surveillance of hospital-acquired infections, including surgical site infections (Cooke et al 2000). This was based on a similar system, the National Nosocomial Infection Surveillance System, that had been operating in the United States for several decades (Gaynes 1997). Participation in the NINSS scheme is voluntary but hospitals are required to use standardized methods of data collection and definitions of infection (Box 8.4) to

---

Box 8.4 Definitions of surgical site infections

Superficial incisional infection
This is defined as a surgical site infection that occurs within 30 days of operation, involves only the skin or subcutaneous tissue of the incision, *and* meets at least *one* of the following criteria:

Criterion 1	Purulent drainage from the superficial incision
Criterion 2	The superficial incision yields organisms from the culture of aseptically aspirated fluid or tissue, or from a swab, and pus cells are present
Criterion 3	At least two of the following symptoms and signs: pain, tenderness, localized swelling, redness or heat *and* a) the superficial incision is deliberately opened by a surgeon to manage the infection, unless the incision is culture negative *or* b) the clinician diagnoses a superficial incisional infection

Deep incisional infection
This is defined as a surgical site infection involving the deep tissues (i.e. muscle and fascial layers) that occurs within 30 days of operation if no implant is in place, or within 1 year if an implant is in place, appears to be related to the surgical procedure, *and* meets at least *one* of the following criteria:

Criterion 1	Purulent drainage from the deep incision
Criterion 2	The deep incision yields organisms from the culture of aseptically aspirated fluid or tissue, or from a swab, and pus cells are present
Criterion 3	A deep incision that spontaneously dehisces or is deliberately opened by a surgeon when the patient has *at least one* of the following symptoms or signs: fever (>38°C), localized pain or tenderness, unless the incision is culture negative
Criterion 4	An abscess or other evidence of infection involving the deep incision that is found by direct examination during reoperation, or by histopathological or radiological examination

Organ or space infection
This is defined as a surgical site infection involving any part of the anatomy other than the incision opened or manipulated during the procedure, that occurs within 30 days of operation if no implant is in place or within 1 year if an implant is in place, appears to be related to the surgical procedure, *and* meets at least *one* of the following criteria:

Criterion 1	Purulent drainage from a drain that is placed through a stab wound into the organ or space
Criterion 2	The organ or space yields organisms from the culture of aseptically aspirated fluid or tissue, or from a swab, and pus cells are present
Criterion 3	An abscess or other evidence of infection involving the organ or space that is found by direct examination, during reoperation, or by histopathological or radiological examination

Source: Nosocomial Infection National Surveillance Scheme (1998)

ensure that data contributed to the scheme are comparable. Participating hospitals are able to compare their results by category of surgical procedure with the results aggregated from all participating hospitals. The ability of hospitals to measure their own performance against others is key to ensuring that poor performance is identified and action taken to review and improve practice (National Audit Office 2000).

One of the problems associated with surgical wound infection surveillance is the difficulty of detecting infections that develop after the patient has been discharged from hospital. The 60% reduction in length of hospital stay that has occurred in the UK and other developed countries over the past two decades exacerbates this problem (Appleby 1997). As many as 50% of wound infections may develop post-discharge and this can result in a significant underreporting of infection rates unless the some form of post-discharge surveillance is included (Mishriki et al 1990, Plownan et al 2000).

WOUNDS HEALING BY SECONDARY INTENTION

The term healing by secondary intention is used to describe the process of healing in wounds when there is tissue loss and the gap must be gradually filled from the base by new tissue. These type of wounds are often referred to as chronic wounds and include ulcers, pressure sores, burns and some surgical wounds in which closure by suture is delayed (e.g. blast injuries, dehisced wounds).

Prevention of infection in chronic wounds

Exposed tissue provides an ideal growth medium for many micro-organisms and the wound rapidly becomes colonized with a variety of bacteria acquired from the patient's own normal flora and the environment. Wounds appear to be able to heal despite the presence of these bacteria, provided they do not invade the tissue and cause infection, although some species have been implicated in the poor healing of ulcers (Hutchinson & Lawrence 1991). Attempting to discourage bacterial growth in a wound by removing exudate and keeping the wound surface dry is inappropriate. Epithelialization, the formation of new granulation tissue and microcirculation are all encouraged in the moist environment provided by an occlusive dressing on the wound (Lydon et al 1989, Winter 1962).

Wound exudate contains white blood cells, which play a major role in destroying bacteria and preventing subsequent infection in the tissues. Their activity is enhanced if the wound is occluded (Buchan et al 1980, Clarke 1985).

The best method of preventing infection in chronic wounds is to ensure that the wound heals as rapidly as possible. Infection is more likely to occur in wounds with a poor blood supply, where the tissue is not well oxygenated and there are fewer white blood cells. **Necrotic tissue** can encourage bacterial multiplication and infection, and delay healing. It should be removed from wounds by surgical means or with dressings that promote desloughing (Hutchinson & Lawrence 1991).

Burns

Burns are always colonized by a variety of micro-organisms. Although most do not usually interfere with healing, some may invade the tissues and cause **septicaemia**, a frequent and serious complication of patients with severe burns. *Streptococcus pyogenes* and *Pseudomonas aeruginosa* may interfere with skin grafting and cause invasive infections which are sometimes fatal (Lowbury & Cason 1985).

Patients with 60% or more of their body surface affected by burns are most vulnerable to infection. Two-thirds will develop infection on the burnt area and most will also develop secondary bloodstream infection (Weber et al 1997). Bacterial multiplication is enhanced because of impaired neutrophil and lymphocyte activity (Dong et al 1993). Pathogens encountered in burn wounds change over time. Initially Gram-negative bacteria predominate, but these are replaced after the first few days by Gram-negative species. Occasionally burns may be infected by fungi such as candida and aspergillus, or viruses (e.g. herpes simplex).

The modern approach to the treatment of burns is prompt excision of the burn wound and covering with a skin graft or skin substitute. This reduces the time during which the wound is exposed and has had a marked effect on the incidence of infection associated with burns (Mozingo et al 1998).

Cross-infection is a major problem in burns units, particularly with *S. aureus*, pseudomonas and other Gram-negative **bacilli** such as acinetobacter. The main risk of transmission is on the hands of staff. Contaminated equipment has also been implicated in outbreaks of infection in burns units. Kolmos et al (1993) reported an outbreak of infection associated with tubes used to irrigate wounds.

All staff should wear appropriate protective clothing for contact with patients, discard it after each use, and wash hands thoroughly between patients.

The large surface area of damaged skin increases the probability of micro-organisms being introduced from an airborne route, particularly those bacteria that are more resistant to desiccation such as staphylococci and acinetobacter. The use of single-bed rooms may help to minimize the risk of cross-infection, but special ventilation is probably not necessary for most types of infection (Mozingo et al 1998). Large numbers of bacteria may be released during dressing changes and the use of a dressing room supplied with filtered air at around 10 changes per hour has been recommended (Ayliffe & Lilly 1985).

For patients who are not critically ill, cleansing is most easily achieved in a shower. Topical antimicrobial solutions are used to control colonization and reduce the mortality rate associated with burns. Commonly used agents are silver nitrate, silver sulphadiazine and chlorhexidine creams, which should be cleansed from the wound and reapplied every 12 hours. These agents are helpful in preventing colonization of burns by *P. aeruginosa* but will not remove it if already established in the burn (Lowbury & Cason 1985). Topical antimicrobial solutions are not recommended for other types of wound.

THE CARE OF WOUNDS

The nurse has a major role to play in preventing the transmission of bacteria in wounds between patients and in minimizing the risk of wound infection developing. However, care of the wound should not be directed solely at the dressing procedure. Encouraging rapid wound healing reduces the possibility of wound infection. Adequate nutrition is essential for wound healing to take place. Collagen, the principal building material for the repair of wounds, is a protein; vitamin C is essential for collagen synthesis; and other trace elements, such as zinc and copper, are also important for the healing process. Nutrition is particularly important to aid wound healing in patients with a poor nutritional state caused by malignancy, malabsorption syndromes or temporary starvation (Westerby 1985).

Promoting a good blood supply to the wound will also aid healing. The relief of pressure from pressure sores is essential if an adequate blood supply is to reach the wound.

The 'aseptic technique'

When the normal defences of the body are breached, the tissues are vulnerable to invasion by micro-organisms. The aseptic technique aims to prevent micro-organisms on hands, surfaces or equipment from being introduced to such a susceptible site. It should also prevent micro-organisms from the patient being transferred to staff or other patients. The aseptic technique has become incorporated into nursing ritual and is often based more on tradition than on rational reason or research evidence. It is frequently performed without reference to the underlying principles of infection prevention or to the requirements of the situation to which it is being applied (Walsh & Ford 1989).

A good example of this is the preparation of the trolley. There is no evidence that bacteria on the trolley are transferred into the wound, or vice versa, and routine cleaning of trolleys with alcohol between patients probably serves no useful purpose (Thompson & Bullock 1992).

The important principles are that the susceptible site should not come into contact with any item that is not sterile and that any items that have been in contact with the wound may be contaminated and should be discarded safely or decontaminated. Because hands are not sterile, forceps have traditionally been used for the procedure, probably because disposable gloves are a relatively recent introduction to medical care. However, forceps are cumbersome to use and do not prevent the transfer of bacteria from the wound to the hands (Tomlinson 1987). The procedure can be performed more easily holding sterile swabs in the hands (Briggs 1994), using gloves to prevent direct contact between hands and a vulnerable site (Box 8.5).

Assessment of the circumstances of individual patients is vital (Briggs et al 1996). In many situations a modified aseptic or 'clean' technique is more appropriate (Box 8.6), for example during the removal of sutures from a sealed surgical wound or the application of dressings to wounds healing by secondary intention. In the latter situation the wound probably already contains large numbers of different bacterial species and will frequently be exposed to new bacteria from the environment. The greatest concern is to ensure that potential pathogens are not transferred to another patient. Clean, rather than sterile, gloves are usually acceptable as when removed from the dispensing box they are likely to be contaminated only by very small numbers of bacteria of low pathogenicity (Rossof et al 1993). If hydrocolloid, alginate or hydrogel dressings have been used, the removal of the dressing is probably best achieved by irrigation with saline or bathing, and the use of a rigorous aseptic technique is unnecessary (Ayliffe et al 1990, Hollinworth & Kingston 1998).

Box 8.5 Aseptic technique

Aim
To minimize the risk of introducing pathogenic organisms into a wound or other susceptible site and to prevent the transfer of pathogens from the wound to other patients or staff.

Indications
Wounds healing by primary intention (before surface skin has sealed)
Intravenous cannulation
Urinary catheterization
Suturing
Vaginal examination during labour
Medical invasive procedures

Principles:
1. Ensure that all equipment required is readily available and there is a clear field in which to carry out the procedure
2. Explain the procedure to the patient, obtain oral consent and position the patient so that the procedure can be performed easily
3. Wash hands or disinfect clean hands with an alcohol handrub
4. Open the sterile pack carefully to prevent contamination of the contents
5. Wear sterile gloves for the procedure to prevent the introduction of pathogenic bacteria to the site or direct contact with body fluids
6. Use aseptic principles to ensure that:
   (a) only sterile items come into contact with the susceptible site
   (b) Sterile items do not come into contact with non-sterile objects
7. After completion, discard waste contaminated with body fluid into a yellow waste bag and sharps into a sharps container.
8. Discard protective clothing and wash hands to prevent cross-infection to others

---

Box 8.6 Clean technique

Aim
To avoid the introduction of pathogens to a susceptible site, and to prevent the transfer of pathogens to other patients or staff

Indications
Dressing of wounds healing by secondary intention
Removal of sutures
Dressing intravenous lines
Removal of drains
Endotracheal suction
Dressing tracheostomy site

Principles
1. Ensure that all equipment required is ready and that a clean area on which to place it is available
2. Explain the procedure to the patient, obtain verbal consent, and position the patient so that the procedure can be performed easily
3. Wash hands and disinfect with alcohol handrub
4. If direct contact with blood or body fluid is anticipated, wear clean gloves and a plastic apron
5. Use sterile swabs to clean the site or irrigate with saline or water, and apply a sterile dressing
6. Avoid touching any unclean area while performing the procedure
7. On completion of the procedure, dispose of all clinical waste into a yellow plastic bag
8. Discard gloves and apron and wash hands to prevent cross-infection to others

---

Surgical wound dressings

The wound dressing should not be disturbed for the first 48 h as bacteria may enter the wound from adjacent skin until the wound surface has sealed. If the dressing is dislodged or cannot contain the wound exudate, it should be changed using an aseptic technique (see Box 8.5).

After 48 h the dressing can be removed and wounds that are not leaking exudate and are not drained can be left exposed or protected with a transparent film dressing; the patient is allowed to shower or bathe (Chrintz et al 1989). Leaving the wound exposed enables the early signs of wound infection to be detected and saves dressing materials and nursing time. However, patients may experience less pain from the wound where a transparent film dressing is used (Briggs 1996). Some wounds continue to seep serous fluid for several days.

These wounds should be covered with a sterile dressing and managed using an aseptic technique, as the superficial layer of the skin will not seal until leakage of fluid has stopped. A dressing will be required to absorb excess exudate on the skin (which is not contributing to the healing process occurring under the skin). The frequency of dressing change should be dictated by the amount of exudate. The site should be cleaned, if necessary with sterile, normal saline.

Wound drains should be attached to a sterile drainage bottle which should be changed when necessary, without touching the connections and washing hands thoroughly before and after the procedure.

Dressings for chronic wounds

Modern dressing materials, such as alginates, hydrocolloids and hydrogels, are designed to absorb excess exudate whilst at the same time providing a warm and moist environment in which healing can take place most effectively (Box 8.7). Research has shown that these dressings can be used safely on wounds without increasing the risk of infection or encouraging the growth of **anaerobic** bacteria (Gilchrist & Reed 1989).

> **Box 8.7** Properties of an ideal wound dressing for wounds healing by secondary intention
>
> - Maintains a high humidity. Epithelial cells require moist conditions to migrate
> - Provides thermal insulation. Tissue repair occurs best at a constant temperature of 37°C
> - Is impermeable to bacteria. Helps to prevent cross-infection
> - Allows gaseous exchange. Promotes healing
> - Removes excess exudate. There is a balance between removal of exudate to prevent tissue maceration whilst maintaining a moist environment. Exudate contains white blood cells, which protect the wound from invasion by bacteria
> - Is non-adherent, preventing the removal of newly formed tissue and capillaries when dressings are changed
> - Is non-toxic and non-allergenic. Avoids interference with healing
> - Comfortable and acceptable to the patient

Removing the dressing reduces the temperature of the wound and may disrupt the delicate new tissue; dressing changes should therefore be kept to a minimum (Lawrence 1982). Because bacteria are not removed from the surface of the wound by cleaning, but are simply redistributed (Tomlinson 1987), dressings should not be changed simply to 'clean' the wound. Dressings on large wounds healing by secondary intention can be removed more easily, and with less damage to the underlying tissue, by irrigation with a syringe of normal saline or by soaking in a bath or shower.

The use of solutions (e.g. hypochlorite, hydrogen peroxide) to debride wounds should be avoided as there is little evidence to support their ability to remove dead tissue and some evidence to suggest that they delay wound healing (Brennan et al 1986, Gruber et al 1975, Leaper 1986). Necrotic tissue or slough may encourage infection and delay healing, and should be removed, for example with a scalpel. Recently, interest in the old remedies of using maggots and leeches to clean wounds of dead and necrotic material has increased. Maggots are bred in sterile conditions and then put into a wound at a ratio of 10 maggots per square centimetre. They use powerful proteolytic enzymes to liquefy dead tissue, which they then digest (Cork 1997).

Preventing cross-infection

Preventing the transmission of micro-organisms from one patient to another is a particular problem with heavily colonized or infected wounds. An organism colonizing the wound of one patient may be transmitted to produce infection in another patient and, as illustrated by Tomlinson (1987), bacteria are easily acquired on the hands whilst cleaning a wound, even if forceps are used.

The use of disposable gloves minimizes the risk of acquiring bacteria on the hands, but hands should still be washed before and after dressing wounds.

Bacteria acquired on the clothing during the procedure may be transferred into the wound of another patient; therefore a clean disposable apron should be used for each dressing procedure.

If dressings are removed by soaking in bathwater or bowls, the bath or bowl should be thoroughly cleaned with detergent and then dried to ensure that pathogens are removed before use by the next patient.

In the past it has been recommended that wounds should not be redressed when cleaning or bedmaking is in progress because of the risk of airborne contamination. However, it has been shown that, although such activities increase the number of bacteria in the air, the increase is not sufficient to present a risk of infection by organisms settling on to a dressing trolley (Ayliffe et al 1990).

Dressing clinics Particular care must be taken to prevent cross-infection between patients attending ulcer treatment or dressing clinics where there are plenty of opportunities for transmission to occur and the rapid turnover of patients may encourage inadequate cleaning of equipment between patients. Bacteria in the wound will have contaminated the dressings and the surrounding skin, and hands must always be washed after touching dressings or skin. Gloves and a plastic apron should be worn for the removal and application of dressings and must be changed after each patient. Creams and dressing materials must be used for one patient only. Equipment such as buckets for soaking off dressings and scissors must be thoroughly cleaned with detergent and water and dried after each patient.

Detection and treatment of wound infection

The diagnosis of wound infection is based on the presence of clinical signs (Box 8.8). The isolation of microorganisms in a wound swab sent for culture does not necessarily indicate that a wound is infected. Surgical wounds should be inspected regularly for signs of **infection** so that prompt treatment with antimicrobial therapy can be initiated (Plate 8.1).

Detection of infection in wounds healing by secondary intention is more difficult. Slough is easily mistaken for pus and in some situations pus collects on the surface of the wound but without evidence of tissue invasion (Plate 8.2). Wound swabs are not a reliable indicator of infection as bacteria may be present even in high numbers in the wound without causing infection. The most important indicator of infection is inflammation spreading from the margins of the wound, local oedema, the patient reporting a marked increase in pain in the wound or a pyrexia where no other focus of infection can be identified (Hutchinson & Lawrence 1991).

Wound infection should always be treated with systemic antibiotics. Topical antiseptic solutions are unlikely to reach organisms that are invading the tissue, and their antibacterial activity is probably lost rapidly in the presence of blood and tissue. Solutions such as hypochlorites are toxic to granulation tissue

Box 8.8   Signs of wound infection
● pain ● inflammation at wound margins ● oedema ● pyrexia ● purulent exudate

and delay healing (Brennan et al 1986) and chlorhexidine and povidone–iodine have been shown to destroy fibroblasts in tissue culture (Gruber et al 1975, Leaper 1986, Neidner & Schopf 1986). Many antiseptic solutions have not been well researched and their effects on wound healing and on bacteria in the wound are unknown.

REFERENCES

Alexander JW, Fischer JE, Boyajian M et al (1983) The influence of hair-removal methods on wound infections. *Arch. Surg.*, **118**: 347–52.

Appleby J (1997) The English patient. *Health Service J.*, **10 April**: 36–7.

Ayliffe GAJ (1991a) Masks in surgery? *J. Hosp. Infect.*, **18**: 165–6.

Ayliffe GAJ (1991b) Role of the environment of the operating suite in surgical wound infection. *Rev. Infect. Dis.*, **13**(10): 5800–4.

Ayliffe GAJ, Lilly HA (1985) Cross-infection and its prevention. *J. Hosp. Infect.*, **6** (Suppl. B): 47–57.

Ayliffe GAJ, Noy ME, Davies JG et al (1983) A comparison of pre-operative bathing with chlorhexidine-detergent and a non-medicated soap in the prevention of wound infection. *J. Hosp. Infect.*, **4**: 237–44.

Ayliffe GAJ, Collins BJ, Taylor LJ (1990) *Hospital Acquired Infection – Principles and Prevention*, 2nd edn. Butterworth, London.

Ayton M (1985) Wounds that won't heal. *Nursing Times*, **81** (46) (Suppl): 16–19.

Barrie D, Wilson JA, Hoffman PN et al (1992) *Bacillus cereus*, meningitis in two neurosurgical patients: an investigation into the source of the organism. *J. Infect.*, **25**: 291–7.

Belkin NL (1997) The evolution of the surgical mask: filtering efficiency versus effectiveness. *Infect. Control Hosp. Epidemiol.*, **18**(1): 49–57.

Brennan SS, Foster ME, Leaper DJ (1986) Antiseptic toxicity in wounds healing by secondary intention. *J. Hosp. Infect.*, **8**: 263–7.

Briggs M (1994) Examining equipment for wound care: the use of forceps and cotton wool in dressing packs. *Accid. Emerg. Nurs.*, **2**(4): 237–9.

Briggs M (1996) Surgical wound pain: a trial of two treatments. *J. Wound Care*, **5**(10): 156–60.

Briggs M, Wilson S, Fuller A (1996) The principles of aseptic technique in wound care. *Prof. Nurse*, **11**(12): 805–8.

Buchan IA, Andrews JK, Lang SM et al (1980) Clinical and laboratory investigation of the composition and

properties of human skin wound exudate under semi-permeable dressings. *Burns*, **7**: 326–34.

Chrintz H, Vibits H, Cordtz TO et al (1989) Need for surgical wound dressing. *Br. J. Surg.*, **76**: 204–5.

Casewell MW (1998) The nose: an underestimated source of *Staphylococcus aureus* causing wound infection. *J. Hosp. Infect.*, **40** (Suppl. B): S3–12.

Clarke RAF (1985) Cutaneous tissue repair: basic biological considerations I. *J. Am. Acad. Dermatol.*, **13**: 701–25.

Cooke EMC, Coello RC, Sedgwick J et al (2000) A national surveillance scheme for hospital-associated infections in England. *J. Hosp. Infect.*, **46**: 1–3.

Cork A (1997) Maggots that munch. *Hosp. Equip. Supplies Suppl.*, **August**: 28.

Cruse PJE (1986) Surgical infection: incisional wounds. In *Hospital Infections*, 2nd edn, pp. 423–36 (JV Bennett, PS Brachman, eds). Little Brown, Boston.

Cruse PJE, Foord R (1973) A five-year prospective study of 23 649 surgical wounds. *Arch. Surg.*, **107**: 206.

Cruse PJE, Foord R (1980) The epidemiology of wound infection – a 10 year prospective study of 62 939 wounds. *Surg. Clin. North Am.*, **60**(1): 27–40.

Culver DH, Horan TC, Gaynes RP et al (1991) Surgical wound infection rates by wound class, operative procedure, and patient risk index. *Am. J. Med.*, **91** (Suppl. 3B): 72–5S.

Dong YL, Abdullah K, Yan TZ et al (1993) Effect of thermal injury and sepsis on neutrophil function. *J. Trauma*, **34**: 417–21.

Drinkwater LJ, Neil MJ (1995) Optimal timing of wound drain removal following joint arthroplasty. *J. Arthroplasty* **10**(2): 185–9.

Elek SD, Conen PE (1957) The virulence of *Staphylococcus pyogenes* for men: a study of the problems of wound infection. *Br. J. Exp. Pathol.*, **38**: 573–86.

Emmerson AM, Enstone JE, Griffin M et al (1996) The second national prevalence survey of infection in hospitals – overview of the results. *J. Hosp. Infect.*, **32**: 175–90.

Gaynes R (1997) Surveillance of nosocomial infections: a fundamental ingredient for quality. *Infect. Control Hosp. Epidemiol.*, **18**(7): 175–8.

Gilchrist B, Reed C (1989) The bacteriology of leg ulcers under hydrocolloid dressings. *Br. J. Dermatol.*, **121**: 337–44.

Gosden PE, MacGowen AP, Bannister GC (1998) Importance of air quality and related factors in the prevention of infection in orthopaedic implant surgery. *J. Hosp. Infect.*, **39**: 173–80.

Gruber RB, Vistnes L, Pardoe R (1975) The effect of commonly used antiseptics on wound healing. *Plast. Reconstr. Surg.*, **55**: 472–6.

Haley RW (1986) *Managing Hospital Infection Control for Cost-effectiveness.* American Hospital Publishing, Chicago.

Haley RW, Culver DH, White JW et al (1985) The efficacy of infection surveillance and control programs in preventing nosocomial infection in US hospitals (SENIC Study). *Am. J. Epidemiol.*, **121**(2): 182–205.

Hambreaus A (1988) Aerobiology in operating rooms. *J. Hosp. Infect.*, **11** (Suppl. A): 68–76.

Heiss MM, Mempel W, Jauch KW et al (1993) Beneficial effect of autologous blood transfusion on infectious complications after colorectal cancer surgery. *Lancet*, **342**: 1328–33.

Henderson B, Poole S, Wilson M (1996) Microbial/host interactions in health and disease: who controls the cytokine network? *Immunopharmacology*, **35**: 1–21.

Hoborn J (1990) Wet strike-through and transfer of bacteria through operating barrier fabrics. *Hyg. Med.*, **15**: 15–20.

Hollinworth H, Kingston JE (1998) Using a non-sterile technique in wound care. *Prof. Nurse*, **13**(4): 226–9.

Holzheimer RG, Haupt W, Thriede A et al (1997) The challenge of post-operative infections. Does the surgeon make a difference? *Infect. Control Hosp. Epidemiol.*, **18**: 449–56.

Howarth FH (1985) Prevention of airborne infection during surgery. *Lancet*, **i**: 386–8.

Hubble MJ, Welae AE, Perez JV et al (1996) Clothing in laminar flow operating theatres. *J. Hosp. Infect.*, **32**: 1–7.

Humphries H, Russell AJ, Marshall RJ et al (1991a) The effect of surgical theatre head-gear on air bacterial counts. *J. Hosp. Infect*, **19**: 175–80.

Humphries H, Marshall RJ, Ricketts VE (1991b) Theatre overshoes do not reduce operating floor bacterial counts. *J. Hosp. Infect.*, **17**: 117–24.

Hutchinson JJ, Lawrence JC (1991) Wound infection under occlusive dressings. *J. Hosp. Infect.*, **17**: 83–94.

Kluytmans J (1997) Surgical infections including burns. In *Prevention and Control of Nosocomial Infection*, 3rd edn, pp. 841–66 (RP Wenzel, ed.). Williams & Wilkins, Baltimore.

Kluytmans J (1998) Reduction of surgical site infections in major surgery by elimination of nasal carriage of *Staphylococcus aureus*. *J. Hosp. Infect.*, **40** (Suppl. B): S25–S30.

Kluytmans JAJW, Moulon JW, Ijzerman EPF et al (1995) Nasal carriage of *Staphylococcus aureus* as a major risk factor for wound infections after cardiac surgery. *J. Infect. Dis.*, **171**: 216–19.

Kolmos HJ, Thuesen B, Nielsen SV et al (1993) Outbreak of infection in a burns unit due to *Pseudomonas aeruginosa* originating from contaminated tubing used for irrigation of patients. *J. Hosp. Infect*, **24**: 11–21.

Korten V, Murray BE (1993) The nosocomial transmission of enterococci. *Curr. Opin. Infect. Dis.*, **6**: 498–505.

Kriezek TJ, Robson MC (1975) Biology of surgical infection. *Surg. Clin. North Am.*, **55**: 1262–7.

Lawrence JC (1982) What materials for dressings? *Injury*, **13**: 500–12.

Leaper DJ (1986) Antiseptics and their effect on healing tissue. *Nursing Times*, **82**(22): 45–7.

Lidwell OM, Lowbury EJL, Whyte W et al (1982) Effect of ultraclean air in operating rooms on deep sepsis in the joint after total hip or knee replacement; a randomised study. *BMJ*, **285**: 10–14.

Lilley HA, Lowbury EJL, Wilkens MD (1979) Limits to progressive reduction of resident skin bacteria by disinfection. *J. Clin. Pathol.*, **32**: 382–5.

Lowbury EJL, Cason JS (1985) Aspects of infection control and skin grafting in burned patients. In *Wound Care*, pp. 170–89 (S. Westerby, ed.). Heinemann Medical, London.

Lydon MJ, Hutchinson JJ, Rippon M et al (1989) Dissolution of wound coagulum and promotion of granulation tissue under DuoDERM™. *Wounds*, **1**: 95–106.

Lynch W, Davey PG, Malek M et al (1992) Cost-effectiveness analysis of the use of chlorhexidine detergent in preoperative whole-body disinfection in wound infection prophylaxis. *J. Hosp. Infect.*, **21**: 179–91.

Mangram AJ, Horan TC, Pearson ML et al (1999) Guideline for the prevention of surgical site infections, 1999. *Am. J. Infect. Control*, **27**: 97–134.

Matthews J, Slater K, Newsom SWB (1985) The effect of surgical gowns made with barrier cloth on bacterial dispersal. *J. Hyg.*, **95**: 123–30.

Millward S (1992) The hazards of communal razors. *Nursing Times*, **88**(6): 58–62.

Mishriki SF, Law DJW, Jeffrey PJ (1990) Factors affecting the incidence of postoperative wound infection. *J. Hosp. Infect.*, **11**: 253–62.

Mitchell NJ, Hunt S (1991) Surgical face masks in modern operating rooms – a costly and unnecessary ritual? *J. Hosp. Infect.*, **18**: 239–42.

Mozingo DW, Mcmanus AT, Pruitt BA Jr (1998) Infections of burn wounds. In *Hospital Infections*, 4th edn, pp. 587–98 (JV Bennett, PS Brachman, eds). Lippencott-Raven, Philadelphia.

National Audit Office (2000) *The Management and Control of Hospital Acquired Infection in Acute NHS Trusts in England. Report of the Comptroller Auditor General.* The Stationery Office, London.

Neidner R, Schopf E (1986) Inhibition of wound healing by antiseptics. *Br. J. Dermatol.*, **115**(S31): 41–4.

Nicholson ML, Dennis MJ, Makin GB et al (1994) Obesity as a risk factor in major reconstructive vascular surgery *Eur. J. Vasc. Surg.*, **8**: 209–13.

Noone MR, Pitt TL, Bedder M et al (1983) *Pseudomonas aeruginosa* colonisation in an intensive therapy unit: role of cross infection and host factors. *BMJ*, **286**: 341–4.

Nosocomial Infection National Surveillance Scheme (1998) *Protocol for Surveillance of Surgical Site Infection. Version 2.* Public Health Laboratory Service, London.

Ojarjärvi J (1976) An evaluation of antiseptics used for hand disinfection in wards. *J. Hyg. (Camb.)*, **76**: 75–82.

Olsen MM, Lee JT Jr (1990) Continuous 10-year wound infection surveillance. Results, advantages and unanswered questions. *Arch. Surg.*, **125**: 794–803.

O'Shaughnessy M, O'Malley VP, Corbett G et al (1991) Optimum duration of surgical scrub-time. *Br. J. Surg.*, **78**: 685–6.

Passaro DJ, Waring L, Armstrong R et al (1997) Postoperative *Serratia marcescens* wound infection traced to an out-of-hospital source. *J. Infect. Dis.*, **175**(4): 992–5.

Pettersson E (1986) A cut above the rest? *Nursing Times*, **31**(5): 68–70.

Plowman R, Graves N, Griffin M et al (1999) *The Socio-economic Burden of Hospital-acquired Infection*. Public Health Laboratory Service, London.

Public Health Laboratory Service (2000) *Surveillance of Surgical Site Infection in English Hospitals 1997–1999*. Nosocomial Infection National Surveillance Scheme, London.

Rossof LJ, Lam S, Hilton E et al (1993) Is the use of boxed gloves in an intensive care unit safe? *Am. J. Med.*, **94**(6): 602–7.

Rotstein C, Ferguson R, Cummings KM et al (1992) Determinants of clean surgical wound infection for breast procedures at an oncology center. *Infect. Control Hosp. Epidemiol.*, **13**: 207–14.

Sanderson PJ (1991) Infection in orthopaedic implants. *J. Hosp. Infect.*, **18** (Suppl A): 367–75.

Schweizer RT (1976) Mask wiggling as a potential source of wound contamination. *Lancet*, **ii**: 1129–30.

Seropian R, Reynolds BM (1971) Wound infections after preoperative depilatory versus razor preparation. *Am. J. Surg.*, **121**: 251–6.

Sethi GK, Copeland JG, Moritz T et al (1991) Comparison of postoperative complication between saphenous vein and IMA grafts to left anterior descending coronary artery. *Ann. Thorac. Surg.*, **51**: 733–8.

Slaughter MS, Olsen MM, Lee JT et al (1993) A 15-year wound surveillance study after coronary artery by-pass. *Ann. Thorac. Surg.*, **56**: 1063–8.

Thompson G, Bullock D (1992) To clean or not to clean? *Nursing Times*, **88**(34): 66–8.

Tokars JJ, Culver DH, Mendelson MH et al (1995) Skin and mucous membrane contact with blood during surgical procedures: risk and prevention. *Infect. Control. Hosp. Epidemiol.*, **16**: 703–11.

Tomlinson D (1987) To clean or not to clean? *Nursing Times*, **83**(9): 71–5.

UK Health Departments (1998) *Guidance for Clinical Health Care Workers: Protection Against Infection with Blood Borne Viruses. Recommendations of the Expert Advisory Group on Hepatitis*. HMSO, London.

Valentine RJ, Weigelt JA, Dryer D et al (1986) Effect of remote infection on clean wound infection rates. *Am. J. Infect. Control*, **14**: 64–7.

Verwaal VJ, Wobbes T, Koopman van Gemert AW et al (1992) Effect of perioperative blood transfusion and cell saver on the incidence of postoperative infective complications in patients with an aneurysm of the abdominal aorta. *Eur. J. Surg.*, **158**: 477–80.

Walsh M, Ford P (1989) *Nursing Rituals, Research and Rational Actions*. Butterworth-Heinemann, Oxford.

Weber JM, Sheridan RL, Pasternack MS et al (1997) Nosocomial infections in pediatric patients with burns. *Am. J. Infect. Control*, **25**: 145–201.

Westerby S (1985) *Wound Care*. Heinemann Medical, London.

Whyte W, Vesley D, Hodgson R (1976) Bacterial dispersion in relation to operating room clothing. *J. Hyg.*, **76**: 367–78.

Whyte W, Hodgson R, Tinkler J (1982) The importance of airborne bacterial contamination of wounds. *J. Hosp. Infect.*, **2**: 349–54.

Whyte W, Hamblen DL, Kelly IG et al (1990) An investigation of occlusive polyester surgical clothing. *J. Hosp. Infect*, **15**: 363–74.

Whyte W, Hambreaus A, Laurell G et al (1991) The relative importance of routes and sources of wound contamination during general surgery. 1. Non-airborne. *J. Hosp. Infect.*, **18**: 93–107.

Williams REO (1963) Healthy carriage of *Staphylococcus aureus*: its prevalence and importance. *Bacteriol. Rev.*, **27**: 56–71.

Winston KR (1992) Hair and neurosurgery. *Neurosurgery* **31**(2): 320–9.

Winter GD (1962) Formation of the scab and the rate of epithelialisation of superficial wounds in the skin of the young domestic pig. *Nature*, **193**: 293–4.

FURTHER READING

Briggs M (1997) Principles of closed surgical wound care. *J. Wound Care*, **6**(6): 288–92.

Dowding CM (1986) Nutrition in wound healing. *Nursing*, **4**: 174–6.

Flanagan M (1997) Wound Management. Churchill Livingstone, Edinburgh.

Humphries H (1993) Infection control and the design of a new operating theatre suite. *J. Hosp. Infect.*, **23**: 61–70.

Little K, Rutherford M, Jenkins M (1999) Ritual or reason? *Nursing Times*, **95**(20): 57–9.

Morison M (1990) Pressure sores: a risk assessment and prevention plan. *Prof. Nurse*, **5**: 12 (Wallchart).

Morison M (1992) *A Colour Guide to the Nursing Management of Wounds*. Wolfe, London.

Nichols RL (1991) Surgical wound infection. *Am. J. Med.*, **91** (Suppl. 3B): 54S–63S.

Orr J, Hain P (1994) Burn wound management: an overview. *Prof. Nurse*, **December**: 153–6.

Public Health Laboratory Service (1997) *Standard Operating Procedure. Investigation of Skin and Superficial Wound*

Swabs. B.SOP 11, Issue 1. PHLS Technical Services, London.

Public Health Laboratory Service (1997) *Standard Operating Procedure. Investigation of Abscesses and of Post-operative Wound and Deep-seated Infections*. B.SOP 14, Issue 1. PHLS Technical Services, London.

Rubio PA (1991) Use of semi-occlusive transparent film dressings for surgical wound protection: experience in 3637 cases. *Int. Surg.*, **76**: 253–4.

Stewart A, Foster M, Leaper D (1985) Cleaning v. healing. *Community Outlook*, **August**: 22–6.

Thomas S (1994) *Handbook of Wound Dressings*. Macmillan Magazines, London.

Van Rijn RR, Kuijper EC, Kreis RW et al (1997) Seven-year experience with a 'quarantine and isolation unit' for patients with burns. A retrospective analysis. *Burns* **23**(4): 345–8.

Williams CM (1986) Wound healing: a nutritional perspective. *Nursing*, **7**: 249–51.

9

Preventing infection associated with intravascular therapy

INTRODUCTION

Intravascular (IV) devices are now an indispensable part of medical care used to administer fluids, blood products and nutritional support, and for haemodynamic monitoring. Over 60% of patients admitted to hospital are likely to receive therapy via an intravascular (IV) device and in the UK almost all patients in intensive therapy units have at least one device inserted into a central vein or artery (Glynn et al 1997, Nystrom et al 1983). The most important infections associated with IV devices are bloodstream infections which, although they affect less than 1% of patients admitted to hospital, are associated with considerable mortality and morbidity especially amongst the critically ill (Emmerson et al 1996, Public Health Laboratory Service 2000).

The management of IV devices has an important effect on the incidence of device-associated infection and there is considerable potential to prevent infections through the application of the best principles of practice (Ena et al 1992, MMWR 2000).

INFECTIONS ASSOCIATED WITH IV DEVICES

Infection associated with intravenous therapy can be difficult to diagnose. IV devices are frequently not recognized as the cause of the symptoms of infection in the patient and it may not be possible to identify the cause of fever in the immunocompromised or critically ill (Maki 1991). A range of infectious complications can be identified.

Infection at the insertion site

Superficial infection may develop at the point where the device enters the skin, indicated by erythema or the presence of pus. There is considerable evidence to suggest a link between the presence of bacteria at the insertion site and subsequent catheter-associated bloodstream infection (Cercenardo et al 1990, Mermel et al 1991). Bacteria colonizing the skin site gain access to the blood vessel by migrating along the outside of the catheter.

Phlebitis, inflammation of the vein where the device is sited, develops in approximately one-third of patients who have a peripheral catheter, but rarely in association with central vascular devices (Maki et al 1991a). The signs include tenderness, erythema, swelling or palpable cord. Usually, phlebitis is caused by the mechanical irritation of the tissues by the device or chemical irritation by the device or infusate. The risk of phlebitis is influenced by the catheter material and size, quality of insertion, and time for which the device remains in place. The presence of phlebitis increases the risk of infection and, if infection develops, the device should be removed. Occasionally a purulent suppurative phlebitis occurs in a peripheral vein. This is an extremely serious infection that requires surgical treatment and is associated with a high mortality rate (Hammond et al 1988).

Bloodstream infections

Bacteria colonizing the surface of the catheter are released into the bloodstream causing bacteraemia. Bacteraemia accounts for 6% of hospital-acquired infections and affects at least three patients in every 1000 admitted to acute hospitals (Emmerson et al 1996, Public Health Laboratory Service 2000). The critically ill are particularly vulnerable, with around 10 infections per 1000 patient-days reported in intensive care units and 6 per 1000 patient-days in haematology departments. IV devices account for at least 38% of these infections, with central vascular catheters presenting the greatest risk (Public Health Laboratory Service 2000). Bloodstream infections are associated with a case fatality rate of at least 20%; in the critically ill this rises to about 35% (Pittet et al 1994, Pittet & Wenzel 1995).

The presence of bacteria in the bloodstream may be accompanied by systemic symptoms such as fever, hypertension, chills or rigors, and this is termed septicaemia. In children aged less than one year, symptoms may include hypothermia, apnoea or bradycardia (Public Health Laboratory Service 1998). Once introduced into the bloodstream from the IV device, bacteria may lodge on other tissues to cause secondary endocarditis or osteomyelitis (Fang et al 1993).

SOURCES OF IV DEVICE-ASSOCIATED INFECTION

The two main routes by which micro-organisms gain access to the bloodstream via an IV device are by migrating along the outside of the catheter from the insertion site and by travelling through the catheter lumen (Fig. 9.1). The importance of the external route is demonstrated by the strong association between catheter-associated infection (CAI), the culture of micro-organisms from the skin at the site of insertion and micro-organisms cultured from the outside of the catheter tip if the device is removed (Maki et al 1973).

Contamination of the internal surface of the catheter usually begins at the hub, and colonized hubs are responsible for a significant proportion of CAI (Linares et al 1985). Bacteria are protected from the immune defences of the host as they migrate through the lumen to the catheter tip; the rate of CAI increases when catheters with more than one hub are used (Clark-Christoff et al 1992, McCarthy et al 1987). Colonization of the internal surface of the catheter increases with the duration of catheterization. Thus, in patients with short-term catheters the skin at the insertion site is the most likely source of CAI, whereas in the long-term catheterized the hub is a more likely source (Raad et al 1993b).

More rarely the source of CAI may be contaminated infusate. Good quality control in manufacturing has reduced the risk from commercially prepared fluids but in-use contamination may still occur, especially where fluids are accessed frequently (Maki et al 1987). In some cases, the external surface of the catheter tip becomes colonized by bacteria circulating in the blood from another focus of infection (e.g. the respiratory or urinary tract). This is called haematogenous seeding. The bacteria may then multiply on the catheter tip and subsequently cause CAI.

Fibrin sheath

In common with other foreign materials inserted into the tissues, IV catheters become coated with proteins soon after insertion (Gristina 1987). These include fibrinogen, collagen and other glycoproteins. Bacteria adhere to these proteins or, in the case of *Staphylococcus epidermidis*, to the surface of the catheter itself. The presence of the device impairs the activity of neutrophils and protects bacteria from the effect of antimicrobial agents. Bacteria are therefore able to multiply freely in the biofilm on the catheter surface from where they are released into the bloodstream.

Microbiology

Most IV device-associated infections are acquired endogenously from micro-organisms colonizing the patient's skin, although micro-organisms may also be introduced into the hub or administration set during manipulation by healthcare staff (Table 9.1). Coagulase-

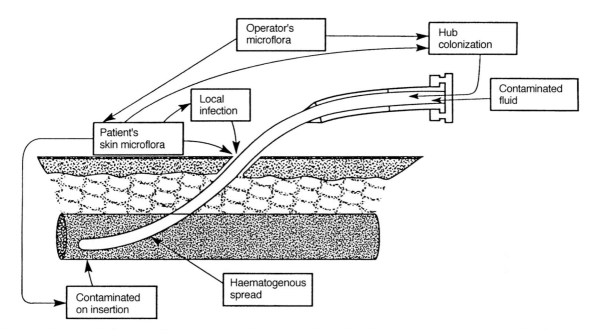

Fig. 9.1 Sources of infection in IV devices. Schematic cross-section of the skin and underlying tissue at the site of catherization. Reprinted with permission from Elliott (1988).

negative staphylococci, predominantly *S. epidermidis*, are the organisms that most commonly colonize IV devices, and when they cause infection are associated with a high mortality rate (Daschner & Frank 1989). The incidence of CAI caused by *S. epidermidis* has increased in the last two decades as a result of the improvement in survival rate of the critically ill, especially neonates (Freeman et al 1990). *Staphylococcus aureus* is less likely to colonize the catheter, but more likely to cause bacteraemia and subsequent osteomyelitis and endocarditis (Richet et al 1990).

S. *epidermidis*, although part of the normal flora of the skin, is not usually pathogenic. Its ability to cause infection in IV devices is related to the production of a glycocalyx called 'slime', which enables the bacteria to adhere to the catheter surface, especially when the surface is irregular (Ishak et al 1985, Davenport et al 1986) (see Fig. 6.1). Gram-negative micro-organisms are less common causes of IV device-associated infection, but may affect the critically ill whose skin flora is altered by antibiotic therapy. Devices such as transducers or heparin pumps may also be a source of these bacteria (Cheeseborough & Catlow 1999). Other pathogens emerging as an important cause of CAI are fungi and enterococci (Beck-Sague & Jarvis 1993, PHLS 2000).

Table 9.1 Micro-organisms most commonly responsible for IV device-related infection

Micro-organism	Source
Staphylococcus epidermidis	Common skin commensal
Staphylococcus aureus	Skin commensal
Enterococcus spp.	Gut flora, colonizes skin sites in the critically ill
Klebsiella	
Pseudomonas	Gram-negative organisms, colonize the skin of hospitalized patients; carried transiently on the hands of staff, may contaminate pumps, transducers, etc.
Eschericia coli	
Serratia	
Candida	May colonize skin when normal flora altered by antibiotic therapy; associated with haemodialysis or parenteral nutrition

DIAGNOSIS OF INFECTION RELATED TO IV DEVICES

One of the difficulties of quantifying the risks of IV devices is the difficulty of defining what constitutes a catheter-related infection. Some studies use the incidence of septicaemia or bacteraemia as a measure; others use the occurrence of phlebitis or colonization of the catheter (Maki & Ringer 1987, Ricard et al 1985, Tager et al 1983, Weightman et al 1988). It is frequently difficult to make a precise diagnosis of catheter-associated bloodstream infection, especially in the ICU when the patient may have more than one site of infection. Often the main indication of a line-associated infection is a pyrexia that has no other apparent cause and is unresponsive to antibiotic therapy (Elliot 1993).

A standard method of diagnosing catheter-related infection is by culture of the catheter tip. The method used is semiquantitative: it involves an estimation of the number of bacteria present and takes account of inadvertent contamination when the catheter is removed (Maki et al 1977). Growth is considered significant when more than 15 bacteria are found, confirming the catheter as the source of clinical symptoms of infection. However, this is not a practical method in many circumstances because it is usually not possible to remove the catheter to confirm it as the source of fever. Skin culture of the insertion site may be a useful alternative as there is a high correlation between skin colonization and catheter-related infection (Raad et al 1995).

Bacteraemia is diagnosed by culturing blood in the laboratory. At least 10 ml of blood must be inoculated into each of the culture bottles, one of which is incubated under anaerobic conditions, the other aerobically (see p. 25). To confirm the IV device as the source of infection, two sets of blood cultures should be taken, one from a peripheral vein and the second through the catheter. New methods of measuring the concentration of micro-organisms in the catheter may enable CAI to be diagnosed by taking blood samples from the lumen without removing the catheter. However, more work on the reliability of these methods is required (Farr 1999).

If the same organism is isolated from both sources, particularly if more organisms are obtained from the catheter specimen, this is suggestive of a device-related infection (Wing et al 1979). Studies on IV devices are difficult to interpret because of the variety of diagnostic methods available. The low incidence of infection also means that significant conclusions are unlikely unless at least 1500 patients are included in the study (Widner 1997).

FACTORS THAT INFLUENCE THE RISK OF INFECTION

Type of device

There are several different types of intravascular device and each is associated with different risks of infection (Table 9.2).

Peripheral catheters Peripheral venous catheters are associated with very few infections, affecting less than 1% of catheters. About one-third of patients develop phlebitis, although the risk of phlebitis is reduced if a vein in the hand is used (Maki et al 1991a, Nystrom et al 1983). Peripheral arterial catheters are used to measure intra-arterial pressure and oxygenation, and frequent manipulation increases the risk of CAI in these devices.

Central vascular catheters These are inserted into the subclavian, internal jugular or femoral vein. Catheters inserted into the jugular vein are more likely to become colonized and are associated with a higher risk of CAI. This increased risk is probably related to the proximity to oropharyngeal secretions, the mechanical effects of head movement, and the difficulty of fixing and dressing the insertion site (Mermel et al 1991). Femoral catheters have a similar risk of CAI to those inserted in the jugular vein, although the risk of catheter colonization may be higher (Goetz et al 1998, Williams et al 1991). Subclavian catheters are associated with fewer infectious complications but are more difficult to insert. They are therefore preferable for patients in intensive care who require prolonged venous access.

Early studies suggested that multilumen catheters increase the risk of CAI (Weightman et al 1988).

Table 9.2 Approximate incidence of IV device-related bloodstream infection based on a combination of published data. From Maki DG, Mermel LA (1998) Infections due to infusion therapy. In *Hospital Infections*, 4th edn (Bennett JV, Brachman PS, eds), Lippincott-Rowen, with permission

Type of device	Incidence (%)	Range (%)
Peripheral		
Venous	<0.2	0–1
Arterial	1	0.56–4.6
Central venous		
General purpose (multilumen)	3	1–7
Pulmonary artery	1	0–5
Haemodialysis	10	3–18
Long-term access		
Peripherally inserted central vascular Catheter	0.2	
Cuffed (Hickman, Broviac)	0.2	0.1–0.5
Subcutaneous port	0.04	0.2–0.1

However, differences in risk are difficult to assess because triple-lumen catheters are more likely to be used for treatment of the seriously ill (Farkas et al 1992, Pearson 1996).

Pulmonary arterial catheters (Swan–Ganz) These balloon-tipped catheters are inserted over the heart valves and are used to manage critically ill patients who are haemodynamically unstable. The trauma they cause to the valves and endocardium increases the risk of endocarditis. The risk of CAI is around 1%, but increases significantly with duration of catheterization.

Pressure monitoring systems Where arterial catheters are used for pressure monitoring, the risk of CAI is increased (Thomas et al 1993). Micro-organisms may be introduced into the fluid-filled system by unsterile transducers, calibrating devices or infusate, or from the hands of the operator when the device is manipulated (Pearson 1996). Stopcocks may also become contaminated (Crow et al 1989). Once in the system micro-organisms can multiply in the fluid and move from the pressure monitoring system into the patient's bloodstream via the IV device. Several outbreaks associated with inadequate decontamination of reusable transducers have been reported. Infections have even occurred when the fluid in the monitoring system is isolated from the patient by a sterile disposable membrane as a result of contamination during manipulation (Beck-Sague et al 1990, Hekker et al 1990).

Tunnelled and totally implanted central venous catheters These types of catheter (e.g. Hickman, Broviac, Porta-Cath) are indicated for use where prolonged venous access of more than 30 days is required, for example for chemotherapy. The catheter is inserted into the subclavian vein, and either tunnelled under the skin to exit on the chest wall or totally implanted under the skin and accessed by inserting a needle through the skin into a subcutaneous self-sealing port. These types of catheter minimize the migration of micro-organisms along the outside of the catheter and are associated with a much lower risk of CAI than conventional venous catheters. The lowest rates of CAI are associated with totally implanted devices (Garden & Sim 1983, Pratt et al 2001, Wurzel et al 1988) (see p. 181).

Peripherally inserted central vascular catheters (PICCs) These are used for medium- to long-term access, especially for outpatient treatment. The risk of CAI is lower than with non-tunnelled central vascular catheters, and similar to that associated with fully implanted devices (Ryder 1995). Insertion is associated with fewer mechanical problems and does not require a surgical procedure (Graham et al 1991). However, as with other peripherally sited catheters, PICCs are associated with phlebitis, although to a lesser extent than other peripheral catheters (Raad et al 1993b).

Duration of catheterization

The length of time for which a catheter is in place probably has most effect on the risk of infection. The longer a device is in place, the more likely it is that an infection will develop (Elliot 1988). To take account of this many studies report infections related to the number of days of catheterization. For example, if 100 catheters are under study and each is in place for 10 days, the total number of days of catheterization is 1000. If two become infected, then the rate of infection is two per 1000 catheter-days. Tager et al (1983) found that the risk of phlebitis related to peripheral catheters increased after 96 h and recommended that the peripheral catheter site should be changed at this time interval. However, other studies have suggested that routine replacement is not necessary (Bregenzer et al 1995). With central vascular catheters there appears to be no difference in rate of CAI whether they are changed routinely or left in place for the duration of catheterization (Cobb et al 1992). The duration of catheterization is particularly important for arterial catheters. Raad et al (1993b) found that for peripheral arterial catheters the risk of CAI was between 3% and 5% for each day of catheterization, and by 21 days the risk of CAI was 60%. In pulmonary arterial catheters the risk of CAI is substantially increased after 5 days; after 14 days the risk is 80%. These catheters should therefore be removed as soon as possible (Mermel et al 1991).

Catheter material

Common pathogens that cause CAI, such as *S. epidermidis*, readily colonize catheters that have irregular surfaces. The smooth surface of Teflon and polyurethane catheters are therefore the most resistant to bacterial adherence.

Most short-term catheters are made of polyurethane, whereas long-term catheters are usually silicone (Pratt et al 2001). Some materials are also more thrombogenic than others. Polyurethane catheters are less likely to cause phlebitis than Teflon catheters (Raad et al 1993a).

Catheters coated with antibacterial substances such as silver sulphadiazine and chlorhexidine have been developed recently. They have been shown significantly to reduce catheter colonization and catheter-related bloodstream infections and are probably cost effective in high-risk patients (Maki et al 1997, Veenstra et al 1999a,b). Catheters coated with two antimicrobial agents, minocycline and rifampicin, have been found to be even more effective (Darouiche et al 1999). Although there is a risk that micro-organisms resistant to these antimicrobials may emerge, they are probably still of benefit in high-risk patients because of the reduction in use of other agents, such as vancomycin, if bloodstream infections are prevented (Mermel 2000, Pratt et al 2001).

PREVENTING INFECTION IN IV DEVICES

Most bloodstream infections associated with IV devices can be prevented by careful management of the device (Maki & Mermel 1998). Clear guidelines for the insertion, management and removal of devices should be established and adhered to, especially in units where patients commonly require a central vascular catheter and where the risks of CAI are relatively high. Of key importance is the use of strict aseptic technique for handling IV devices and handwashing before and after contact with the device (Pratt et al 2001, Ward et al 1997). Education and training is an essential part of this process and several studies have demonstrated a substantial reduction in the numbers of infections where IV devices have been maintained by specially trained personnel (Keohane et al 1983, Puntis et al 1990).

Insertion of the catheter

The catheterization procedure may introduce bacteria from the skin into the vein. These bacteria may be derived either from the patient or from the hands of the person inserting it. The catheter site has been described as 'not unlike an open wound containing a foreign body' (Maki et al 1973) and insertion should therefore be considered a minor surgical procedure carried out with a high standard of asepsis and preceded by thorough handwashing. Asepsis is particularly important for the insertion of central catheters, which is a more invasive procedure associated with a greater risk of infection. Raad et al (1994) showed that it was the use of a high level of barrier precautions for insertion that was important rather than the place of insertion (operating theatre or ward). Swan–Ganz catheters inserted in the ICU using high-level barrier precautions (sterile gloves, gowns, masks, large drapes) were much less likely to become infected than those inserted in the operating theatre with a lesser level of barrier precautions. This was despite the fact that catheters inserted in ICU stayed in place for longer and were used more frequently for parenteral nutrition.

The catheter should be firmly anchored to prevent movement, which may both carry micro-organisms

---

> **Guidelines for practice: insertion of an intravenous catheter**
>
> - Use a Teflon or polyurethane catheter for peripheral cannulation
> - Wash hands before insertion. Use sterile gloves, masks, gowns and drapes to insert central venous and arterial catheters
> - Use chlorhexidine to clean skin and allow to dry before insertion
> - Avoid shaving the site of insertion
> - Secure catheter but do not cover the insertion site with non-sterile tape

---

from the skin into the wound and increase the risk of mechanical phlebitis (Maki et al 1973). Tape has been implicated as a source of infection, and tape that is in direct contact with the insertion site should be sterile (Sheldon & Johnson 1979).

Skin preparation

A study by Maki et al (1991a) suggested that cleaning the site with chlorhexidine before insertion of a central or arterial catheter is associated with a lower rate of infection than 10% povidone–iodine or 70% alcohol. Although the 2% solution of chlorhexidine used in this study is not commercially available, 0.5% solutions have also been shown to be effective (Garland et al 1995). To ensure maximum disinfection of the skin, the disinfectant should be applied for about 30 s and allowed to dry before starting the procedure.

Effective skin preparation will remove bacteria from hair as well as the skin. Shaving the skin causes microscopic damage, which can increase microbial colonization. Shaving around the insertion site should therefore be avoided. See practice guidelines for the insertion of a catheter.

Catheter replacement

A marked increase in the incidence of phlebitis and catheter colonization when peripheral catheters are left in place for more than 72 h has been reported (Band & Maki 1980). Routine replacement of peripheral catheter every 48–72 h has therefore been recommended (Pearson 1996). However, other studies have shown no difference in rate of phlebitis when peripheral catheters were left in for 96 h, and others have suggested that routine replacement is not necessary (Bregenzer et al 1995, Lai 1998).

With central vascular catheters the situation is more complex. Although the risk of CAI associated with central vascular catheters increases with duration of catheterization, the daily risk of infection appears to remain constant and the rate of catheter colonization and CAI is not reduced by routine replacement (Cobb et al 1992, Eyer et al 1990, Stenzel et al 1989). With pulmonary artery catheters the risk of CAI increases after 3 days of catheterization, and these should be replaced at least every 5 days (Mermel et al 1991, Pearson 1996).

If the patient develops a CAI, central vascular catheters should be removed and a new catheter inserted at a different site. If a central catheter requires replacement because of malfunction, it can be exchanged over a guidewire rather than be removed completely; however, this should be avoided if there is evidence of infection at the insertion site (Cook et al 1997, Pearson 1996). If infection is suspected, the catheter tip should be cultured and, if the result is positive, a new catheter inserted at a different site (Pratt et al 2001).

Care of the insertion site

The conventional method of protecting the insertion site is with a dressing but there is considerable controversy about which type of dressing is most effective. Gauze dressings do not protect the site from moisture and do not allow the insertion site to be visualized easily. Transparent film dressings enable the insertion site to be viewed easily to detect early signs of phlebitis or infection, allow the patient to bathe, and require less frequent attention. An accumulation of bacteria on the skin under transparent film dressings has been reported, although most studies have not demonstrated an increased risk of device-related infection. In a major study comparing transparent dressings and gauze used on peripheral catheters, Maki & Ringer (1987) found no significant difference in the rate of catheter colonization or phlebitis between the two types of dressing. There was also no increase in risk if transparent dressings were left on for the lifetime of the catheter. Ricard et al (1985) also found no difference in skin colonization or catheter-related infection between films left on for 7 days and gauze changed every 2–3 days.

Studies on central vascular catheters have reported an increased rate of site infections and bacteraemia associated with transparent films (Conly et al 1989). However, a meta-analysis by Hoffman et al (1992) indicated that, although transparent films were associated with an increase in catheter-tip colonization, there was no significant increase in CAI. This finding was confirmed by Maki et al (1994) in a study on pulmonary

arterial catheters in which gauze dressings (changed every 2 days) were compared with polyurethane transparent film (changed every 5 days). Other studies on pulmonary arterial catheters have shown a large increase in risk of CAI when transparent films are used. This may be related to the collection of blood at the insertion site, which provides a rich medium for bacterial growth (Maki & Will 1984). One explanation for the conflicting information is the variation in moisture vapour permeability of dressings made by different manufacturers. New transparent films with a high vapour permeability may reduce skin colonization by allowing moisture to escape (Maki et al 1991b).

Skin disinfectants used to clean the skin when the dressing is changed may reduce the rate of infection associated with central venous and arterial catheters, for example an aqueous solution of chlorhexidine, which has a residual antibacterial effect on the skin for several hours after application (Maki & Ringer 1987, Maki et al 1991a). See practice guidelines for care of the insertion site.

Topical antimicrobial agents applied to insertion sites have been recommended but are prone to encourage the growth of fungi such as candida or other resistant micro-organisms. They should therefore not be used routinely (Maki & Mermel 1998). Povidone–iodine ointment applied to subclavian haemodialysis catheters has been shown to reduce the incidence of CAI (Levin et al 1991). A chlorhexidine-impregnated disc pressed on to the skin at the insertion site has also been reported to reduce the risk of CAI significantly in central vascular catheters (non-tunnelled), PICC and arterial catheters for short- or medium-term use. The effect is not apparent for long-term catheters where the intralumen route is an important source of the infections (Maki et al 2000).

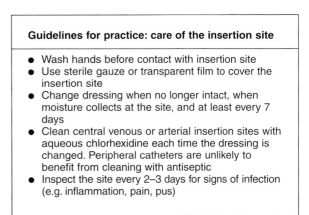

Guidelines for practice: care of the insertion site

- Wash hands before contact with insertion site
- Use sterile gauze or transparent film to cover the insertion site
- Change dressing when no longer intact, when moisture collects at the site, and at least every 7 days
- Clean central venous or arterial insertion sites with aqueous chlorhexidine each time the dressing is changed. Peripheral catheters are unlikely to benefit from cleaning with antiseptic
- Inspect the site every 2–3 days for signs of infection (e.g. inflammation, pain, pus)

Management of catheters and fluid administration sets

The aseptic management of the catheter hub, connection ports and administration sets is essential to prevent contamination of the system and subsequent infection.

Contamination of stopcocks used to administer drugs or infusates is common, although a causal relationship between colonization and subsequent infection is difficult to demonstrate (Cheeseborough & Finch 1985, Grabe & Jakobsen 1983, Pearson 1996). Hub contamination is increased by prolonged catheterization and frequent manipulation (Mermel 2000). The number of access points and catheter lumens should be kept to a minimum, and access points should be disinfected with alcohol, chlorhexidine or povidone–iodine before use (Maki et al 1997, Pearson 1996, Pratt et al 2001).

Piggy-back systems, where a needle is inserted into a rubber membrane, may be beneficial (Inoue et al 1992), but needle-less systems may increase the incidence of CAI where high-risk fluids such as parenteral nutrition are being administered (Danzig et al 1995).

Bacteria may also be introduced in the infusion fluid. Some bacteria, notably klebsiella and enterobacter, are able to grow even in simple IV solutions, such as 5% dextrose (Centers for Disease Control 1971). A number of outbreaks of infection in the 1970s were caused by IV fluids contaminated during manufacture, but improvements in quality control methods have now made this an unlikely source of infection.

Infusion fluids may also become contaminated during use when drugs are added, or when infusion fluids or administration sets are changed. Units of blood or platelets may contain bacteria, which can contaminate the infusion set (Walsh et al 1993).

The extent to which fluids are accessed affects the risk of infection (Table 9.3). Administration sets in intensive care units, where lines are frequently manipulated for haemodynamic monitoring and drug administration, are more likely to become contaminated (Maki et al 1987, Mermel et al 1991). Bacteria introduced from contaminated infusate or during manipulation of the line will multiply over time and to prevent this administration sets should be changed regularly (Maki et al 1987, Syndman et al 1987). Several studies have shown that replacing administration sets every 72 h is safe. However, they should be replaced more frequently if used to administer fluids that readily support the growth of bacteria, such as parenteral nutrition, lipid emulsions, blood and blood products (Pratt et al 2001).

Hands should be washed thoroughly before manipulating IV devices or fluid administration sets. In most circumstances gloves are unnecessary but it may be preferable to use sterile gloves to attach new bags of parenteral nutrition fluid because of the high risk of infection (see p. 181).

Where systems are used for pressure monitoring, the tubing, flush device and transducer should be replaced every 96 h. Disposable transducers and closed flush systems are preferable. Dextrose should not be used in a pressure monitoring system because it supports the growth of micro-organisms, and the system should not be used for obtaining blood samples as this will increase the risk of contamination (Pearson 1996).

Flush solutions

The use of anticoagulants to flush IV devices is intended to maintain patency, to prevent bacteria from adhering to the catheter, and thrombosis. Current evidence suggests that in peripheral catheters heparin flushes were no more beneficial than saline in maintaining patency and preventing infection. In central venous and arterial catheters, routine flushing with heparin reduces thrombus formation and may prevent CAI (Pratt et al 2001, Randolph et al 1998). Glyceryl trinitrate applied on the skin near to the insertion site encourages vasodilation and reduces the incidence of phlebitis (O'Brien et al 1990).

IV filters

A filter placed between the catheter and the fluid administration set may reduce the incidence of phlebitis and can be used to prevent bacteria and endotoxins in the fluid from gaining access to the bloodstream. Filters may be cost effective with administration sets that are frequently accessed (Spencer 1990). Filters cannot be used on Swan–Ganz catheters or where blood, blood products, lipid emulsion and amphotericin are being infused (Quercia et al 1986).

Table 9.3 Contamination of infusion fluids. From Maki et al (1987) JAMA 258: 2396–403 Copyrighted 1987, American Medical Association

Type or location of IV device	Infusions contaminated (%)
Peripheral	0.6
Central venous	1.5
Central – total parenteral nutrition	3.6
Devices on the intensive care unit	2.5
Devices on general wards	0.9

Guidelines for practice: care of the administration set	Guidelines for practice: management of parenteral nutrition
<ul><li>Wash hands before accessing IV devices. Do not touch IV line connections or allow them to come into contact with non-sterile surfaces. Sterile gloves are not usually necessary provided sterile connections are not touched by hand</li><li>Keep the number of access points on an intravenous line to a minimum. If a tap or stopcock is not in use then remove it</li><li>Use single-lumen central vascular catheters if possible</li><li>Administer IV drugs through the latex membrane on peripheral lines to avoid the use of ports</li><li>Change administration sets every 72 h (24–48 h if accessed frequently) and always after the infusion of blood products</li><li>Consider use of IV filters where lines are accessed frequently</li><li>Remove device as soon as clinically indicated</li></ul>	The risks of infection associated with the infusion of parenteral nutrition are much greater than with other fluids and extreme care must be taken to avoid contamination.<ul><li>The catheter should be inserted under maximal aseptic conditions in the theatre or treatment room by an experienced doctor</li><li>Designate the catheter for PN only (avoid using multilumen catheters). Do not add drugs or withdraw blood from the line</li><li>Do not connect ports, stopcocks or taps</li><li>Change the PN fluid and administration set every 24 h using sterile gloves and a no-touch technique</li><li>Inspect the insertion site daily for signs of infection and clean with chlorhexidine when dressing is changed</li><li>Record temperature and pulse 4 hourly to detect early signs of sepsis</li><li>Take blood cultures through the line and from a peripheral vein if the patient becomes pyrexial</li></ul>

There is no evidence that wrapping hub joints with gauze soaked in antiseptic prevents infections, and alcohol-based solutions may damage the catheter material (Medical Devices Directorate 1993). Practice guidelines for the care of administration sets are described above.

Parenteral nutrition

The administration of elemental nutrients into a vein is used to feed patients who are unable to meet their nutritional requirements by oral or nasogastric feeding. Conventionally, parenteral nutrition is administered via a central venous catheter where the high blood flow reduces the thrombophlebitic effects of glucose. Bacteria can multiply easily in parenteral nutrition (PN) fluid and infection is a frequent complication of PN therapy, with an infection rate of around 14% (Mughal 1989). Particular care must therefore be taken to avoid contamination of the fluids and devices used to administer PN. Fluids are usually prepared in the pharmacy using strict asepsis and under laminar flow ventilation to minimize the risk of contamination. Ideally, a single catheter should be designated for administering PN, and this should not be used to take blood or give drugs. Triple-lumen catheters should not be used for PN, because the risk of sepsis has been reported to be four times that of single-lumen catheters (Clark-Christoff et al 1992). A high level of asepsis should be used for manipulating the administration set and fluids (see practice guidelines).

Peripherally inserted central catheters have been used successfully for short-term feeding using a lower concentration of glucose and are associated with a lower risk of infection (Hansell 1989). The use of glyceryl trinitrate patches may prolong the life of peripheral devices used for PN (Khawaja et al 1988).

Hickman and subcutaneous lines

Intravenous catheters made from an inert material, silicone elastomer, were pioneered by Broviac and developed by Hickman. These catheters are inserted into a central vein and tunnelled under the skin to exit on the chest wall (Fig. 9.2). Tissue grows into a Dacron cuff positioned in the skin tunnel, and this stabilizes the catheter so that a securing suture is not necessary and prevents bacteria migrating from the skin into the vein. Cuffs added to conventional central catheters reduce the incidence of infection (Flowers et al 1989).

Hickman catheters are used extensively in the management of patients requiring prolonged venous access, particularly for chemotherapy. They are associated with low rates of infection considering the length of time they are in the vein. The incidence of infection is estimated at 1.4 infections per 1000 catheter-days, compared with more than 3 infections per 1000 catheter-days with non-tunnelled central vascular devices (Clark & Raffin 1990, Widner 1997). Neutropenia or other forms of immunosuppression increase the risk of CAI related to tunnelled catheters (Howell et al 1995, Raviglione et al 1989).

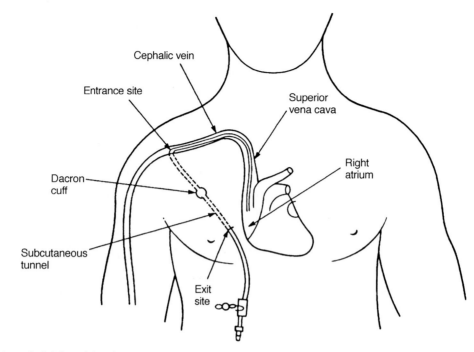

Fig. 9.2 A tunnelled right atrial catheter.

Infection of the exit site or tunnel may occur, and both may result in bloodstream infection. Bacteraemia associated with these long-term catheters occurs frequently but is usually asymptomatic and caused by coagulase-negative staphylococci. If the line is suspected to be a source of a symptomatic infection, antibiotics may be instilled into the device to eliminate colonization whilst avoiding removal of the catheter (Widner 1997).

Initially insertion site care should be the same as for other central catheters, but approximately 10 days after insertion the Dacron cuff has been secured by tissue ingrowth and the exit site suture can be removed. Some then recommend leaving the site exposed without a dressing, but transparent dressings left in place for 5–7 days have also been used with no increase in risk of CAI (Johnstone 1982, Shivnan et al 1991). In common with other central catheters, provided that a good no-touch technique is used, gloves are not necessary to manipulate the administration set or to administer intravenous drugs, except perhaps where PN is being infused and the risk of introducing infection through line manipulation is much greater.

Totally implanted or subcutaneous central venous catheters (e.g. Port-a-Cath) with a self-sealing septum are being used increasingly, particularly for patients cared for in their own home. These devices have the lowest risk of infection (approximately 0.2 infections

per 1000 catheter-days; Groeger et al 1993). Occasionally infection of the subcutaneous pocket occurs (Decker & Edwards 1988).

IV therapy teams

The impact of high-quality IV device care has been demonstrated by a number of studies in which trained IV therapy teams have been used to insert catheters and provide follow-up care: this approach is associated with substantially lower rates of CAI (Faubion et al 1986, Keohane et al 1983). Others have used intensive education of staff and catheter care protocols to achieve reductions (Lange et al 1997, Parras et al 1994). As with many aspects of infection control, the provision of a high standard of IV device care is dependent on patient–nurse ratios, and understaffing in the ICU can have a major impact on the risk of CAI (Fridkin et al 1996).

Surveillance of CAI in high-risk units such as the ICU, neonatal intensive care and haematology can provide essential information with which to evaluate practice, motivate change and encourage adherence to local protocols (Stonehouse & Butcher 1996). In the USA, hospitals that participate in the national surveillance system have achieved reductions in the incidence of CAI during the past decade (MMWR 2000).

Management of IV devices in the home

It is often difficult to translate the care of IV devices in hospital to the environment of the home, where the patient may be responsible for most of the care and the facilities and equipment available are less sophisticated. The risks of introducing infection may be lower because cross-infection from other patients is unlikely to occur. However, patients are still at risk of endogenous infection from their own skin flora. Thorough training of the patient or carers on the management of the device, in particular the importance of asepsis, is therefore essential (Willis 1996). The plan of care should be as simple as possible, although considerable distress can be caused by forcing patients to adopt unfamiliar procedures and is unnecessary, provided the general principles of infection control are adhered to.

Written instructions are preferable as detailed information may not be retained after discharge. Advice given by healthcare workers involved in care must be consistent.

REFERENCES

Band JD, Maki DG (1980) Steel needles used for intravenous therapy. Morbidity in patients with hematologic malignancy. *Arch. Intern. Med.*, **140**: 31–4.

Beck-Sague CM, Jarvis WR (1993) Secular trends in the epidemiology of nosocomial fungal infections in the United States, 1980–1990. *J. Infect. Dis.*, **167**: 1247–51.

Beck-Sague CM, Jarvis WR, Brook JH et al (1990) Epidemic bacteremia due to *Acinetobacter baumannii* in five intensive care units. *Am. J. Epidemiol.*, **132**: 723–33.

Bregenzer T, Widmer AF, Conen D (1995) Routine replacement of peripheral catheters is not necessary: a prospective study. *Can. J. Infect. Dis.*, **6** (Suppl. C): 247C.

Centers for Disease Control (1971) Nosocomial bacteremias associated with intravenous fluid therapy. *MMWR*, **20** (Suppl. 9): 1–2.

Cercenardo E, Ena J, Rodriguez-Creixems M et al (1990) A conservative procedure for the diagnosis of catheter-related infections. *Arch. Intern. Med.*, **150**: 1417–20.

Cheeseborough JS, Catlow R (1999) Contamination of intravenous heparin infusions. *J. Hosp. Infect.*, **43**(3): 248–9.

Cheeseborough JS, Finch RG (1985) Studies on the microbiological safety of the valved side-port of the 'Venflon' cannula. *J. Hosp. Infect.*, **6**: 201–8.

Clark-Christoff N, Watters VA, Sparks W et al (1992) Use of triple-lumen subclavian catheters for administration of total parenteral nutrition. *J. Parenter. Enteral Nutr.*, **16**: 403–7.

Clarke DE, Raffin TA (1990) Infectious complications of indwelling long-term central venous catheters. *Chest*, **97**: 966–72.

Cobb DK, High KP, Sawyer RG et al (1992) A controlled trial of scheduled replacement of central venous and pulmonary artery catheters. *N. Engl. J. Med.*, **327**: 1062–8.

Conly JM, Grieves K, Peters B (1989) A prospective randomised study comparing transparent and dry gauze dressings for central venous catheters. *J. Infect. Dis.*, **159**: 310–19.

Cook D, Randolph A, Kemerman P et al (1997) Central venous catheter replacement strategies: a systematic review of the literature. *Crit. Care Med.*, **25**(8): 1417–24.

Crow S, Conrad SA, Chaney-Rowell C et al (1989) Microbial contamination of arterial infusions used for hemodynamic monitoring: a randomised trial of contamination with sampling through conventional stopcocks versus a novel, closed system. *Infect. Control Hosp. Epidemiol.*, **10**: 557–61.

Danzig LE, Short L, Collins K et al (1995) Bloodstream infections associated with a needles intravenous infusion system and total parenteral nutrition. *JAMA*, **273**: 1862–4.

Daschner FD, Frank U (1989) Intravenous catheter and device-related infection. *Curr. Opin. Infect. Dis.*, **2**: 663–7.

Davenport DS, Massanari RM, Pfaller MA et al (1986) Usefulness of a test for slime production as a marker for clinically significant infections with coagulase-negative staphylococci. *J. Infect. Dis.*, **153**: 332–9.

Darouiche RO, Raad I, Heard SO et al (1999) A comparison of two antimicrobial-impregnated central venous catheters. *N. Engl. J. Med.*, **340**: 1–8.

Decker MD, Edwards KM (1988) Central venous catheter infections. *Pediatr. Clin. North Am.*, **14**: 503–9.

Elliot TSJ (1988) Intravascular device infections. *J. Med. Microbiol*, **27**: 161–7.

Elliot TSJ (1993) Line-associated bacteraemias. *Commun. Dis. Rep.*, **3**(7): R91–5.

Emmerson AM, Enstone JE, Griffin M et al (1996) The second national prevalence survey of infection in hospitals – overview of the results. *J. Hosp. Infect.*, **32**: 175–90.

Ena J, Cerenardo E, Martinez D et al (1992) Cross-sectional epidemiology of phlebitis and catheter-related infections. *Infect. Control Hosp. Epidemiol.*, **13**: 15–20.

Eyer S, Brummitt C, Crossley K et al (1990) Catheter-related sepsis: prospective randomised study of three methods of long-term catheter maintenance. *Crit. Care Med.*, **18**(10): 1073–9.

Fang G, Keys TF, Gentry LO et al (1993) Prosthetic valve endocarditis resulting from nosocomial bacteremia: a prospective, multicenter study. *Ann. Intern. Med.*, **111**: 560–7.

Farkas JK, Liu N, Bleriot JP et al (1992) Single versus triple-lumen central catheter-related sepsis: a prospective randomized study in a critically ill population. *Am. J. Med.*, **93**: 277–82.

Farr BM (1999) Accuracy and cost-effectiveness of new tests for diagnosis of catheter-related bloodstream infections. *Lancet*, **354**: 1487–8.

Faubion WC, Wesley JR, Khalidi N et al (1986) Total parenteral nutrition catheter sepsis: impact of the team approach. *J. Parenter. Enteral Nutr.*, **10**: 642–5.

Flowers RH, Schwezer KJ, Kopel RJ et al (1989) Efficacy of an attachable subcutaneous cuff for the prevention of intravascular catheter-related infection. *JAMA*, **261**: 878–883.

Freeman J, Goldmann DA, Smith NE et al (1990) Association of intravenous lipid emulsion and coagulase-negative staphylococcal bacteraemia in neonatal intensive care units. *N. Engl. J. Med.*, **323**: 301–8.

Fridkin SK, Pear SM, Williamson et al (1996) The role of understaffing in central venous catheter-associated bloodstream infections. *Infect. Control Hosp. Epidemiol.*, **17**: 150–8.

Garden OJ, Sim AJW (1983) A comparison of tunnelled and non-tunnelled subclavian catheters: a prospective study of complications during parenteral feeding. *Clin. Nutr.*, **2**: 51–4.

Garland JS, Buck RK, Maloney P (1995) Comparison of 10% povidone iodine and 0.5% chlorhexidine gluconate for the prevention of peripheral IV catheter colonization in neonates: a prospective trial. *Pediatr. Infect. Dis. J.*, **14**: 510–16.

Glynn A, Ward V, Wilson J et al (1997) *Hospital-acquired Infection: Surveillance, Policies and Practice.* Public Health Laboratory Service, London.

Goetz A, Wagener M, Miller J et al (1998) Risk of infection due to central venous catheters: effect of site of placement of catheter type. *Infect. Control Hosp. Epidemiol.*, **19**(11): 842–5.

Grabe N, Jakobsen CJB (1983) Bacterial contamination of Venflon intravenous cannulae with valved injection sideport. *J. Hosp. Infect.*, **4**: 291–5.

Graham DR, Keldermans MM, Klemm LW et al (1991) Infectious complications among patients receiving home intravenous therapy with peripheral, central or peripherally placed central venous catheters. *Am. J. Med.*, **91** (Suppl. B): 95S–101S.

Gristina AG (1987) Biomaterial-centered infection: microbial adhesion versus tissue integration. *Science*, **237**: 1588–95.

Groeger JS, Lucas AB, Thaler HT et al (1993) Infectious morbidity associated with long-term use of venous access devices in patients with cancer. *Ann. Intern. Med.*, **119**: 1168–74.

Hammond JS, Varas R, Ward CG (1988) Suppurative thrombophlebitis: a new look at a continuing problem. *South Med. J.*, **81**: 969–71.

Hansell DT (1989) Intravenous nutrition: the central or peripheral route? *Intravenous Therapy and Clinical Monitoring*, **July**: 184–90.

Hekker TA, van Overhagen W, Schneider AJ (1990) Pressure transducers: an overlooked source of sepsis in the intensive care unit. *Intensive Care Med.*, **16**: 511–12.

Hoffman KK, Weber DJ, Samsa GP et al (1992) Transparent polyurethane film as an intravenous catheter dressing: a meta-analysis of the infection risks. *JAMA*, **267**: 2072–6.

Howell PB, Walter PE, Doncwitz GR et al (1995) Risk factors for infection of adult patients with cancer who have tunnelled central venous catheters. *Cancer*, **75**: 1367–75.

Inoue Y, Nezu R, Matsuda H et al (1992) Prevention of catheter-related sepsis during parenteral nutrition: effect of a new connection device. *J. Parenter. Enteral Nutr.*, **16**: 581–5.

Ishak MA, Groschel DHM, Mandell GI et al (1985) Association of slime with pathogenicity of coagulase-negative staphylococci causing nosocomial septicaemia. *J. Clin. Microbiol.*, **22**: 1025–9.

Johnstone JD (1982) Infrequent infections associated with Hickman catheters. *Cancer Nursing*, **April**: 125–9.

Keohane PP, Jones BJM, Attrill H et al (1983) Effect of catheter tunnelling and a nutrition nurse on catheter sepsis during parenteral nutrition. A controlled trial. *Lancet*, **ii**: 1388–90.

Khawaja HT, Campbell MJ, Weaver PC (1988) Effect of transdermal glyceryl trinitrate on the survival of peripheral intravenous infusions: a double-blind prospective clinical study. *Br. J. Surg.*, **75**: 1212–15.

Lai KK (1998) Safety of prolonging peripheral cannula and IV tubing use from 72 hours to 96 hours. *Am. J. Infect. Control*, **26**: 66–70.

Lange BJ, Weiman M, Feuer EJ et al (1997) Impact of changes in catheter management on infectious complication among children with central venous catheters. *Infect. Control Hosp. Epidemiol.*, **18**: 326–32.

Levin A, Mason AJ, Jindal KK et al (1991) Prevention of hemodialysis subclavian vein catheter infections by topical povidone–iodine. *Kidney Int.*, **40**: 934–8.

Linares J, Sitges-Serra A, Garau J et al (1985) Pathogenesis of catheter sepsis: a prospective study with quantitative and semiquantitative cultures of catheter hub and segments. *J. Clin. Microbiol.*, **21**: 357–60.

Maki DG (1991) Infection caused by intravascular devices: pathogenesis, strategies for prevention. In *Improving Catheter Site Care.* Proceedings of a symposium, Series 179, March 1991. Royal Society of Medicine Services, London.

Maki DG, Mermel LA (1998) Infections due to infusion therapy. In *Hospital Infections*, 4th edn, pp. 659–725 (JV Bennett, PS Brachman, eds). Lippincott-Raven, Philadelphia.

Maki DG, Ringer M (1987) Evaluation of dressing regimens for prevention of infection with peripheral intravenous catheters, gauze, a transparent polyurethane dressing and an iodophor-transparent dressing. *JAMA*, **258**: 2396–403.

Maki DG, Will L (1984) Colonisation and infection associated with transparent dressings for central venous, arterial and Hickman catheters: a comparative trial. In *24th Interscience Conference on Antimicrobial Agents and Chemotherapy.*, Abstract 991. American Society for Microbiology, Washington.

Maki DG, Goldman DA, Rhame FS (1973) Infection control in intravenous therapy. *Ann. Intern. Med.*, **79**: 867–87.

Maki DG, Hassemer C, Sarafini HW (1977) A semi-quantitative culture method for identifying intravenous catheter-related infection. *N. Engl. J. Med.*, **296**: 1305–9.

Maki DG, Botticelli JT, Le Roy ML et al (1987) Prospective study of replacing administration sets for intravenous therapy at 48 hour versus 72 hour intervals. 72 hours is safe and cost-effective. *JAMA*, **258**: 1777–81.

Maki DG, Ringer M, Alvarado CJ (1991a) Prospective randomised trial of povidone–iodine, alcohol and chlorhexidine for prevention of infection associated with central venous and arterial catheters. *Lancet*, **338**: 339–43.

Maki DG, Stolz S, Wheeler S (1991b) A prospective, randomised, three-way clinical comparison of a novel, highly impermeable, polyurethane dressing with 206 Swan–Ganz pulmonary artery catheters: Opsite IV3000 vs Tegaderm v gauze and tape. I. Cutaneous colonisation under the dressing, catheter-related infection. In *Improving Catheter Site Care.* Proceedings of a symposium, Series 179, pp. 61–6. Royal Society of Medicine Services, London.

Maki DG, Stolz SS, Wheeler S et al (1994) A prospective, randomised trial of gauze and two polyurethane dressings for site care of pulmonary artery catheters: implications for catheter management. *Crit. Care Med.*, **32**: 1729–37.

Maki DG, Stolz SS, Wheeler S et al (1997) Prevention of central venous catheter-related bloodstream infection by use of an antiseptic-impregnated catheter. A randomized controlled trial. *Ann. Intern. Med.*, **127**: 257–66.

Maki DG, Narans LL, Knasinski V et al (2000) Prospective, randomized, investigator-masked trial of a novel chlorhexidine-impregnated disk (Biopatch) on central venous and arterial catheters. *Infect. Control Hosp. Epidemiol.*, **21**(2): 96.

McCarthy MC, Shives JK, Robison RJ et al (1987) Prospective evaluation of single and triple lumen catheter in total parenteral nutrition. *J. Parenter. Enteral Nutr.*, **11**: 259–62.

Medical Devices Directorate (1993) *Degradation of Silicone Tubing by Alcohol-based Antiseptics.*, HN(93) 7. Medical Devices Directorate, 22 March. Department of Health, Wetherby, UK.

Mermel LA (2000) Prevention of intravascular catheter-related infections. *Ann. Intern. Med.*, **132**(5): 391–402.

Mermel L, Stolz S, Maki DG (1991) Epidemiology and pathogenesis of infection with Swan–Ganz catheters. A prospective study using molecular epidemiology. *Am. J. Med.*, **91**(3b): 197.

Morbidity and Mortality Weekly Report (2000) Monitoring hospital-acquired infections to promote patient safety – United States, 1990–1999. *MMWR*, **49**(2): 149–52.

Mughal MM (1989) Complications of intravenous feeding catheters. *Br. J. Surg.*, **76**: 15–21.

Nystrom B, Larson SO, Dankert J et al (1983) Bacteraemia in surgical patients with intravenous devices: a European multicentre incidence study. The European Working Party on the Control of Hospital Infections. *J. Hosp. Infect.*, **4**: 338–49.

O'Brien BJ, Buxton MJ, Khawaja HT (1990) An economic evaluation of transdermal glyceryl trinitrate in the prevention of intravenous infusion failure. *J. Clin. Epidemiol.*, **43**: 757–63.

Parras F, Ena J, Bouza E et al (1994) Impact of an educational program for the prevention of colonisation of intravascular catheter. *Infect. Control Hosp. Epidemiol.*, **15**: 335–7.

Pearson ML (1996) Guideline for prevention of intravascular device-related infections. *Am. J. Infect. Control*, **24**: 262–93.

Pittet D, Wenzel RP (1995) Nosocomial bloodstream infections. Secular trends in rates, mortality and contribution to total hospital deaths. *Arch. Intern. Med.*, **155**: 1177–84.

Pittet D, Tarara D, Wenzel RP (1994) Nosocomial bloodstream infections in critically ill patients: excess length of stay, extra costs and attributable mortality. *JAMA*, **271**: 1598–607.

Pratt RA, Pellowe CM, Loveday HP et al (2001) The Epic project: developing national evidence-based guidelines for preventing healthcare associated infections. *J. Hosp. Infect.*, **47**: Suppl. A.

Public Health Laboratory Service (1998) *Protocol for Surveillance of Hospital-acquired Bacteraemia.* Nosocomial Infection National Surveillance Scheme, PHLS, London.

Public Health Laboratory Service (2000) *Surveillance of Hospital-acquired Bacteraemia in English Hospitals, 1997–1999.* PHLS, London.

Puntis JWL, Holden CE, Smallman S (1990) Staff training: key factor in reducing intravascular catheter sepsis. *Arch. Dis. Child.*, **65**: 335–7.

Quercia RA, Hills SW, Klimek JJ et al (1986) Bacteriologic contamination of intravenous infusion delivery systems in an intensive care unit. *Am. J. Med.*, **80**: 364–8.

Raad I, Davies S, Becker M et al (1993a) Low infection rate and long durability of nontunnelled silastic catheters. A safe cost-effective alternative for long-term venous access. *Arch. Intern. Med.*, **153**: 1791–96.

Raad II, Umphrey J, Khan A et al (1993b) The duration of placement as a predictor of peripheral and pulmonary arterial catheter infections. *J. Hosp. Infect.*, **23**: 17–26.

Raad II, Hohn DC, Gilbreath BJ et al (1994) Prevention of central venous catheter-related infections by using maximal sterile barrier precautions during insertion. *Infect. Control Hosp. Epidemiol.*, **15**: 231–8.

Raad II, Baba M, Bodey GP (1995) Diagnosis of catheter-related infections: the role of surveillance and targeted quantitative skin cultures. *Clin. Infect. Dis.*, **20**: 593–7.

Randolph AG, Cook DJ, Gonzales CA et al (1998) Benefit of heparin use in central venous and pulmonary artery catheters: a meta-analysis of randomized controlled trials. *Chest*, **113**: 165–71.

Raviglione MC, Battan R, Pablos-Mendez A et al (1989) Infections associated with Hickman catheters in patients with acquired immune deficiency syndrome. *Am. J. Med.*, **86**: 780–6.

Ricard P, Martin R, Marcoux JA (1985) Protection of indwelling vascular catheters; incidence of bacterial contamination and catheter-related sepsis. *Crit. Care Med.*, **13**: 541–3.

Richet H, Hubert B, Nitemberg G et al (1990) Prospective multicenter study of vascular catheter-related complications and risk factors for positive central-catheter cultures in intensive care unit patients. *J. Clin. Microbiol.*, **28**: 2520–5.

Ryder MA (1995) Peripheral access. *Opin. Oncol. Clin. North Am.*, **4**: 395–427.

Sheldon DL, Johnson WC (1979) Cutaneous mucomycosis: two documented cases of suspected nosocomial infection. *JAMA*, **241**: 1032–3.

Shivnan JC, McGuire D, Freeman S et al (1991) Comparison of transparent adherent and dry sterile gauze dressings for long-term central catheters in patients undergoing bone marrow transplant. *Oncol. Nurse Forum*, **18**: 1349–56.

Spencer RC (1990) Use of in-line filters for intravenous infusions in intensive care units. *J. Hosp. Infect.*, **16**: 281.

Stenzel JP, Green TP, Fuhrman BP et al (1989) Percutaneous central venous catheterization in a pediatric intensive care unit: a survival analysis of complications. *Crit. Care Med.*, **17**: 984–8.

Stonehouse J, Butcher J (1996) Phlebitis associated with peripheral cannulae. *Prof. Nurse*, **12**(1): 51–4.

Syndman DR, Donnelly-Reidy M, Perry WC et al (1987) Intravenous tubing containing burettes can be safely changed at 72-hour intervals. *Infect. Control*, **8**: 113–16.

Tager IB, Ginsberg MB, Ellis SE (1983) An epidemiologic study of the risks associated with peripheral intravenous catheters. *Am. J. Epidemiol.*, **118**(6): 839–51.

Thomas A, Lalitha MK, Jesudason MV et al (1993) Transducer related *Enterobacter cloacae* sepsis in post-operative cardiothoracic patients. *J. Hosp. Infect.*, **25**: 211–14.

Veenstra DL, Saint S, Saha S et al (1999a) Efficacy of antiseptic-impregnated central venous catheter in preventing catheter-related bloodstream infection: a meta-analysis. *JAMA*, **281**(3): 261–6.

Veenstra DL, Saint S, Sullivan S (1999b) Cost-effectiveness of antiseptic-impregnated central venous catheter for the prevention of catheter-related bloodstream infection. *JAMA*, **282**(6): 554–60.

Walsh R, Gurevich R, Cunha SA (1993) *Listeria*: a potential cause of febrile transfusion reactions. *J. Hosp. Infect.*, **24**: 81–2.

Ward V, Wilson J, Taylor L et al (1997) *Preventing Hospital-acquired Infection. Clinical Guidelines*. Public Health Laboratory Service, London.

Weightman NC, Simpson EM, Speller DCE et al (1988) Bacteraemia related to indwelling central venous catheters: prevention, diagnosis, and treatment. *Eur. J. Clin. Microbiol. Infect. Dis.*, **7**(2): 125–9.

Widner AF (1997) Intravenous-related infections. In *Prevention and Control of Nosocomial Infections*, 3rd edn, pp. 771–806 (RP Wenzel, ed.). Williams & Wilkins, Baltimore.

Williams JF, Seneff MG, Freidman BC et al (1991) Use of femoral venous catheters in critically ill adults: prospective study. *Crit. Care Med.*, **19**: 550–3.

Willis J (1996) Home parenteral nutrition. *Nursing Times*, **92**(47): 50–1.

Wing EJ, Norden CW, Shadduck RK et al (1979) Use of quantitative bacteriological techniques to diagnose catheter-related sepsis. *Ann. Intern. Med.*, **139**: 482.

Wurzel CL, Halom K, Feldman JG et al (1988) Infection rates of Broviac–Hickman catheters and implantable venous devices. *Am. J. Dis. Child.*, **142**: 536–40.

FURTHER READING

Elliot TSJ, Faroqui MH (1992) Infection and intravascular devices. *Br. J. Hosp. Med.*, **48**(8): 496–503.

Fletcher SJ, Bodenham AR (1999) Catheter-related sepsis: an overview – part 1. *Br. J. Intensive Care*, **9**(2): 46–53.

Henry L (1997) Parenteral nutrition. *Prof. Nurse*, **13**(1): 39–41.

Mermel LA, Maki DG (1994) Infectious complications of Swan–Ganz pulmonary artery catheters. Pathogenesis, epidemiology, prevention and management. *Am. J. Respir. Crit. Care Med.*, **149**: 1020–36.

Sitges–serra A, Linares J, Perez JL et al (1985) A randomised trial on the effect of tubing changes on hub contamination and catheter sepsis during parenteral nutrition. *J. Parenter. Enteral Nutr.*, **9**: 322–5.

Wille JC, Blusse A, Van Oud Ablas et al (1993) A comparison of two transparent film-type dressings in central venous therapy. *J. Hosp. Infect.*, **23**: 113–22.

10

Preventing infection associated with urethral catheters

INTRODUCTION

Urinary tract infections (UTIs) are the most common infection acquired in hospital, affecting approximately 2.5% of patients admitted to hospital and accounting for over 20% of all such infections (Emmerson et al 1996, Glynn et al 1997, Plowman et al 1999).

The normal bladder has a number of defences against infection: the urethra provides an obstacle that is difficult for micro-organisms to traverse, the epithelial cells lining the bladder are resistant to bacterial adherence, and the process of urination ensures that bacteria that do manage to gain access are diluted by fresh urine and removed by the next urination. The presence of a urethral catheter interferes with these defences and as a result it is a major predisposing factor for hospital-acquired UTIs, three-quarters of which are related to indwelling urethral catheters. UTI is also a major problem in nursing homes and rehabilitation centres where the elderly, debilitated and others catheterized for prolonged periods are at greater risk of acquiring recurrent UTIs and of developing the long-term complications associated with the infection (Warren et al 1982).

SYMPTOMS, DIAGNOSIS AND TREATMENT OF URINARY TRACT INFECTION

In a non-catheterized individual the diagnosis of a UTI is usually based on clinical symptoms: frequency of micturition, pain on micturition (dysuria), fever, and sometimes loin or suprapubic pain. These symptoms reflect an inflammatory process in the bladder or kidneys caused by the invasion of the tissues by micro-organisms. In the catheterized patient diagnosis of UTI is more complex; frequency and dysuria will not be apparent unless the catheter is removed, and other symptoms may be absent, particularly in elderly or confused patients (Warren et al 1987).

The diagnosis of UTI may be confirmed in the microbiology laboratory by culturing a specimen of urine. In the non-catheterized patient, the specimen is readily contaminated by micro-organisms colonizing the periurethral area and therefore only the isolation of a single micro-organism in high concentration (more than 10^5 organisms per mL) is considered indicative of infection. In catheterized patients urine samples should be taken from the sampling sleeve on the catheter or drainage system (see p. 22). These specimens are less prone to contamination and a lower concentration of micro-organisms (10^2 per mL) may be considered significant (Stark & Maki 1984), as they are likely to reach a much higher concentration within a few days (Garibaldi et al 1982). Where bacteria are found to be present in urine this is termed bacteriuria; in the catheterized patient bacteriuria is commonly asymptomatic. The presence of white blood cells (pyuria) in the urine of bacteriuric patients is usually suggestive of host infection, although the cells may equally represent a response to the catheter or to urological surgery (Stamm 1983).

The micro-organisms that commonly cause UTI are found colonizing the periurethral area. In the non-catheterized patient virulent strains of *Escherichia coli* cause the most serious infections. These carry genes coding for fimbriae, adhesions and haemolysin that enable them to adhere to uroepithelial cells, invade and damage tissue (Johnson 1991). In catheterized patients in whom normal host defences are compromised these strains rarely cause infection; instead, a wide range of different species is responsible. Mostly these are Gram-negative bacilli, but yeasts are an increasingly frequent cause of catheter-associated UTI, especially when the patient has received antimicrobial agents (Bronsema et al 1993).

If more than one type of bacterium is found in the urine of a non-catheterized patient, this is often attributed to contamination of the specimen by bacteria from the skin or perineum. In the catheterized patient, two or more types of bacteria are frequently identified. The longer the catheter is in situ the greater the variety of bacteria isolated from the urine (Warren et al 1982a).

THE EFFECT OF URINARY TRACT INFECTIONS

Bacteriuria in catheterized patients is generally asymptomatic with no evidence of bacteria invading the bladder tissues, ureters or kidneys. However, in up to 30% of catheterized patients with bacteriuria, the bacteria invade the tissues and the patient develops symptoms of UTI (Garibaldi et al 1982) such as fever, flank pain and haematuria. Patients with long-term catheters have approximately one episode of unexplained fever every 100 days and UTI is responsible for two-thirds of these febrile episodes. Most of these fevers are low grade, resolve rapidly without antibiotic treatment, and do not appear to increase the mortality rate (Peterson & Roth 1989, Warren et al 1987).

A study by Platt et al (1982) demonstrated that catheterized patients who acquired a UTI in hospital were three times more likely to die than those who did not, even if other factors such as age, duration of catheterization and the severity of the illness were taken into account. This increased mortality rate is probably related to subsequent infections such as bacteraemia or damage to the urinary tract.

Bacteraemia The invasion of the bloodstream by bacteria colonizing the urinary tract is the most serious outcome of bacteriuria. Bacteraemia develops in approximately 5% of catheter-associated UTIs (Bryan & Reynolds 1984, Krieger et al 1983). As approximately 10% of patients admitted to hospital are catheterized, the urinary tract is an important source of hospital-acquired bacteraemia, responsible for 9% of these infections (Crow et al 1988, Public Health Laboratory Service 2000). Infections caused by Gram-negative bacilli, the most common uropathogen, are often severe and in about one-third of cases the patient dies as a result (Bryan & Reynolds 1984).

Bacteraemia probably goes unrecognized in many catheterized patients. It is particularly likely to occur during catheterization, when trauma to the mucosa during the procedure enables bacteria to enter the bloodstream.

Secondary infections Bacteria originating from the urinary tract may also circulate around the body to cause secondary infections at other sites, for example wounds and central venous cannulas (Garibaldi 1993).

Damage to the urinary tract Evidence from autopsies suggests that chronic inflammation of the kidneys occurs in more than one-third of patients who have been catheterized for a prolonged period. These patients are also at risk of developing urinary tract stones, and other periurethral infections such as urethritis and prostatitis (Bryan & Reynolds 1984, Warren et al 1988).

THE ROUTES OF INFECTION

Bacteria enter the bladder of the catheterized patient in one of three ways: first, they may be introduced with the catheter at the time of insertion; second, they may travel along the outside of the catheter; and third, they may travel along the inside lumen of the catheter

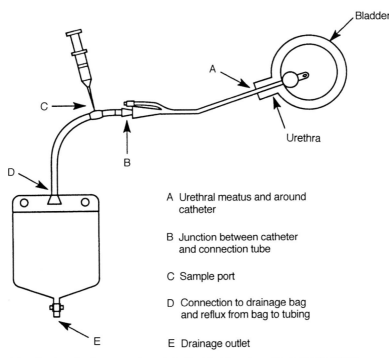

A Urethral meatus and around
   catheter

B Junction between catheter
   and connection tube

C Sample port

D Connection to drainage bag
   and reflux from bag to tubing

E Drainage outlet

Fig. 10.1 Potential points of entry of micro-organisms into the bladder of a catheterized patient.

(Fig. 10.1). There are important differences between men and women in the significance of each route of infection. The perineum is frequently colonized by potential uropathogens from the intestinal tract, especially Gram-negative bacilli. In women the vagina can also be an important source of uropathogens. If the lactobacilli that normally live in the vagina are eliminated by antibiotic therapy or changes in vaginal pH, faecal flora may establish and subsequently invade the urinary tract. In postmenopausal women vaginal pH is affected by the decline in oestrogen production and contributes to the increased incidence of UTI in this group (Nicolle 1997, Stamey & Timothy 1975). In women the relatively short urethra enables bacteria from the perineum to reach the bladder more easily than in men. Garibaldi et al (1974) demonstrated that the risk of bacteriuria increased fourfold in women and twofold in men, 72 h after meatal colonization was established. Kass & Schneiderman (1959) demonstrated that in the presence of a catheter *Serratia marcescens* inoculated on to the urethral meatus travelled along the outside of the catheter and could be recovered in urine from the bladder a few days later. This route probably accounts for a significant proportion of UTI in catheterized women (Daifuku & Stamm 1984). Elderly institutionalized populations are particularly vulnerable to perineal colonization, and

asymptomatic bacteriuria is prevalent in up to 35% of men and 50% of women (Nicolle 1987, 1997).

In men, infection from perineal flora is less important because the urethra is longer and further away from the rectum. Generally, bacteria gain access to the bladder via the lumen of the catheter, frequently as a result of cross-infection from enteric bacteria carried on the hands of staff which enter the urine system when it is emptied, disconnected or handled (Daifuku & Stamm 1984). Bacteria introduced into the drainage bag take only a few days to reach the bladder via the drainage tubing. Some 15–20% of patients with bacteriuria have the same micro-organism in their drainage bag before it reaches the bladder (Garibaldi et al 1974).

Nickel et al (1985) suggested that, in the patient catheterized for less than 7 days, most bacteria enter the drainage system from the drainage tap or following disconnection of the system. As the duration of catheterization increases, bacteria are more likely to enter the bladder alongside the catheter.

The duration of catheterization

Garibaldi et al (1974) demonstrated the strong relationship between the length of time the catheter was in place and the risk of UTI. They found that the risk of

Table 10.1 Urinary catheter use by specialty in 19 hospitals

Specialty	Patients catheterized (%)		Duration of catheterization (days)	
Medicine	11.6	(5–7)	5	(3–9)
Surgery	34.4	(16–50)	3.5	(2–5)
Gynaecology	40.4	(21–72)	2	(0–3)
Orthopaedics	17.3	(10–26)	6	(3–11)
Overall rate	26.3	(12–35)	3	(2–4)

Values are median with range in parentheses.

acquiring infection increased by 5% for each additional day of catheterization and that after 10 days 50% of patients have bacteria in the urine. It is therefore not surprising that virtually all chronically catheterized patients have bacteria in their urine (Warren et al 1982a). This illustrates the importance of early catheter removal as a means of preventing catheter-associated UTI. Although indwelling catheters are no longer in common use as a means of managing incontinence, they are used in the management of surgical procedures and for the measurement of urine output. Glynn et al (1997), in a study of 19 hospitals in England and Wales, found considerable variation between hospitals in the proportion of patients catheterized in different specialties. This suggests that there is potential to reduce catheter-associated UTI by reducing catheter insertion and duration of use (Table 10.1).

Patients who require a permanent or long-term catheter will inevitably acquire bacteria in the urine. Catheter management should therefore be focused on preventing both the introduction of new uropathogens and cross-infection to other patients. Treatment of bacteriuria in these patients is usually not indicated unless the infection is accompanied by symptoms such as fever.

Disruption of host defences

In addition to enhancing the passage of micro-organisms from the perineum to the bladder via the urethra, the presence of an indwelling urine catheter has important effects on other defences against infection. The presence of a foreign body in the bladder diminishes the activity of white blood cells, damages the mucosa and interferes with mechanisms that prevent adherence of bacteria to uroepithelial cells (Daifuku & Stamm 1986). Micro-organisms may accumulate on the surface of the catheter, protected from urine flow, host defences and antibiotics by the formation of a biofilm (Box 10.1). Finally, the residual volume of urine that forms below the level of the drainage channels enables micro-organisms to multiply in the bladder.

Box 10.1 Biofilms

Micro-organisms commonly coat the surfaces of foreign materials inserted into the body by forming biofilms. These are sheets of micro-organisms that adhere to the surface by secreting an extracellular substance called glycocalyx. On urinary catheters biofilms form on the inner surface; they incorporate urinary proteins and salts, and accumulate crystals of struvite and apatite. Eventually the biofilm becomes so thick that it obstructs the flow of urine. Some bacteria present in the urine, particularly proteus and pseudomonas, promote the formation of biofilms (Mobley & Warren 1987).

TREATMENT OF URINARY TRACT INFECTION

Asymptomatic bacteriuria does not usually require treatment unless the patient is at high risk of renal infection or bacteraemia (e.g. neutropenia, pregnancy or urological disorder) or is undergoing urological surgery. In the catheterized patient antibiotic therapy has no effect on the bacteriuria or incidence of febrile episodes while the catheter is in situ, and is likely to encourage antibiotic-resistant strains to emerge (Nicolle 1997, Warren et al 1982b). Symptoms of infection usually resolve spontaneously if the catheter is removed and may be treated after removal if they persist (Stamm 1998). As bacteria embedded in the biofilm on the surface of the catheter may be protected from antimicrobials, the catheter should be changed if treatment is commenced (Garibaldi 1993).

Although UTIs are usually easily treated at relatively low cost, they are associated with an increased hospital stay and the high frequency with which they occur makes their overall costs high in comparison with other hospital-acquired infections (Plowman et al 1999).

MEASURES TO PREVENT INFECTION IN THE CATHETERIZED PATIENT

As the urethral catheter has become a routine feature of medical care it is easy to forget the importance of prevention of infection in its management. The impact of good catheter management has been demonstrated by the reduction in catheter-associated UTI over the last few decades. In the 1960s urethral catheters drained into open buckets or bottles and more than 90% of catheterized patients developed bacteriuria. In the 1970s, the system of closed drainage system into a plastic bag was introduced and the rate dropped to 25%. In the 1980s and 1990s even lower rates of around 10% have been reported, reflecting improved infection control and decreasing duration of catheterization (Stamm 1991). The key practices for preventing catheter-associated infection are minimizing the duration of catheterization and ensuring that the closed drainage system remains closed (Warren 1997). Glynn et al (1997) demonstrated that the rates of UTI associated with urinary catheters varied considerably between different specialties and different hospitals, even when the duration of device use was taken into account by calculating the rate per 1000 device-days (Table 10.2). This suggests that the incidence of catheter-associated UTI could be reduced further by improvements in the management of urinary catheters.

Practices to prevent infection, based on research evidence, should be applied to the insertion of the catheter, the management of the urine drainage system and the care of the urethral meatus. Recommended practices are summarized in the Guidelines for practice and are discussed in more detail below.

Insertion of the catheter

The risk of developing bacteriuria after a single insertion and removal of a catheter ranges from 0.5% to 30% in the severely debilitated (Garibaldi 1993). As the risk of infection increases with each additional day for which the catheter remains in place, catheterization should be avoided wherever possible but discontinued at the earliest opportunity before bacteriuria develops (see Table 10.1). Evidence suggests that in many cases this does not happen (Glynn et al 1997, Hartstein et al 1981).

Table 10.2 Device-day rates of urinary tract infection in catheterized patients by specialty in 19 hospitals

Specialty	Infections per 1000 device-days	
Medicine	2.8	(0–9)
Surgery	3.9	(0–9.6)
Gynaecology	16.7	(1.4–33.4)
Orthopaedics	3.5	(0.8–10.3)
Overall rate	5.0	(2.5–11)

Values are median with range in parentheses.

> **Guidelines for practice: insertion of a urethral catheter**
>
> - Wash hands and use sterile gloves
> - Prepare the patient and position comfortably
> - Instil anaesthetic lubricating gel into the urethra
> - Clean perineum and external meatus with saline, water, or soap and water
> - Use sterile equipment
> - Insert catheter directly into urethra
> - Select catheter appropriately
> - Inflate balloon with correct amount of sterile water
> - Remove the catheter as soon as possible

To minimize the risk of infection the catheter should be inserted directly into the urethra without touching other parts of the perineum, which may be heavily colonized with bacteria. This is probably an important factor in explaining why catheters inserted in the operating theatre, where the procedure is more easily performed, are associated with fewer infections (Castle & Osterhout 1974). It is impossible to remove the perineal flora completely prior to the procedure but the number of bacteria may be reduced by washing with water, saline, or soap and water before insertion. Antiseptic solutions confer no additional benefit (Pratt et al 2001, Kunin 1997). A thorough explanation to the patient improves compliance. The risk of contaminating the catheter or causing trauma to the urethra will be reduced if the procedure is clearly explained to the patient and the healthcare worker performing it has been properly trained and is competent. Trauma and discomfort are also likely to be reduced if a sterile single-use lubricant is applied to the urethra (Boore 1978, Pratt et al 2001).

Securing the catheter to the patient's thigh has been recommended to prevent it moving in the urethra (Jenner 1983). There is no evidence that this reduces the infection rate but for some patients it may be more comfortable.

Intermittent catheterization In patients who need long-term catheterization, periodic emptying of the bladder by the insertion of a sterile or clean catheter every few hours has been shown to be effective in reducing the risk of infection (Perkush & Giroux 1993). Although patients managed in this way still usually become bacteriuric after 2–3 weeks, they have a reduced risk of developing bacteraemia, fever, stone formation and renal deterioration (Wyndaele & Maes 1990). The patient can be taught to self-catheterize safely using a clean reusable catheter washed between each use and stored in a clean covered container (Lapides et al 1975). Self-catheterization is an accepted form of management for many patients with spinal injury, enabling them to lead a more normal life in the community. If hospitalized, these patients should be helped to manage their catheterization using the technique with which they are familiar. The use of intermittent catheterization in other groups of patients has been recommended, for example following hip replacement or fracture repair, and may be a useful technique for managing postoperative urinary retention (Michelson et al 1988).

Suprapubic catheterization The risk of bacteria entering the bladder along the outside of the catheter may be avoided by insertion of a catheter directly into the bladder through the abdominal wall. The catheters are inserted under local or general anaesthesia, and may be self-retaining or stitched to the abdominal wall. There is some evidence to suggest that suprapubic catheters are less frequently associated with bacteriuria (Sethia et al 1987). Intraurethral catheters are devices placed inside the urethra to relieve urinary retention associated with enlarged prostate gland and may be left in place for months with a reduced risk of infection (Neilsen et al 1990).

Penile sheaths Drainage of urine into a penile sheath attached to a drainage bag reduces the risk of bacteria entering the bladder alongside the catheter. However, uropathogens may colonize the skin beneath the condom and result in local skin infection and bacteriuria. They may also provide a reservoir for the spread of hospital pathogens (Fierer & Ekstrom 1981). The risk of bacteriuria may be reduced by ensuring the condom is changed frequently (Waites et al 1993).

Type of catheter

Urinary catheters are available in a wide range of sizes and materials. Appropriate selection is essential to minimize trauma to the delicate mucosa of the bladder and urethra (Pomfret 1996).

Catheter size The diameter of a catheter is measured in Charrière: 8–10 Ch for paediatric catheters and 12–30 Ch for adult catheters. The lumen of even the smallest catheter is sufficient to cope with the volume of urine produced and the larger catheters are indicated only where the lumen may become blocked by an unusual amount of debris (e.g. following bladder or prostate gland surgery). To minimize trauma to the urethra only 12- and 14-Ch catheters should be used for routine catheterization in adults, unless the urine contains a considerable amount of debris. Whistle-tip catheters have large drainage holes to accommodate clots and debris. The Conformacath catheter is designed to conform to the slit-like shape of the normal urethra to reduce discomfort and trauma to the mucosa. Pomfret (1992) found it offered a useful alternative method of catheterization for patients who could not tolerate a conventional catheter.

Catheters are now also available in a shorter length for female patients. Male length catheters used in female patients result in a considerable amount of excess tubing, which is more likely to kink and cannot be easily concealed under skirts when used with leg bags.

The most common sizes of retention balloon are 10 and 30 ml. Large balloons irritate the bladder mucosa, causing pain and discomfort to the patient (Roe & Brocklehurst 1987). They also increase the volume of urine remaining in the bladder, providing nutrients in which bacteria can multiply (Fig. 10.2). The 30-ml balloon is therefore usually indicated only after prostate surgery where its size and weight may reduce bleeding from the prostatic bed. All other catheters should be retained in the bladder with a 10-ml balloon. It is also essential to inflate the balloon with the correct amount of sterile water. Balloons that are underinflated or overinflated become misshapen and increase the risk that the bladder mucosa will be traumatized (Fig. 10.3).

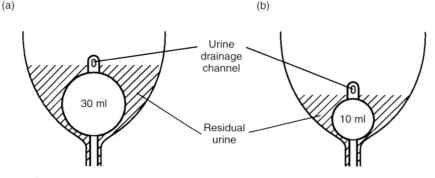

(a)   (b)

Urine drainage channel

30 ml

10 ml

Residual urine

Fig. 10.2 The urinary catheter retention balloon. (a) A 30-ml balloon. (b) A 10-ml balloon.

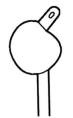

Fig. 10.3 An underinflated retention balloon. The distorted balloon is more likely to damage the bladder mucosa.

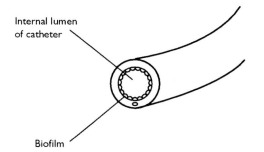

Internal lumen
of catheter

Biofilm

Fig. 10.4 Biofilm formation inside a urethral catheter.

Catheter material Bacteria attach to the internal surface of the catheter, forming a **biofilm** (Box 10.1). This biofilm, commonly referred to as encrustation, builds up over time and may eventually obstruct the lumen of the catheter, preventing the flow of urine (Fig. 10.4). Patients who are expected to have a catheter in place for more than 3 weeks require a catheter that will be resistant to encrustation and cause the minimum of irritation (Pomfret 1996) (Table 10.3).

Urinary catheters are made of plastic, latex coated with inert materials such as silicone or Teflon, or all-silicone. The bladder mucosa tolerates these materials to a variable extent and the material also influences the rate at which biofilms develop. Plastic catheters are associated with bladder spasm, urethral pain and leakage, and their use should be avoided (Blannin & Hobden 1980). Silicone is a very inert material, causes minimal irritation and is fairly resistant to encrustation (Kunin 1997). Latex is a highly irritant material but when coated with a more inert material, such as silicone, can be tolerated for longer. Hydrogel coating absorbs liquid to become soft and slippery and therefore causes minimal damage to the urethral mucosa and is resistant to encrustation (Cox et al 1988). Various types of antimicrobial-impregnated catheters have been tried. Silver has generated the most interest as silver ions are antibacterial, non-toxic and do not encourage the emergence of antibiotic-resistant strains. Early studies on silver oxide-coated catheters did not demonstrate any benefit. However, more recently silver alloy-coated catheters have been shown to reduce the incidence of bacteriuria, although they are not widely available (Johnson et al 1990, Leidberg & Lindeberg 1990, Saint et al 1998).

Frequency of catheter replacement A transient bacteraemia may occur during recatheterization and long-term catheters should therefore not be changed unless necessary (Bryan & Reynolds 1984). Provided

Table 10.3 Selection of urinary catheters

Catheter material	Indication	Comments
Plastic	Very short-term use only; avoid if possible	Rigid material, irritates mucosa and causes trauma
Latex (thin silicone coat)	Short-term use, up to 14 days	Prone to encrustation, associated with trauma and strictures
Latex coated with Teflon	Short-term use, up to 28 days	Minimal mucosal irritation, resistant to encrustation
Latex with bonded silicone coating	Long-term use, up to 12 weeks	Minimal mucosal irritation, resistant to encrustation
Latex with hydrogel coating	Long-term use, up to 12 weeks	Minimal mucosal irritation, resistant to encrustation
All silicone	Long-term use, up to 12 weeks	Minimal mucosal irritation, but D-shaped lumen prone to encrustation

Note: examine the packaging carefully for a description of the catheter material.

the most appropriate size and type of catheter has been selected, the main indication for catheter change is blockage of the lumen by debris or encrustation. The rate at which the catheter encrusts depends on the catheter material and the urine. An alkaline urine which contains high concentrations of proteins and calcium salts causes biofilms to develop more rapidly (Kunin et al 1987). The presence of certain types of bacteria in the urine, especially proteus and pseudomonas, also encourages the formation of biofilms. Some solutions are recommended for regular instillations into the bladder to prevent biofilm formation, but the efficacy of these solutions has not been demonstrated (Roe 1989).

A catheter blocked by encrustation may cause urine to leak around the side of the catheter. Bladder spasm caused by irritation of the mucosa may also force urine out of the bladder around the catheter. Large catheters are particularly associated with irritation and leakage (Blannin & Hobden 1980). Catheter blockage affects a large proportion of long-term catheterized patients and is associated with bladder stones (Kohler-Ockmore & Feneley 1996).

Reducing colonization of the perineum

A considerable amount of advice about the management of urinary catheters relates to preventing bacteria that colonize the perineum from gaining access to the bladder from the urethral opening. Regular cleansing with an antiseptic solution has been recommended (Seal et al 1982) and used to be practised widely (Crow et al 1986). However, the controlled trial by Burke et al (1981) found that catheterized patients who received no meatal cleansing had the lowest infection rate and that cleansing with soap was associated with fewer infections than with povidone–iodine. The conclusion to be drawn from this study is that bacteria are more likely to be introduced to the urethra during the cleaning procedure and a specific meatal cleansing procedure should be avoided. Meatal care using soap and water and clean wipes should therefore be based on the usual hygiene requirements of individual patients.

There is little evidence that bathing increases the incidence of UTI in catheterized patients. Degroot (1979) in a study on 10 catheterized patients, used a dye in the bathwater to indicate that the water did not pass into the bladder during bathing.

Although antimicrobial creams applied to the urethral opening may postpone bacteriuria, the additional costs of cream and nursing time do not make this procedure cost effective (Classen et al 1991).

Guidelines for practice: perineal cleansing

- Routine bathing or showering as part of daily hygiene is sufficient
- The perineum should be cleaned after an episode of faecal incontinence
- Clean underneath the prepuce
- Use soap and water and clean wipes
- Wash hands before and after the procedure
- Antimicrobial creams are not necessary

Management of the drainage system

Bacteria enter the drainage system in the drainage bag or at the junction between the catheter and the drainage bag. These bacteria reach the bladder along the tubing after a few days (Garibaldi et al 1974).

The significance of a closed system of urinary drainage to the prevention of UTI was not really appreciated until the 1960s. Prior to this time, catheter urine had commonly flowed into an open container and infection rates as high as 95% within 24 h of catheterization were common. The plastic, drainable, urine drainage bags with which we are now familiar were introduced in the early 1970s and have had a significant impact on reducing the rate of UTI (Thornton & Andriole 1970).

Breaks in the closed system have been reported to occur frequently (Burke et al 1986). Crow et al (1988) found that the catheter–drainage bag junction was disconnected in 42% of patients, and in 52% the bag was not properly positioned to ensure downward flow of urine.

The importance of not opening the drainage system was demonstrated in a study by Platt et al in 1983, who used catheters that had been presealed to a drainage bag. The seals could be removed and the bag disconnected but, none the less, a 17% reduction in disconnection was recorded. The control group of patients whose catheters were not sealed had three times more UTI than the group with sealed catheters. These studies highlight deficiencies in the management of urine drainage systems which, if prevented, may reduce the incidence of bacteriuria in the short-term catheterized. The drainage system should not be opened to take specimens: these should be taken aseptically from the sampling port with a needle. The drainage bag should be emptied when necessary to avoid reflux of urine. A clean pair of gloves should be worn for emptying the drainage bag and discarded on completion of the procedure. When the bag is emptied, care should be taken to ensure that micro-organisms are not introduced on to the tap by contact with a contaminated container or other surface. Observational studies have shown that containers used for urine collection are commonly not decontaminated properly between use (Glynn et al 1997). Containers should be decontaminated in a bedpan washer or autoclaved after each use.

Bacteria easily gain access to the drainage bag from the tap and multiply very rapidly in urine at room temperature (Bradley et al 1986). Bacteria remaining in the bag after it is emptied inoculate fresh urine entering the bag. The bacterial biofilm that adheres and spreads over the surface of the catheter and drainage bag enables bacteria in the bag to travel through non-return valves in the bag and along the lumen of the catheter into the bladder (Nickel et al 1985). Flutter valves, drip chambers or airlocks are of no value in preventing bacteriuria.

Incorrect positioning of the drainage bag can assist the transfer of bacteria to the bladder. Roberts et al (1965) found that bacteria could be transported distances of 0.9–1.2 m in rising air bubbles, often generated when the tubing is kinked and columns of urine are formed. Drainage bags should therefore be positioned so that backflow is avoided and on a stand that prevents contact with the floor. If downward flow of urine cannot be maintained, the tubing should be clamped for a short period until the correct drainage can be resumed (Pratt et al 2001).

Bacteria grow less readily in dilute urine which has scarce nutrients (Asscher et al 1966). Encouraging the catheterized patient to drink plenty of fluid has the practical value of maintaining a constant downward flow of urine and reducing bacterial multiplication in the drainage bag. Some fluids (e.g. cranberry juice) are considered to reduce the number of bacteria in the urine by changing its acidity (Rogers 1991).

Catheter valves have also been proposed as a method of preventing bacteria from gaining access to the bladder via the drainage bag. They enable the bladder to fill and to be emptied intermittently without the use of a drainage system. They may benefit the catheterized patient by reducing the incidence of infection, restoring bladder tone and improving the quality of life (Roe 1990a).

Cross-infection between catheterized patients has been frequently reported but the extent of the problem is probably underestimated. Schaberg et al (1980) showed that a significant proportion of nosocomial UTIs occur in clusters, particularly those caused by serratia and pseudomonas. Bacteria contaminating the drainage bag and the junction between catheter and bag are easily transferred to the hands when the bag is emptied or the drainage system is handled. The design

---

> **Guidelines for practice: maintenance of the drainage system**
>
> - Use a bag with an integral measuring chamber if monitoring of urine output is required
> - Do not change the bag routinely
> - Do not disconnect the catheter from the drainage bag unless absolutely necessary
> - Empty the bag as infrequently as possible
> - Wash hands before and after handling the drainage system
> - Use clean gloves to handle the drainage system and discard afterwards
> - Empty urine into a clean container and disinfect after use
> - Take urine specimens from the sample port, not the drainage bag
> - Ensure urine always flows downwards
> - Avoid kinks in tubing
> - Hang bag evenly on stand
> - Do not change leg bags at night but connect to an overnight drainage bag
> - Avoid use of bladder instillations

of the tap influences the extent to which urine contaminates the hands during the emptying of the bag (Glenister 1987). Inadequately cleaned collection containers may also transmit infection between catheterized patients. Antibiotic-resistant strains of bacteria, which often have an ability to survive and transmit easily in the hospital environment, are commonly associated with outbreaks of infection amongst catheterized patients. The insertion of antiseptic solutions into urine drainage bags, although probably not effective or practical for routine use, may have a role in preventing transmission of nosocomial pathogens, for example in outbreaks of antibiotic-resistant strains, by reducing their concentration in the bag urine (Thompson et al 1984, Warren 1997).

Bladder instillations The administration of a bladder instillation involves disconnection of the closed drainage system which, as illustrated above, has been clearly demonstrated to increase the incidence of UTI. Such instillations should therefore be used only if a clear benefit can be demonstrated.

There is some evidence that antiseptics instilled in the bladder may prevent infection in patients who have had urological surgery, but they are ineffective in treating established infections (Slade & Gillespie 1985). There is no evidence that they are of benefit in preventing bacteriuria in the long-term catheterized and extensive use of these solutions has been associated with the emergence of resistant bacteria (Davies et al 1987, Schneeberger et al 1992, Stickler 1990).

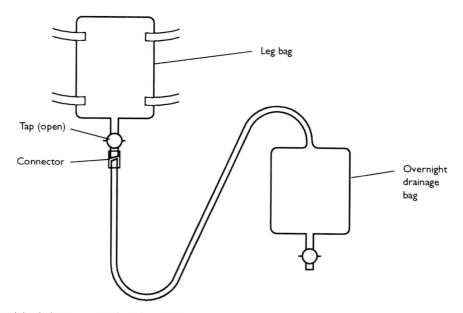

Fig. 10.5 Overnight drainage system for a leg drainage bag.

Instillation of antiseptic solutions such as chlorhexidine and noxythiolin should therefore not be used as part of routine management of the catheterized patient. A catheter blocked with debris should be flushed with saline, taking great care not to contaminate the connections (Pomfret 1996).

Other bladder instillations containing weak acids are intended to remove or control crystal formation (e.g. Suby-G). These are indicated only for patients who have particular problems with rapidly encrusting catheters where they may remove or prevent encrustation and may reduce the need for frequent recatheterization (Roe 1990c).

Leg drainage bags In the past patients using a bag attached to the leg for collecting urine changed it for a larger overnight drainage bag to hold the volume of urine produced at night, but required frequent disconnection of the drainage system. Leg bag systems that enable an overnight drainage bag to be connected directly to the leg bag without incurring a break in the closed system (Fig. 10.5) are preferred to minimize disconnection and reduce the risk of introducing micro-organisms. The overnight bag should be discarded after each use.

Patient education

In hospital, encouraging patients to care for their own urinary catheters can minimize the risk of cross-infection. The long-term catheterized patient in the community can benefit from education on how to manage the catheter and minimize the risk of introducing bacteria. Instructions should include advice on careful hand hygiene, perineal cleansing, positioning of the drainage bag and recognizing symptoms of infection (Roe 1990b).

REFERENCES

Asscher AW, Sussman M, Waters WE et al (1966) Urine as a medium for bacterial growth. *Lancet*, 1: 1039–41.

Blannin JP, Hobden J (1980) The catheter of choice. *Nursing Times*, 76: 2092–3.

Boore JRP (1978) *Prescription for Recovery*. Nursing Research Series. Royal College of Nursing, London.

Bradley C, Babb J, Davies J et al (1986) Taking precautions. *Nursing Times*, **5 March**: 70–3.

Bronsema D, Adams J, Pallares R et al (1993) Secular trends in rates and etiology of nosocomial urinary tract infections at a university hospital. *J. Urol.*, **150**: 414–16.

Bryan CS, Reynolds KL (1984) Hospital-acquired bacteremic urinary tract infection. Epidemiology and outcome. *J. Urol.*, **132**: 494–8.

Burke JP, Garibaldi RA, Britt MR et al (1981) Prevention of catheter-associated urinary tract infections – efficacy of daily meatal care regimes. *Am. J. Med.*, **70**: 655–8.

Burke JP, Larsen RA, Stevens LE (1986) Nosocomial bacteriuria: estimating the potential for prevention by closed sterile urinary drainage. *Infect. Control,* **7**: 96–9.

Castle M, Osterhout S (1974) Urinary tract catheterisation and associated infection. *Nurs. Res.,* **23**: 170–4.

Classen DC, Larsen RA, Burke JP et al (1991) Daily meatal care for prevention of catheter-associated bacteriuria: results using frequent applications of polyantibiotic cream. *Infect. Control Hosp. Epidemiol.,* **12**: 157–62.

Cox A, Hukins D, Sutton T (1988) Comparison of in vitro encrustation on silicone and hydrogel-coated latex catheters. *Br. J. Urol.,* **61**: 156–61.

Crow RA, Chapman RG, Roe BH, Wilson JA (1986) *A Study of Patients with an Indwelling Urethral Catheter and Related Nursing Practice.* Nursing Practice Research Unit, University of Surrey, Guildford.

Crow RA, Mulhall A, Chapman RG (1988) Indwelling catheterisation and related nursing practice. *J. Adv. Nurs.,* **13**: 489–95.

Daifuku R, Stamm W (1984) Association of rectal and urethral colonisation with urinary tract infection in patients with indwelling urethral catheters. *JAMA,* **252**: 2028–30.

Daifuku R, Stamm W (1986) Bacterial adhesion to bladder uroepithelial cells in catheter-associated urinary tract infection. *N. Engl. J. Med.,* **3145**: 1208–13.

Degroot JE (1979) Entrance of water into the bladder during Sitz bath in elderly catheterised and non-catheterised females. *Invest. Urol.,* **117**: 207–8.

Emmerson AM, Enstone JE, Griffin M et al (1996) The second national prevalence survey of infection in hospitals – overview of the results. *J. Hosp. Infect.,* **32**: 175–90.

Fierer J, Ekstrom M (1981) An outbreak of *Providencia stuartii* urinary tract infection. Patients with condom catheters are a reservoir of the bacteria. *JAMA,* **245**: 1553–5.

Garibaldi RA (1993) Hospital-acquired urinary infections. In *Prevention and Control of Nosocomial Infections,* pp. 600–13, 2nd edn (RP Wenzel, ed.). Williams & Wilkins, Baltimore, MD.

Garibaldi RA, Burke JP, Dickman ML et al (1974) Factors predisposing to bacteriuria during indwelling urethral catheterisation. *N. Engl. J. Med.,* **291**: 215–19.

Garibaldi RA, Mooney BR, Epstein BJ et al (1982) An evaluation of daily bacteriologic monitoring to identify preventable episodes of catheter-associated urinary tract infection. *Infect. Control,* **3**: 466–70.

Getliffe K (1990) Catheter blockage in the community. *Nursing Standard,* **5**(9): 33–6.

Glenister H (1987) The passage of infection. *Nursing Times,* **83**(22): 68–73.

Glynn A, Ward V, Wilson J et al (1997) *Hospital-acquired Infection. Surveillance, Policies and Practice.* Public Health Laboratory Service, London.

Hartstein AJ, Garber SB, Ward TT et al (1981) Nosocomial urinary tract infection: a prospective evaluation of 108 catheterised patients. *Infect. Control,* **2**: 380–6.

Jenner EA (1983) Prevention of catheter associated urinary tract infection. *Nursing,* **2**(13) (Suppl.): 1–3.

Johnson JR (1991) Virulence factors in *Escherichia coli* urinary tract infection. *Clin. Microbiol. Rev.,* **4**: 80.

Johnson JR, Roberts PL, Olsen RJ et al (1990) Prevention of catheter-associated urinary tract infections with a silver oxoid-coated urinary catheter: clinical and microbiological correlates. *J. Infect. Dis.,* **162**: 1145–50.

Kass EH, Schneiderman LJ (1959) Entry of bacteria into the urinary tract of patients with inlying catheters. *N. Engl. J. Med.,* **256**: 556–7.

Kohler-Ockmore J, Feneley RCI (1996) Long-term catheterisation of the bladder: prevalence and morbidity. *Br. J. Urol.,* **77**: 347–51.

Krieger JN, Kaiser DL, Wenzel RP (1983) Nosocomial urinary tract infections: secular trends, treatment and economics in a university hospital. *J. Urol.,* **130**: 102–6.

Kunin CM (1997) *Urinary Tract Infections: Detection, Prevention and Management,* 5th edn. Williams & Wilkins, Baltimore.

Kunin CM, Chin QF, Chambers S (1987) Formation of encrustations on indwelling urinary catheters in the elderly: a comparison of different types of catheter materials in blockers and non-blockers. *J. Urol.,* **138**: 899–902.

Lapides J, Diokono AC, Gould FR et al (1975) Further observations on self-catheterisation. *Transactions of the American Association of Genito-urinary Surgeons,* **67**: 15–17.

Leidberg LP, Lindeberg T (1990) Silver alloy coated catheters reduce catheter-associated bacteriuria. *Br. J. Urol.,* **65**: 379–81.

Michelson JD, Lotke PA, Steinberg ME (1988) Urinary-bladder management after total joint-replacement surgery. *N. Engl. J. Med.,* **319**: 321–6.

Mobley HLT, Warren JW (1987) Urease-positive bacteriuria and obstruction of long-term urinary catheters. *J. Clin. Microbiol.,* **25**: 2216.

Neilsen KK, Klarskov P, Nordling J et al (1990) The intraprostatic spiral. New treatment for urinary retention. *Br. J. Urol.,* **65**: 500–3.

Nickel JC, Grant SK, Costerton JW (1985) Catheter-associated bacteriuria an experimental study. *Urology,* **36**: 369–75.

Nicolle LE (1987) Urinary tract infections in long-term care facilities. *Infect. Control Hosp. Epidemiol.,* **14**: 220–5.

Nicolle LE (1997) Asymptomatic bacteriuria in the elderly. *Infect. Dis. Clin. North Am.,* **11**(3): 647–63.

Perkush I, Giroux J (1993) Clean intermittent catheterisation in spinal cord injury patients. A follow-up study. *J. Urol.,* **149**(5): 1068–71.

Peterson JR, Roth EJ (1989) Fever, bacteriuria and pyuria in spinal cord injured patients with indwelling urethral catheters. *Arch. Phys. Med. Rehabil.,* **70**: 839–41.

Platt R, Polk BF, Murdock B et al (1982) Mortality associated with nosocomial urinary tract infection. *N. Engl. J. Med.,* **307**: 939–43.

Platt R, Murdock B, Polk BF (1983) Reduction of mortality associated with nosocomial urinary tract infection. *Lancet,* i: 1893–7.

Plowman R, Graves N, Griffin M et al (1999) *The Socio-economic Burden of Hospital-acquired Infection.* PHLS, London.

Pomfret IJ (1992) Conformacath update. *J. Commun. Nurse,* **6**(8): 14–16.

Pomfret IJ (1996) Continence clinic catheters: design, selection and management. *Br. J. Nurs.,* **5**: 245–51.

Pratt RA, Pellowe CM, Loveday HP et al (2001) The Epic project: developing national evidence-based guidelines for preventing healthcare associated infections. *J. Hosp. Infect.,* **47**: Suppl. A.

Public Health Laboratory Service (2000) *Surveillance of Hospital-acquired Bacteraemia in English Hospitals, 1997–1999.* Nosocomial Infection National Surveillance Scheme, PHLS, London.

Roberts JMB, Linton KB, Pollard BR et al (1965) Long term catheter drainage in the male. *Br. J. Urol.,* **37**: 63–72.

Roe BH (1989) Use of bladder washouts: a study of nurses' recommendations. *J. Adv. Nurs.,* **14**: 494–500.

Roe B (1990a) Do we need to clamp catheters? *Nursing Times,* **86**(43): 66–7.

Roe BH (1990b) Study of the effects of education on the management of urine drainage systems by patients and carers. *J. Adv. Nurs.*, **15**: 223–31.

Roe B (1990c) Bladder instillations. *Nursing Standard*, **4**(51): 25–7.

Roe BH, Brocklehurst JC (1987) Study of patients with indwelling catheters. *J. Adv. Nurs.*, **12**: 713–18.

Rogers J (1991) Pass the cranberry juice. *Nursing Times*, **87**: 36–7.

Saint S, Elmore JG, Sullivan SD et al (1998) The efficacy of silver alloy-coated urinary catheters in preventing urinary tract infection: a meta-analysis. *Am. J. Med.*, **105**: 236–41.

Schaberg DR, Haley RW, Highsmith AK et al (1980) Nosocomial bacteriuria: a prospective study of case clustering and antimicrobial resistance. *Ann. Intern. Med.*, **93**: 420–4.

Schneeberger PM, Vreede RW, Bogdanowicz JF et al (1992) A randomised study on the effect of bladder irrigation with povidone–iodine before removal of an indwelling catheter. *J. Hosp. Infect.*, **21**: 223–9.

Seal DU, Wood S, Barret S et al (1982) Evaluation of aseptic techniques and chlorhexidine on the rate of catheter-associated urinary-tract infection. *Lancet*, **i**: 89–92.

Sethia KK, Selkon JB, Berry AR et al (1987) Prospective randomised controlled trial of urethral versus suprapubic catheterisation. *Br. J. Surg.*, **74**: 624–5.

Slade N, Gillespie WA (1985) *The Urinary Tract and the Catheter: Infection and Other Problems.* John Wiley, Chichester.

Stamey TA, Timothy MM (1975) Studies of introital colonisation in women with recurrent urinary infections. I: The role of vaginal pH. *J. Urol.*, **114**: 261.

Stamm WE (1983) Measurement of pyuria and its relation to bacteriuria. *Am. J. Med.*, **75** (Suppl.): 53.

Stamm WE (1991) Catheter-associated urinary tract infections: epidemiology, pathogenesis and prevention. *Am. J. Med.*, **91** (Suppl. 3B): 65S–71S.

Stamm WE (1998) Urinary tract infection. In: *Hospital Infections*, 4th edn, pp. 477–86 (JV Bennett, PS Brachman, eds). Lippincott-Raven, Philadelphia.

Stark RP, Maki D (1984) Bacteriuria in the catheterised patient. What quantitative level of bacteriuria is relevant? *N. Engl. J. Med.*, **311**: 560–4.

Stickler DJ (1990) Antiseptics in bladder catheterization. *J. Hosp. Infect.*, **16**: 89–108.

Thompson RL, Haley CE, Searcy MA et al (1984) Catheter-associated bacteriuria. Failure to reduce attack rates using periodic instillations of a disinfectant into urinary drainage systems. *JAMA*, **251**: 747–51.

Thornton GF, Andriole VT (1970) Bacteriuria during indwelling catheter drainage II: effect of a closed sterile drainage system. *JAMA*, **214**: 339–42.

Waites K, Canupp K, DeVivo M (1993) Epidemiology and risk factors for urinary tract infection following spinal cord injury. *Arch. Phys. Med. Rehabil.*, **74**: 691–5.

Warren JW (1997) Catheter-associated urinary tract infections. Infect. *Dis. Clin. North Am.*, **11**(3): 609–17.

Warren JW, Antony WC, Hoopes JM et al (1982b) Cephalexin for susceptible bacteriuria in afebrile, long-term catheterised patients. *JAMA*, **248**: 454–8.

Warren JW, Tenney JH, Hoopes JM, Muncie HL (1982a) A prospective microbiological study of bacteriuria in patients with chronic indwelling urethral catheters. *J. Infect. Dis.*, **146**: 719–23.

Warren JW, Damron D, Tenney JH (1987) Fever, bacteraemia and death as complications of bacteriuria in women with long-term urethral catheters. *J. Infect. Dis.*, **155**: 1151–8.

Warren JW, Muncie HL, Hall-Craggs M (1988) Acute pyelonephritis associated with bacteriuria during long-term catheterisation: a prospective clinicopathological study. *J. Infect. Dis.*, **158**: 1341–6.

Wyndaele J-J, Maes D (1990) Clean intermittent self-catheterisation: a 12-year followup. *J. Urol.*, **143**: 906–8.

FURTHER READING

Berman P, Hogan DB, Fox RA (1987) The atypical presentation of infection in old age. *Age Ageing*, **16**: 201–7.

Cowan T (1997) Catheters designed for intermittent use. *Prof. Nurse*, **12**(4): 297–302.

Saint S, Lipsky BA (1999) Preventing catheter-related bacteriuria. Should we? Can we? How? *Arch. Intern. Med.*, **159**: 800–8.

Vinder A (1990) Intermittent self-catheterisation. *Nursing Times*, **86**(43): 63–4.

11

Preventing infection of the respiratory tract

INTRODUCTION

The respiratory tract is divided into the upper part, from the nostrils to the larynx, and the lower part, from the larynx to the alveoli (Fig. 11.1).

Infections of the upper respiratory tract are usually minor; most are caused by viruses and are commonly acquired in the community (e.g. influenza, respiratory syncytial virus). Occasionally they may progress to more serious lower respiratory tract infection, particularly in the very young or the elderly (Breuer & Jeffries

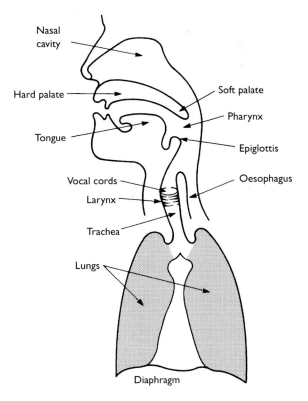

Fig. 11.1   The respiratory tract.

1990). Cross-infection between hospitalized patients and staff may occur.

Infections of the lower respiratory tract, in particular pneumonia, are more serious and frequently life threatening. Micro-organisms enter the lower respiratory tract from the oropharynx by aspiration or are inhaled on minute particles. When they reach the lungs an inflammatory response is initiated. This causes the mucous membranes lining the alveoli and bronchi to swell and pus to collect in the alveoli, interfering with ventilation and gas exchange. The accumulation of pus in the alveoli that occurs in pneumonia is termed 'consolidation'.

Primary pneumonia may develop in healthy people in the community, although most commonly it affects those with pre-existing pulmonary disease, the immunocompromised or immobile, young children and the elderly. *Streptococcus pneumoniae, Haemophilus influenzae* and *Moraxella catarrhalis* are the most common micro-organisms associated with these community-acquired infections.

In hospitals other factors predispose to pneumonia. The micro-organisms colonizing the upper respiratory tract are frequently replaced by hospital pathogens within a few days of admission, and most pneumonia acquired in hospital is caused by aspiration of these micro-organisms (Torres et al 1993). Underlying illness in the patient may promote oropharyngeal colonization. Intubation, mechanical ventilation and other invasive procedures disrupt the normal defences of the lung against invasion by pathogens and markedly increase susceptibility to pneumonia (Tablan et al 1994). Hospital-acquired pneumonia is therefore rarely caused by the same pathogens as community-acquired infection: half are caused by Gram-negative bacilli and 20% by *Staphylococcus aureus* (Emori & Gaynes 1993).

Pneumonia is the second most common hospital-acquired infection, accounting for 23% of such infections (Emmerson et al 1996). It is associated with considerable mortality, particularly in the seriously ill. In intensive care units up to 50% of patients who acquire pneumonia die, and in nearly one-third of cases death is directly attributable to the pneumonia (Fagon et al 1993). Similarly, 50% of deaths in patients undergoing bone marrow transplantation are due to pneumonia (Pannuti et al 1992). The costs associated with hospital-acquired pneumonia are also high, with estimates of more than £2000 per patient, and an increased length of stay in hospital of 12 days (Plowman et al 1999). Some cases of hospital-acquired pneumonia are caused by inhalation of micro-organisms (e.g. legionella, aspergillus and respiratory viruses) from the environment or from infected individuals.

NATURAL DEFENCES AGAINST INFECTION OF THE RESPIRATORY TRACT

Micro-organisms can enter the respiratory tract on particles of dust or droplets of moisture carried in the air. Hairs in the nose filter some of the particles as they are breathed in. Most of the respiratory tract is lined by ciliated cells covered with sticky mucus. The mucus traps small particles, preventing micro-organisms from reaching the lungs. The **cilia**, which are hair-like structures, beat rhythmically in a coordinated fashion, propelling mucus upwards towards the larynx from the lower respiratory tract and downwards from the nasal passages towards the larynx. When the mucus reaches the pharynx it is swallowed or coughed out of the respiratory system. If very small particles reach the alveoli they are engulfed by **phagocytic** cells of the immune system.

The cough reflex is stimulated by larger particles on the larynx or trachea and is an important mechanism for the expulsion of micro-organisms.

DIAGNOSIS OF PNEUMONIA

Amongst patients who are not critically ill, the diagnosis of pneumonia is based on fever, purulent respiratory secretions and the identification of new lung infiltrates by radiography. In the critically ill, the diagnosis is more complex and less precise. It may be difficult to establish the cause of a fever; purulent respiratory secretions are common; the significance of positive microbiology may be difficult to establish in incubated patients; and other underlying conditions such as oedema may cause infiltrates seen by radiography. Sampling of the respiratory tract by means of fibreoptic bronchoscopy or bronchial lavage is a more reliable method of obtaining microbiological specimens, but not recommended for routine use (Flanagan 1999).

FACTORS PREDISPOSING TO HOSPITAL-ACQUIRED PNEUMONIA

The risk of a patient developing pneumonia depends on the number of bacteria that enter the respiratory tract, the susceptibility of the patient to infection and the **virulence** of the organism. There are several key factors that influence the acquisition of hospital-acquired pneumonia: host factors that increase susceptibility to the infection (Box 11.1), factors that facilitate colonization of the oropharynx by pathogens, conditions that promote aspiration of oropharyngeal secretions, and exposure to pathogens as a result of

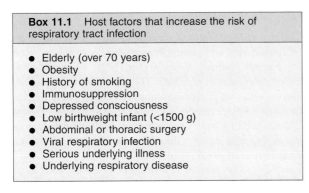

Box 11.1   Host factors that increase the risk of respiratory tract infection

- Elderly (over 70 years)
- Obesity
- History of smoking
- Immunosuppression
- Depressed consciousness
- Low birthweight infant (<1500 g)
- Abdominal or thoracic surgery
- Viral respiratory infection
- Serious underlying illness
- Underlying respiratory disease

respiratory therapy. These factors are summarized in Fig. 11.2 and discussed in more detail below.

Aspiration

The most common cause of bacterial pneumonia is the aspiration of **pathogens colonizing** the surface of the oropharyngeal mucosa (Pugliese & Lichtenberg 1987). Some 45% of healthy people aspirate secretions from the oropharynx whilst they are asleep; however, the natural defences are usually able to remove bacteria introduced to the respiratory system in this way (Huxley et al 1978).

In hospital patients the risk of aspiration is increased by invasive procedures that bypass the natural defences, for example endotracheal and tracheostomy tubes and instrumentation of either the respiratory or gastrointestinal tract. Aspiration is also more likely in patients with reduced levels of consciousness, for

example following cerebrovascular accidents or drug overdose, and during general anaesthesia. Subsequent infection will be caused by the micro-organisms that are colonizing the oropharynx (Tablan et al 1994).

Colonization of the oropharynx

In healthy people the oropharynx is often colonized by *S. pneumoniae* and *H. influenzae*, and these two organisms are responsible for most pneumonia acquired in the community.

In hospitalized patients, particularly those with serious underlying illness and who have been exposed to **antibiotics**, the **normal flora** of the oropharynx is replaced with **Gram-negative bacilli** such as pseudomonas, klebsiella and enterobacter soon after admission (Torres et al 1993). These account for approximately 50% of the infections (Table 11.1). For colonization to establish, micro-organisms must be able to adhere to the epithelial cells. After operation or during severe illness, levels of fibronectin, a protein that prevents bacteria from adhering to cells in the oropharynx, appear to be depleted. In the absence of fibronectin, Gram-negative bacteria are able to establish. Virulence factors such as fimbriae, capsules or enzymes produced by micro-organisms may also be important determinants of colonization. The degree of colonization is particularly high in critically ill patients and is strongly associated with the development of pneumonia (Johanson et al 1972).

Various approaches have been tried to prevent Gram-negative micro-organisms from colonizing the

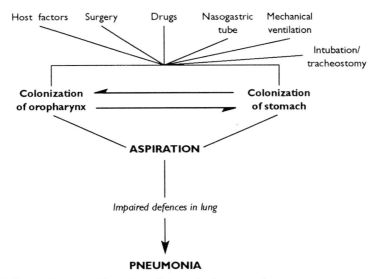

Fig. 11.2   Factors that influence the acquisition of hospital-acquired pneumonia.

Table 11.1 Pathogens associated with hospital-acquired pneumonia. From Emori & Gaynes (1993), by permission of the American Society for Microbiology

Pathogen	Percentage of pneumonias
Gram-negative bacilli	48
Pseudomonas aeruginosa	16
Enterobacter spp.	11
Klebsiella pneumoniae	7
Escherichia coli	4
Other	10
Gram-positive cocci	48
Staphylococcus aureus	20
Streptococcus pneumoniae	5

oropharynx. Aerosolized antimicrobial agents eradicate the pathogens but the risks of infection with other more resistant micro-organisms have discouraged the use of this method. Selective decontamination of the digestive tract (SDD) in mechanically ventilated patients has also been recommended (Stoutenbeek et al 1984). This aims to eliminate Gram-negative bacilli and candida from the oropharynx and stomach without affecting the normal anaerobic flora. Currently, there is insufficient evidence to demonstrate a clear benefit in terms of reduction of nosocomial pneumonia (Tablan et al 1994, Ward et al 1997).

Colonization of the stomach

In healthy people the stomach is normally sterile because the hydrochloric acid destroys micro-organisms entering with ingested food. If the acidity is reduced to a pH of around 4, the stomach rapidly becomes colonized by large numbers of Gram-negative bacilli which subsequently colonize the oropharynx and cause pneumonia (Craven et al 1986, Du Moulin et al 1982). Bacterial colonization of the stomach is also more likely to occur in the elderly or malnourished and in those with gastrointestinal disease. Once in the stomach, bacteria may ascend the oesophagus to colonize the oropharynx and subsequently cause pneumonia.

Drugs such as antacids and H_2 blockers are used to reduce gastric pH and prevent the formation of stress ulcers in critically ill or postoperative patients. Their use has been associated with high levels of micro-organisms colonizing the stomach (Prodham et al 1994). Sulcralfate, a cryoprotective agent that has minimal effect on gastric pH, has been recommended as an alternative, but clear benefits have yet to be demonstrated (Pickworth et al 1993, Tablan et al 1994).

Nasogastric intubation

The presence of a nasogastric tube is associated with an increased risk of pneumonia, particularly when used for enteral feeding (Craven et al 1991, Methany et al 1986, Pingleton et al 1986). The nasogastric tube may favour reflux of gastric contents or enable micro-organisms to migrate along the tube to the upper airway. Enteral feeding may increase microbial colonization of the stomach by raising the pH or by introducing micro-organisms in feed solutions contaminated during handling. The rise in intragastric pressure may also increase reflux from the stomach (Jacobs et al 1990). The reflux may be reduced by ensuring the patient lies in a semirecumbent position and by not administering feeds when the stomach is full or there is no evidence of bowel motility (Torres et al 1992).

Mechanical ventilation and respiratory equipment

The highest incidence of hospital-acquired pneumonia occurs amongst patients who have received respiratory therapy (Cross & Roup 1981). Intubated patients are more likely to acquire pneumonia than those without such a device. The tube impedes the cough reflex and clearance mechanisms, damages the mucosal lining, and allows bacteria to colonize the secretions that accumulate above the cuff (Holzapfel et al 1993). If a patient is mechanically ventilated the risk of acquiring ventilator-associated pneumonia is 1% for each day of ventilation (Fagon et al 1989).

Several factors combine to increase the risk of pneumonia significantly in these patients, including an increase in oropharyngeal colonization, impairment of the mechanisms that normally clear the airway and inhalation of contaminated aerosols (Garibaldi et al 1981).

The endotracheal and tracheostomy tubes cause irritation and injury to the mucosa, enhancing the ability of Gram-negative bacilli to colonize the oropharynx. They also bypass the nose filter and allow respiratory secretions to pool in the trachea above the tube cuff. These heavily contaminated secretions may leak around the cuff, particularly when it is deflated, or enter the bronchi during suctioning procedures (Fig. 11.3). Like other types of invasive tubing, endotracheal tubes are susceptible to the formation of **biofilms**, a sheet of bacteria and proteins that adheres firmly to the surface of the tube (Sottile et al 1986).

Respiratory therapy equipment may become contaminated and deliver bacteria directly into the lungs. This is a particular problem when gases are mixed

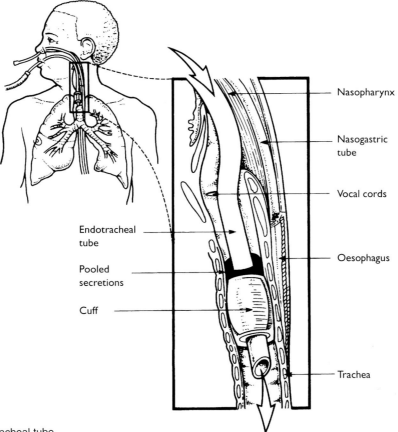

Fig. 11.3   An endotracheal tube.

with aerosolized water from nebulizers or humidifiers because bacteria, particularly Gram-negative bacilli, are able to survive and multiply in the moist environment (Figs 11.4, 11.5).

Epidemics of hospital-acquired pneumonia related to contaminated nebulizers have been reported since the introduction of respiratory therapy equipment in the 1950s (Reinarz et al 1965). *Legionella* spp. thrive in water and are relatively resistant to heat. Outbreaks of infection associated with humidifiers and nebulizers, related to the use of tap water to fill the chamber or inadequate decontamination measures, have been reported (Arnow et al 1982, Mastro et al 1991). Nebulizers are especially hazardous as they create an aerosol of small droplets, 1–2 μm in diameter, that can be inhaled into the lower respiratory tract. The large-volume nebulizers used in intermittent positive pressure breathing (IPPB) machines or room air humidifiers present the greatest risk because of the quantity of aerosol generated. Contamination of small-volume medication nebulizers has been reported and has been associated with increased oropharyngeal colonization and ventilator-associated pneumonia (Botman & de Krieger 1987, Craven et al 1984a).

Humidifiers increase the amount of water vapour in the inhaled gas but, unlike nebulizers, should not produce an aerosol of water droplets. Therefore, although the humidification reservoir may become contaminated with bacteria, the organisms are not as likely to be inhaled into the respiratory tract. None the less, humidified circuits are prone to the condensation of water in the tubing. Bacteria from the patient may colonize and multiply in this moisture and if the tubing is inadvertently raised the condensate will drain into the patient's trachea and increase the risk of pneumonia (Craven et al 1984b). Stucke & Thompson (1980) found that 45% of ventilator tubing was contaminated before the same organism appeared in the tracheal aspirates, implicating cross-infection as the source of contamination of the tubing.

The development of heat–moisture exchange filters, which recycle the moisture in exhaled air, has

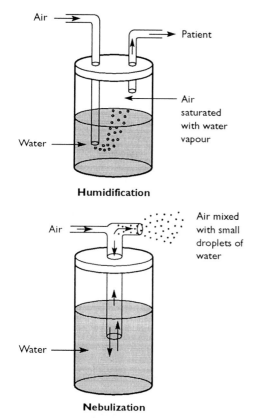

Fig. 11.4 Humidification and nebulization.

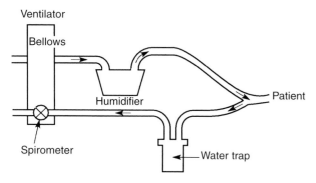

Fig. 11.5 Ventilator tubing with a heated-water humidifier.

eliminated the need for a humidifier in the ventilation of many patients and these filters have the added advantage of eliminating the collection of condensate in the tubing (Make et al 1987).

Surgery

Three-quarters of cases of hospital-acquired pneumonia have been found to occur in patients who have under-gone surgery. The risk is especially high in those who have had abdominal or thoracic procedures (Haley et al 1985). This increased risk is related to several factors. The defences of the respiratory tract can be impaired by endotracheal intubation, the surgical procedure and anaesthetic gases. Aspiration is more likely to occur during anaesthesia and oropharyngeal colonization with Gram-negative bacilli commonly establishes within 48 h of major surgery (Johanson et al 1980). Coughing is often difficult and painful after an operation, especially procedures involving the abdominal or thoracic cavity, and respiration may be depressed by the use of sedatives and narcotic drugs for pain control. Effective pain control after surgery has been shown to reduce the incidence of pneumonia (Wasylak et al 1990).

PREVENTION OF HOSPITAL-ACQUIRED PNEUMONIA

Management of the patient

Positioning of vulnerable patients is a simple measure that can have an important effect on the aspiration of oropharyngeal secretions. Torres et al (1992) demons-trated that intensive care patients positioned semi-recumbently (45° angle) were 10 times less likely to aspirate oropharyngeal secretions. Positioning is also important to minimize the risk of reflux of fluid from the stomach of patients with nasogastric tubes, especially those receiving enteral feeding. For patients at risk of developing pneumonia after operation (see Box 11.1), a programme of breathing exercises to encourage lung expansion and coughing should be implemented before operation. Lung expansion will also be helped by early ambulation. Some patients may need postural drainage and percussion after surgery to assist expectoration of sputum. Incentive spirometry and IPPB may also be of value, especially for patients with abnormal lung func-tion (Tablan et al 1994). Pain that interferes with deep breathing or coughing should be controlled with anal-gesics together with appropriate wound support.

If oxygen therapy is required, it should always be humidified to prevent drying of respiratory secretions and subsequent impairment of the normal clearance mechanisms.

Management of respiratory therapy equipment

Contaminated respiratory equipment has frequently been incriminated in outbreaks of respiratory tract infection and an effective and organized approach to its decontamination is essential (Cefai et al 1990,

Gorman et al 1993). For most equipment, high-level **disinfection** is required to remove or substantially reduce microbial contamination. This can be achieved by **autoclave**, automated washing machine or, when these are unavailable, by chemical **disinfectants** (see Ch. 13). Tap water can be used to rinse off chemical disinfectants, provided the equipment can be dried completely to prevent the growth of any bacteria remaining after cleaning. This may not be possible for tubing or some types of nebulizer (Tablan et al 1994).

Mechanical ventilators

The ventilator itself is not an important source of micro-organisms, and filters placed between the breathing circuit and the machine can be used to protect it. Routine disinfection or sterilization of ventilators is not usually necessary (Gallagher et al 1987). Condensate that collects in the breathing circuits of humidified systems rapidly becomes colonized with bacteria from the patient's oropharynx (Craven et al 1984b). This may be directed into the upper respiratory tract of the patient when the tubing is moved and should therefore be drained periodically, although not into the humidification reservoir or the patient's trachea. Staff handling the breathing circuit readily acquire the contaminating bacteria on their hands and can transfer them to other patients. Hands should therefore always be washed after the tubing is handled (Gorman et al 1993). Conventionally, these circuits are changed at 48 h intervals, although there is evidence that the risk of pneumonia is not increased if they are not changed for longer periods, including the entire period of use on an individual patient (Craven et al 1982, Dreyfuss et al 1991, Kollef et al 1995, Stamm 1998). If a heat–moisture exchange filter is fitted on the inspiratory tubing, humidification is not required; condensate does not collect in the tubing and only the exchange filter needs to be changed every 48 h. The tubing of anaesthetic machines may also be protected with heat–moisture exchange filters.

Ventilator and anaesthetic breathing circuits may be decontaminated by washing, but thorough drying is a key part of the process. This is achieved most effectively in a washing machine specifically designed for washing and drying tubing (Das & Fraise 1997). An outbreak reported by Gray et al (1999) illustrates the hazards associated with the decontamination of ventilator circuits. Six preterm neonates acquired *Bacillus cereus* respiratory tract infection when circuits were contaminated by the organism in a washing machine. Although subsequently subjected to low temperature steam, these spore-forming bacteria were able to survive this disin-

---

Guidelines for practice: prevention of hospital-acquired pneumonia

Handwashing and gloves
- Wear clean gloves for all contact with the respiratory tract secretions (including oral hygiene)
- Wash hands after every contact with an intubated patient even if gloves are worn

Maintenance of respiratory therapy equipment
- Replace ventilator breathing circuits every 48 h or protect with a filter
- Fill nebulizers and humidifiers with sterile water
- Replace all opened fluid containers daily
- Decontaminate cascade humidifiers and nebulizers every 48 h (unless disposable)
- Clean and dry medication nebulizers between each treatment and discard between patients
- Change oxygen masks and tubing between patients, and more frequently if soiled

Suctioning
- Use clean gloves and wash hands before and after procedures
- Use sterile suction catheters and sterile fluid to flush catheters
- Insert the catheter directly into the airway and discard after each use
- Change suction collection canisters between patients (or daily in short-term care units)
- Change suction tubing between patients

Postoperative care
- Implement breathing exercises before operation
- Early ambulation following surgery
- Control pain with analgesia
- Support wound to aid coughing

---

fection process and inadequate drying afterwards enabled them to multiply inside the tubing.

Spirometers and rebreathe bags have been associated with the transmission of infection and should be changed with the ventilator circuits (Irwin et al 1980, Weber et al 1990, Weems 1993, Woo et al 1986). Rebreathe bags may be protected from contamination by the use of a filter. Alternatively they should be autoclaved, preferably in a sterile supply department where porous-load autoclaving will ensure decontamination of the inside of the bag.

Nebulizers and humidifiers

Nebulizers and humidifiers should always be filled with sterile water to prevent colonization by legionella or other bacteria that will withstand the temperature of the water (Arnow et al 1982). They may become contaminated by backflow of condensate from the delivery tubing and should be decontaminated every 48 h by washing with detergent and water and drying thoroughly (Ayliffe et al 1993, Craven et al 1982). In cascade humidifiers bacteria will usually be prevented from multiplying as the temperature of the water is maintained at over 50°C (Christopher et al 1983). Large-volume room air humidifiers or nebulizers (e.g. IPPB machines and ultrasonic room humidifiers) should be filled only with sterile water and decontaminated daily. Medication nebulizers have been reported to become easily contaminated and should be cleaned with detergent and thoroughly dried after each treatment (Tablan et al 1994). This is also important for patients receiving respiratory therapy in their own home (Pitchford et al 1987). Wall humidifiers can probably be used safely between patients provided the manufacturer's instructions are followed (Golar et al 1993).

Nebulizers and humidifiers should always be stored clean and dry when not in use and, together with delivery tubing and mask, changed between patients.

Disposable humidification systems have not been shown to reduce the incidence of pneumonia but are a useful alternative when access to autoclaving facilities is not possible (Daschner et al 1988).

Respiratory suction

Bacteria colonizing the oropharynx are easily acquired on the hands and catheter during suctioning. To minimize the risk of cross-infection a sterile suction catheter should be used, inserted directly into the trachea or pharynx, and discarded after each use. Hands should be washed thoroughly before and after the procedure but clean gloves should also be worn to protect hands from contamination. There is no evidence that bacteria in suction canisters can reach the suction catheter, although a filter should be used on the canister to prevent release of bacteria into the environment. Canisters, and the tubing between the canister and the patient, should be changed between patients in units where they are in regular use (Tablan et al 1994). Multi-use closed-suction catheter systems are now available. In these systems the catheter is contained inside a sterile sheath and incorporated into the ventilator circuit. This reduces the risk of introducing bacteria with the suction catheter and prevents condensate and tracheal secretions from contaminating the environment (Blackwood & Webb 1998, Cobbley et al 1991). However, although they do not appear to influence the risk of acquiring pneumonia, these systems have been associated with extensive hand contamination and difficulties with secretions

removal (Blackwood & Webb 1998, Deppe et al 1990). Studies comparing multi-use closed-suction systems with the conventional single-use suction catheter system suggest that there is little difference in risk of pneumonia between the two (Deppe et al 1990).

Cross-infection

Bacteria that colonize the oropharynx of one patient may easily be transferred on the hands of staff to other patients (Lowbury et al 1970). This is a particular problem in intensive care or neonatal units where contact with respiratory excretions is extensive and where colonization of the oropharynx with Gram-negative bacteria is very common. In one study, the hands of staff were found to be contaminated with Gram-negative bacilli after changing ventilator tubing and were rarely washed before new tubing was attached (Cadwallader et al 1990). The routine use of gloves in intensive care units for contact with respiratory secretions has been associated with a decreased incidence of hospital-acquired pneumonia (Green et al 1987). Gloves and plastic aprons must be discarded and hands washed after contact with respiratory secretions. The same protective clothing should never be worn for contact with other patients because of the risk of transferring Gram-negative bacilli. Alcohol handrubs provide a rapid and effective means of removing transient flora from the hands and are particularly useful in intensive care settings where frequent handwashing is required.

Often outbreaks of infection are caused by bacteria resistant to a number of antibiotics. Controlling their spread usually requires isolation of colonized patients and rigorous use of protective clothing and handwashing to interrupt spread (Sakata et al 1989).

Equipment must be decontaminated between patients. The level of decontamination required depends on the type of equipment; for example, low-risk items such as reusable oxygen masks should be washed with detergent and water, and dried after each use. Other items that may be contaminated by blood or body fluid (e.g. laryngoscopes, endotracheal tubes) should be decontaminated by autoclaving or washing at a temperature of at least 70°C. See Chapter 13 for further information on methods of decontamination.

Monitoring the incidence of hospital-acquired pneumonia

Awareness of the problem of hospital-acquired pneumonia and the need to consider its prevention when planning postoperative care and the management of respiratory therapy can significantly reduce the incidence of infection. Regular feedback of information to clinical staff on the incidence of hospital-acquired pneumonia in their ward has been shown to reduce the infection rate considerably (Haley et al 1985).

Kelleghan et al (1993) achieved a 57% reduction in the incidence of ventilated associated pneumonia as result of a continuous quality improvement programme focused on surveillance, feedback of pneumonia rates, and increased awareness of infection prevention and control procedures.

OTHER CAUSES OF HOSPITAL-ACQUIRED PNEUMONIA

Most reported cases of hospital-acquired pneumonia are caused by bacteria and are not transmitted by an airborne route. Airborne transmission is of significance in the spread of respiratory viruses, tuberculosis and, on rare occasions, legionella. Severely **immunocompromised** patients may be susceptible to a range of unusual respiratory pathogens, notably aspergillus and atypical mycobacterium, which may be associated with outbreaks of **hospital-acquired infection** in certain circumstances (see Ch. 6). Tuberculosis is transmitted by the inhalation of airborne droplets expelled from the lungs of an infected person, but prolonged, close contact is usually necessary for transmission to occur (see p. 106).

Respiratory viruses

Viral respiratory infections are commonly not diagnosed because the laboratory techniques that such diagnosis requires are frequently not requested by clinical staff. However, viruses have been found to be responsible for 20% of lower respiratory tract infections acquired in hospital (Valenti et al 1981). They often reflect the prevalence of the virus in the community and, in contrast to bacterial infections, most are acquired **exogenously** from other patients, staff or visitors. Viral respiratory infections are not particularly associated with debilitated patients, although they may result in serious disease in this group.

A large proportion of hospital-acquired viral pneumonias are caused by respiratory syncytial virus (RSV), influenza and parainfluenza viruses (Hall 1981). RSV commonly affects children, and community epidemics occur regularly in winter. Children admitted to hospital with the infection act as a source of infection to other patients in the ward (Madge et al 1992). Outbreaks of nosocomial influenza usually occur when the infection is epidemic in the community. Secondary bacterial pneumonia may develop as result of severe influenza, especially in the very young, elderly immunocompromised or people with underlying heart or lung disease. Elderly residents of nursing homes are particularly vulnerable and annual vaccination of people at high risk of developing severe infection is recommended (Communicable Disease Report 1998, Department of Health 1996).

These respiratory viruses are spread by droplets expelled from the respiratory tract and deposited on to the eyes, nose or mouth (Hall 1983). However, virus may also be acquired on the hands either directly from respiratory secretions or indirectly via contaminated surfaces or equipment (Ansari et al 1991). In addition, influenza may be spread by small droplet aerosols and the virus may be shed for up to seven days after the onset of symptoms (Breese-Hall et al 1980, Tablan et al 1994).

To prevent transmission, patients admitted with suspected viral respiratory infection should be nursed in a single room with isolation precautions or cohorted with other affected patients (see Ch. 14). Masks are not necessary as they are unlikely to protect the wearer. The greatest risk is from direct contact with secretions from the mouth and nose; gloves and aprons should be used to handle respiratory secretions and hands should always be washed before leaving the patient's room. In units caring for immunocompromised or cardiac patients additional measures are required to ensure early identification and isolation of infected patients. Contact with visitors under 12 years of age should also be restricted (Garcia et al 1997, Madge et al 1992).

Staff with respiratory infections also present a risk to patients and they should not care for patients who could develop serious illness if they acquired the infection.

Legionnaires' disease

Legionella pneumophila is commonly found in natural sources of water and in water supply systems. Under some conditions it multiplies in water systems and can be transmitted by an aerosol or spray of water from water cooling towers, whirlpool spas or humidifiers (Communicable Disease Report 2000, Joseph et al 1994). *L. pneumophila* has been responsible for a number of outbreaks of nosocomial pneumonia, principally affecting the elderly or **immunosuppressed**. Twenty-two outbreaks were reported between 1980 and 1982 (Joseph et al 1994, Timbury et al 1986).

Infection is thought to be acquired by inhalation of legionella in small water droplets. The risk from legionella infection can be minimized by chlorination of the water supply, regular cleaning of the system, prevention of water stagnation in pipework and ensuring water is kept at temperatures at which the organism cannot multiply (less than 20°C or more than 60°C). Unfortunately, this means that the temperature of the hot water supply in hospitals must not fall below 50°C and care must be taken to avoid scalds to patients or staff. Showerheads do not require disinfecting if the water supply system is properly maintained (NHS Estates 1993).

Respiratory therapy equipment has also been implicated in hospital-acquired legionellosis. Humidifiers or nebulizers contaminated with tap water can result in inhalation of aerosolized legionella (Arnow et al 1982). Other studies have implicated rebreathe bags attached to ventilators as a source of legionella if rinsed with tap water (Woo et al 1986) and ice-making machines (Medical Services Directorate 1993). There is no evidence that legionella can be transmitted from person to person and therefore isolation of infected patients is not necessary.

Aspergillosis

Aspergillus may cause pneumonia in the severely immunocompromised or people with pre-existing lung disease such as cystic fibrosis. Aspergillus is found in soil, water and vegetation, and its spores become airborne particularly when the soil is disturbed, for example during construction. Systems to filter air are frequently used to try to protect the most vulnerable patients (Barnes & Rogers 1989, Tablan et al 1994).

Cystic fibrosis

Cystic fibrosis (CF) is caused by a defect in a gene that controls the regulation of salt and water movement across cell membranes. It results in a build-up of mucous secretions that obstruct many organs of the body including the lungs. The abnormally thick secretions in the lungs impair the activity of the ciliary escalator and obstruct the bronchioles. As a result the lungs become colonized and infected with a range of pathogenic bacteria. *Staphylococus aureus* is a common cause of infection, especially in infants (Branger et al 1994). By 10 years of age most patients will have *Pseudomonas aeruginosa* in their sputum. This organism has a range of toxic effects on the lung tissue but is rarely transmitted between patients and can usually be treated with aerosol or oral antimicrobial therapy (Pitt 2000). Recently, another Gram-negative bacterium, *Burkholderia cepacia*, has been isolated from the lungs of patients with CF. In many patients colonization is asymptomatic, but in 15–20% it results in a fatal fulminant pneumonia and septicaemia. Some strains of *B. cepacia* are transmissible and outbreaks of infection have been reported, although the outcome of acquisition of an outbreak stain appears to be mediated by host factors. Patients colonized with *B. cepacia* should take precautions to minimize the risk of spread to others. These include covering the nose and mouth when coughing, immediate disposal of tissues, keeping sputum pots covered, not sharing nebulizers or eating utensils, not sleeping in the same room as other patients with CF, and frequent and thorough handwashing (Pitt 2000).

REFERENCES

Ansari SA, Springthorpe S, Sattar SA et al (1991) Potential role of hands in the spread of respiratory viral infections: studies with human para-influenza virus 3 and rhinovirus 14. *J. Clin. Microbiol.*, **29**: 2115–19.

Arnow P, Chou T, Weil D (1982) Nosocomial Legionnaires disease caused by aerosolised tap water from respiratory devices. *J. Inf. Dis.*, **146**: 460–7.

Ayliffe GAJ, Coates D, Hoffman PN (1993) *Chemical Disinfection in Hospitals*. Public Health Laboratory Service, London.

Barnes RA, Rogers TR (1989) Control of an outbreak of nosocomial aspergillosis by laminar air-flow isolation. *J. Hosp. Infect.*, **14**: 89–94.

Blackwood B, Webb CH (1998) Closed tracheal suctioning systems and infection control in the intensive care unit. *J. Hosp. Infect.*, **39**(4): 315–22.

Botman MJ, de Krieger RA (1987) Contamination of small volume medication nebulisers and its association with oropharyngeal colonisation. *J. Hosp. Infect.*, **10**: 204–8.

Branger C, Fournier JM, Loulergue J et al (1994) Epidemiology of *Staphylococcus aureus* in patients with cystic fibrosis. *Epidemiol. Infect.*, **112**: 489–500.

Breese-Hall C, Doughlas RG, Gelman JM (1980) Possible transmission by fomites of respiratory syncytial virus. *J. Infect. Dis.*, **141**: 98–102.

Breuer J, Jeffries DJ (1990) Control of viral infections in hospital. *J. Hosp. Infect.*, **16**: 191–221.

Cadwallader HL, Bradley CR, Ayliffe GAJ (1990) Bacterial contamination and frequency of changing ventilator circuitry. *J. Hosp. Infect.*, **15**: 65–72.

Cefai C, Richards J, Gould FK et al (1990) An outbreak of *Acinetobacter* respiratory tract infection resulting from incomplete disinfection of ventilatory equipment. *J. Hosp. Infect.*, **15**: 177–82.

Christopher KL, Saravoltatz LD, Bush TL et al (1983) The potential role of respiratory therapy equipment in cross-infection. *Am. Rev. Respir. Dis.*, **128**: 271.

Cobbley M, Atkins M, Jones PL (1991) Environmental contamination during tracheal suctioning. *Anaesthesia*, **44**: 957–61.

Communicable Disease Report (1998) An outbreak of influenza in four nursing homes in Sheffield. *CDR Weekly*, **8**(16): 139.

Communicable Disease Report (2000) Legionella from guests of Welsh hotel indistinguishable from humidifier isolates. *CDR Weekly*, **10**(16): 141.

Craven DE, Connolly MG, Lichtenberg DA et al (1982) Contamination of mechanical ventilator with tubing changes every 24 or 48 hours. *N. Engl. J. Med.*, **306**: 1505–8.

Craven DE, Lichtenberg DA, Goularte TA (1984a) Contaminated medication nebulisers in mechanical ventilatory circuits: a source of bacterial aerosols. *Am. J. Med.*, **77**: 834–8.

Craven DE, Goularte TA, Make BJ (1984b) Contaminated condensate in mechanical ventilator circuits: a risk factor for nosocomial pneumonia? *Am. Rev. Respir. Dis.*, **129**: 625–8.

Craven DE, Kunches LM, Kilinsky V et al (1986) Risk factors for pneumonia and fatality in patients receiving continuous mechanical ventilation. *Am. Rev. Respir. Dis.*, **133**: 792–6.

Craven DE, Steiger KA, Barber TW (1991) Preventing nosocomial pneumonia: state of the art and perspectives for the 1990s. *Am. J. Med.*, **91** (Suppl. 3B): 44S–53S.

Cross AS, Roup B (1981) Role of respiratory assistance devices in endemic nosocomial pneumonia. *Am. J. Med.*, **70**: 681–5.

Das I, Fraise AP (1997) How useful are microbial filters in respiratory apparatus? *J. Hosp. Infect.*, **37**(4): 263–72.

Daschner FD, Kappstein I, Schuster F et al (1988) Influence of disposable ('Conchapak') and reusable humidifying systems on the incidence of ventilation pneumonia. *J. Hosp. Infect.*, **11**: 161–8.

Department of Health (1996) *Immunisation Against Infectious Disease.* HMSO, London.

Deppe SA, Kelly JW, Thoi LL et al (1990) Incidence of colonization, nosocomial pneumonia and mortality in critically ill patients using TrachC are closed suction system versus open suction system: prospective randomised study. *Crit. Care Med.*, **18**: 1389–93.

Dreyfuss D, Djedaini K, Weber P et al (1991) Prospective study of nosocomial pneumonia and of patients and circuit colonisation during mechanical ventilation with circuit changes every 48 hours versus no change. *Am. Rev. Respir. Dis.*, **143**: 738–43.

Du Moulin GC, Paterson DG, Hedley-White J et al (1982) Aspiration of gastric bacteria in antacid treated patients: a frequent cause of post-operative contamination of the airway. *Lancet*, **i**: 242–5.

Emmerson AM, Enstone JE, Griffin M et al (1996) The second national prevalence survey of infection in hospitals – overview of the results. *J. Hosp. Infect.*, **32**: 175–90.

Emori TG, Gaynes RP (1993) An overview of nosocomial infections, including the role of the microbiology laboratory. *Clin. Microbiol. Rev.*, **6**(4): 428–42.

Fagon JY, Chastre J, Domart Y et al (1989) Nosocomial pneumonia in patients receiving continuous mechanical ventilation: prospective analysis of 52 episodes with use of a protected specimen brush and quantitative culture techniques. *Am. Rev. Respir. Dis.*, **139**: 877–84.

Fagon JY, Chastre J, Hance AJ et al (1993) Nosocomial pneumonia in ventilated patients: a cohort study evaluating attributable mortality and hospital stay. *Am. J. Med.*, **94**(3): 281–8.

Flanagan PG (1999) Diagnosis of ventilator-associated pneumonia. *J. Hosp. Infect.*, **41**: 87–99.

Gallagher J, Strangeways JEM, Allt-Graham J (1987) Contamination control in long-term ventilation. *Anaesthesia*, **42**: 476–81.

Garcia R, Raad I, Abi-Said D et al (1997) Nosocomial respiratory syncitial virus infections: prevention and control in bone marrow transplant patients. *Infect. Control Hosp. Epidemiol.*, **18**: 412–16.

Garibaldi RA, Britt MR, Coleman ML et al (1981) Risk factors for post-operative pneumonias. *Am. J. Med.*, **70**: 677–80.

Golar SD, Sutherland LLA, Ford GT (1993) Multi-patient use of pre-filled disposable oxygen humidifiers for up to 30 days: patient safety and cost analysis. *Respir. Care*, **38**: 343–7.

Gorman LJ, Sanai L, Notman W et al (1993) Cross-infection in an intensive care unit by *Klebsiella pneumoniae* from ventilator condensate. *J. Hosp. Infect.*, **23**: 17–26.

Gray J, George RH, Durbin GM et al (1999) An outbreak of *Bacillus cereus* respiratory tract infection on a neonatal unit due to contaminated ventilator circuits. *J. Hosp. Infect.*, **41**: 19–22.

Green SL, Overton S, Procter C (1987) The effect of glove wearing on the ICU nosocomial infection rates. *14th Annual APIC Educational Conference.* Abstract 1.

Haley RW, Culver DH, White JW et al (1985) The efficacy of infection surveillance and control programs in preventing nosocomial infections in US hospitals *Am. J. Epidemiol.*, **121**: 182.

Hall CB (1981) Nosocomial viral respiratory infections: perennial weeds on pediatric wards. *Am. J. Med.*, **70**: 670–6.

Hall CB (1983) The nosocomial spread of respiratory syncitial viral infections. *Ann. Rev. Med.*, **34**: 311–19.

Holzapfel L, Chevret S, Madinier O et al (1993) Influence of long-term oro- or nasopharyngeal intubation on nosocomial maxillary sinusitis and pneumonia. *Crit. Care Med.*, **21**(8): 1132–8.

Huxley EJ, Viroslav J, Gray WR et al (1978) Pharyngeal aspiration in normal adults and patients with depressed consciousness. *Am. J. Med.*, **64**: 564–8.

Irwin RS, Demars RR, Pratter MR et al (1980) An outbreak of *Acinetobacter* infection associated with the use of a ventilator spirometer. *Respir. Care*, **25**: 232–7.

Jacobs S, Chang RWS, Lee B et al (1990) Continuous enteral feeding; a major cause of pneumonia among ventilated intensive care unit patients. *J. Parenter. Enteral Nutr.*, **14**: 353–86.

Johanson WG, Pierce AK, Sanford JP et al (1972) Nosocomial respiratory infections with Gram negative bacilli: the significance of colonisation of the respiratory tract. *Ann. Intern. Med.*, **77**: 701–6.

Johanson WG, Higuchi JG, Chaudhuri TR et al (1980) Bacterial adherence to epithelial cells in bacillary colonisation of the respiratory tract. *Am. Rev. Respir. Dis.*, **121**: 55–63.

Joseph CA, Watson JM, Harrison TG et al (1994) Nosocomial legionnaire's disease in England and Wales, 1980–1992. *Epidemiol Infect.*, **112**: 329–45.

Kelleghan SI, Salemi C, Padillo S et al (1993) An effective continuous quality improvement approach to the prevention of ventilator-associated pneumonia. *Am. J. Infect. Control*, **21**(6): 322–30.

Kollef MH, Shapiro SD, Fraser VJ et al (1995) Mechanical ventilation with or without 7-day circuit changes: a randomised controlled trial. *Ann. Intern. Med.*, **123**: 168–74.

Lowbury EJL, Thorn BT, Lilly HA et al (1970) Sources of infection with *Pseudomonas aeruginosa* in patients with tracheostomy. *J. Med. Microbiol.*, **3**: 39–56.

Madge P, Payton JY, McColl JH et al (1992) Prospective controlled study of four infection control procedures to prevent nosocomial infection with respiratory syncitial virus. *Lancet*, **340**: 1079–83.

Make BJ, Craven DE, O'Donnell C et al (1987) Clinical and bacteriologic comparison of hydroscopic and cascade humidifiers in ventilated patients. *Am. Rev. Respir. Dis.*, **135**: A212.

Mastro TD, Fields BS, Breiman RF et al (1991) Nosocomial legionnaire's disease and use of medication nebulisers. *J. Infect. Dis.*, **163**: 667–70.

Medical Services Directorate (1993) *Ice Cubes: Infection Caused by* Xanthomonas maltophta. HN(93)42. Department of Health, Wetherby, UK.

Methany NA, Eisenberg P, Spies M (1986) Aspiration pneumonia in patients fed through nasoenteral tubes. *Heart Lung*, **15**: 256–61.

NHS Estates (1993) *The Control of Legionella in Healthcare Premises – a Code of Practice*. Health Technical Memorandum 240. HMSO, London.

Pannuti C, Gingrich R, Pfaller MA et al (1992) Nosocomial pneumonia in patients having bone marrow transplant: attributable mortality and risk factors. *Cancer*, **69**(11): 2653–62.

Pickworth KK, Falcone RE, Hooge-boom JE et al (1993) Occurrence of nosocomial pneumonia in mechanically ventilated trauma patients: a comparison of sucralfate and ranitidine. *Crit. Care Med.*, **21**: 1856–62.

Pingleton SK, Hinthorn DR, Liu C (1986) Enteral nutrition in patients receiving mechanical ventilation: multiple sources of tracheal colonisation include the stomach. *Am. J. Med.*, **80**: 827–32.

Pitchford KC, Corey M, Highsmith AK et al (1987) *Pseudomonas* species contamination of cystic fibrosis patients' home inhalation equipment. *J. Pediatr.*, **111**: 212–16.

Pitt TL (2000) *Burkholderia cepacia* in cystic fibrosis. *Br. J. Infect. Control*, **1**(3): 5–7.

Plowman R, Graves N, Griffin M et al (1999) *The Socio-economic Burden of Hospital-acquired Infection*. Public Health Laboratory Service, London.

Pratt RA, Pellowe CM, Loveday HP et al (2001) The Epic project: developing national evidence-based guidelines for preventing healthcare associated infections. *J. Hosp. Infect.*, **47**: suppl. A.

Prodham G, Leuenberger P, Koerfer J et al (1994) Nosocomial pneumonia in mechanically ventilated patients receiving antacid, ranitidine, or sucralfate as prophylaxis for stress ulcer. A randomised controlled trial. *Ann. Intern. Med.*, **120**(8): 653–62.

Pugliese G, Lichtenberg DA (1987) Nosocomial bacterial pneumonia: an overview. *Am. J. Infect. Control*, **15**: 249–65.

Reinarz JA, Pierce AK, Mays BB et al (1965) The potential role of inhalation therapy equipment in nosocomial pulmonary infections. *J. Clin. Invest.*, **44**: 831–9.

Sakata H, Fujita K, Maruyama S et al (1989) *Acinetobacter calcoaceticus* biovar *anitratus* septicaemia in a neonatal

intensive care unit: epidemiology and control. *J. Hosp. Infect.*, **14**: 15–22.

Sottile FD, Marrie TJ, Prough DS et al (1986) Nosocomial pulmonary infection: possible etiologic significance of bacterial adhesion to endotracheal tubes. *Crit. Care Med.*, **14**: 265–70.

Stamm AM (1998) Ventilator-associated pneumonia and frequency of circuit changes *Am. J. Infect. Control*, **26**: 71–3.

Stoutenbeek CP, Van Saene HKF, Miranda DR et al (1984) The effect of selective decontamination of the digestive tract on colonisation and infection rate in multiple trauma patients. *Intensive Care Med.*, **10**: 185–92.

Stucke VA, Thompson REM (1980) Infection transfer by respiratory condensate during positive pressure respiration. *Nursing Times*, **76**(9): 3–4.

Tablan OC, Anderson LJ, Arden NH et al (1994) Guideline for the prevention of nosocomial pneumonia. *Am. J. Infect. Control*, **22**: 247–92.

Timbury MC, Donaldson JR, McCartney AC et al (1986) Outbreak of legionnaires' disease in Glasgow Royal Infirmary: microbiological aspects. *J. Hyg. (Camb.)*, **97**(3): 393–403.

Torres A, Serra-Batlles J, Ros E et al (1992) Pulmonary aspiration of gastric contents in patients receiving mechanical ventilation: the effect of body position. *Ann. Intern. Med.*, **116**(7): 540–3.

Torres A, el-Ebiary M, Gonzales J et al (1993) Gastric and pharyngeal flora in nosocomial pneumonia acquired during mechanical ventilation *Am. Rev. Respir. Dis.*, **148**(2): 352–7.

Valenti WM, Hall CB, Douglas RG et al (1981) Nosocomial viral infections I: epidemiology and significance. *Infect. Control*, **1**: 33–7.

Ward V, Wilson J, Taylor L et al (1997) *Preventing Hospital-acquired Infection. Clinical Guidelines*. Public Health Laboratory Service, London.

Wasylak TJC, Abbott FV, English MJM et al (1990) Reduction of postoperative morbidity following patient-controlled morphine. *Can. J. Anaesth.*, **37**: 726–31.

Weber DJ, Wilson MB, Rutala WA et al (1990) Manual ventilation bags as a source for bacterial colonisation of intubated patients. *Am. Rev. Respir. Dis.*, **142**: 892–4.

Weems JJ (1993) Nosocomial outbreak of *Pseudomonas cepacia* associated with contamination of reusable electronic ventilator temperature probes. *Infect. Control Hosp. Epidemiol*, **14**: 583–6.

Woo AH, Yu VL, Goetz A et al (1986) Potential in-hospital modes of transmission of *Legionella pneumophila*. Demonstration experiments for dissemination by showers, humidifiers and rinsing of ventilation bag apparatus. *Am. J. Med.*, **80**: 567–73.

FURTHER READING

Hall CB, Douglas RG Jr (1981) Modes of transmission of respiratory syncytial virus. *J. Pediatr.*, **99**: 100.

Harrison L (1993) Factors influencing the frequency of ventilator circuit changes. *Br. J. Nurs.*, **2**(16): 793–801.

Hovig B (1981) Lower respiratory tract infection associated with respiratory therapy and anaesthetic equipment. *J. Hosp. Infect.*, **2**: 301.

Hutchinson DN (1990) *Nosocomial legionellosis. Rev. Med. Microbiol.*, **1**: 108–15.

Tablan OC (1997) Nosocomial pneumonia. In *Infection Control and Applied Epidemiology. Principles and Practice*, pp. 10.1–10.13. Association for Professionals in Infection Control and Epidemiology–Mosby, St Louis.

Taylor D, Littlewood S (1998) Respiratory system part 1: pneumonia. *Nursing Times*, **94**(7): 48–51.

12

Preventing gastrointestinal infection: the principles of food hygiene

INTRODUCTION

Gastrointestinal infections can be acquired directly through the ingestion of contaminated food or water, or may be spread from person to person through contact with infected body fluids such as faeces or vomit. Hospital patients may be particularly susceptible to such infections, because illness or old age can reduce the production of gastric acid in the stomach. In addition, the very young, the elderly or the debilitated are likely to develop more serious disease, and the infection may cause or accelerate their death (Cowden et al, 1995).

Poor personal hygiene or food-handling practices in the kitchens of a hospital or nursing home can cause outbreaks of infection affecting large numbers of patients and staff. Measures to prevent cross-infection are also particularly important as contact with body fluids and the movement of staff and equipment between patients may greatly facilitate the transmission of gastrointestinal infections.

This chapter focuses on micro-organisms that cause foodborne infection and how the principles of food hygiene should be used to prevent infection. It also considers other gastrointestinal pathogens associated with outbreaks of infection in hospitals, and the infection control precautions required to prevent their transmission.

FOODBORNE INFECTION

Food is an important source of infection. Around 50 000 cases of food poisoning are reported in England and Wales every year and there has been a marked increase in notifications during the past two decades. Some of these cases are sporadic, isolated infections but many occur as part of outbreaks of foodborne illness, several hundred of which occur every year. Most outbreaks (43%) are associated with commercial food production in restaurants, pubs, etc., but 17%

occur as a result of domestic food preparation and 13% are associated with catering in hospitals or residential institutions (Cowden et al, 1995).

There has been a marked increase in the number of reported cases of foodborne illness since the 1990s, a pattern that has been seen in many European countries and in North America. The reasons for this increase are not entirely clear, but factors such as increasing use of restaurants, availability of a wide range of convenience foods and changes in farming methods have probably all played a part (Sharp 1992). The upward trend in reported cases of foodborne illness rose particularly sharply in the 1980s. This was largely due to a dramatic increase in cases of salmonella, and has been associated with the development of factory farming in the poultry industry which uses intensive methods of chicken rearing, processing and egg production (Cooke 1990, Sharp 1992). Table 12.1 illustrates the pathogens most commonly responsible for foodborne infections in the UK, the sources of infection and associated symptoms.

Table 12.1 Pathogens that cause foodborne illness

Micro-organism	Source of infection	Route of transmission	Symptoms
Aeromonas	Aquatic environments	Ingestion of contaminated water, shellfish or raw foods washed in contaminated water	Vomiting, diarrhoea
Bacillus B. cereus B. subtilis	Commonly found in the environment Contaminated cereals, dried food Contaminated dairy and meat products, especially pastries	Spores not always destroyed by cooking, germinate and release toxin if food stored in warm temperatures for prolonged periods	Emetic toxin causes rapid onset of vomiting (within 5 h). B. cereus also produces a diarrhoeal toxin which causes abdominal pain and diarrhoea 8–16 h after ingestion
Campylobacter	Gastrointestinal tract of birds (poultry), cattle, other animals	Undercooked poultry and meat; contaminated water; unpasteurized milk; cross-contamination of cooked and raw food. Infective dose low. Person-to-person spread possible but unusual	Severe abdominal pain, profuse diarrhoea, 2–5 days after ingestion
Clostridium perfringens	Gastrointestinal tract of animals	Spores on contaminated meat not destroyed by cooking and germinate if food kept warm and not reheated thoroughly. Symptoms caused by toxin produced in the gut during sporulation	Diarrhoea and abdominal pain, usually 12–18 hrs after ingestion
Escherichia coli Verocytotoxin producing (VTEC) Serotype O157 most common in UK	Gastrointestinal tract of animals, especially cattle	Undercooked beef and beef products, milk and vegetables. Also acquired by direct contact with infected animals and people	Bloody diarrhoea, abdominal pain 1–6 days after ingestion; 5% of patients develop haemolytic uraemic syndrome (HUS)
Enterotoxigenic (ETEC)	Gastrointestinal tract of animals and humans	Major cause of traveller's diarrhoea, acquired through ingestion of contaminated food and water	Diarrhoea, 12–72 h after exposure
Salmonella Typhi/paratyphi	Gastrointestinal tract of humans	Food washed in sewage-contaminated water or contaminated by infected food handler. Person-to-person spread uncommon	Fever, malaise, nausea. Constipation followed by diarrhoea 1–3 weeks after infection
Other species	Gastrointestinal tract of animals, birds (poultry) and occasionally humans	Undercooked meat, especially poultry; eggs; dairy products. Close contacts may spread infection from person to person	Diarrhoea, vomiting, fever, 12–72 h after infection

cont.

Table 12.1 (*cont.*)

Micro-organism	Source of infection	Route of transmission	Symptoms
Shigella	Gastrointestinal tract of humans	Occasionally spread by contaminated water or raw foods washed in contaminated water. Most cases spread by faecal–oral contact	Bloody diarrhoea caused by a toxin occurs 1–7 days after infection
Staphylococcus aureus	Infected or colonized skin lesions, fingers or nose of food handlers	Cooked food (e.g. meat, poultry, fish) and dairy products, handled and stored at warm temperatures for several hours before eating. Symptoms caused by an ingested toxin	Vomiting and abdominal pain, usually within 4 h of ingestion
Viruses (e.g. small round structured viruses; SRSVs)	Gastrointestinal tract of humans	Contaminated water and food, especially shellfish; cold foods contaminated by a food handler. Very low infective dose. Most cases spread from person to person by contact with faeces or vomit	Vomiting, diarrhoea, fever 24–48 h after infection
Yersinia enterocolitica	Gastrointestinal tract of animals and birds	Infection particularly associated with pork, but milk and milk products also implicated. Will grow at 4°C and may withstand pasteurization. Person-to-person spread may occur	Watery diarrhoea, abdominal pain, fever and arthritis 3–7 days after ingestion

The Food Safety Act 1990

This Act governs the production of food and drink from preparation to the point of sale and provides local authorities with the necessary powers to register food premises, enforce their compliance with Regulations and deal with unsafe food. Any premises involved in the production, supply or storage of food must be registered with the local authority. Environmental health officers employed by the local authority have the right to inspect premises, check their records and take samples of food. They can issue warnings: *improvement notices*, which specify remedial action to be taken within a given period, or *prohibition notices*, which require the immediate closure of the premises. They may also prosecute those responsible where breaches in the food legislation are identified.

The General Food Hygiene Regulations came into force in 1995 and aim to ensure that common food hygiene rules are applied across the European Community. There are also a range of product-specific Regulations covering, for example, poultry, meat, fishery and dairy products. The General Food Hygiene Regulations apply to anyone who sells food, whether for profit or fundraising, publicly or privately, and requires those preparing, transporting or selling food to identify and control food safety risks systematically (see p. 218) and to ensure that premises are hygienic. They also specify the mandatory training of people who handle food. The Food Safety (Temperature Control) Regulations 1995 provide specific guidance on temperatures at which certain foods must be kept.

Specific guidance on food handling in healthcare establishments can be found in *Hospital Catering: Delivering a Good Service* (NHS Executive 1996a) and HSG(96)20 (NHS Executive 1996b).

PRINCIPLES OF FOOD HYGIENE

As food in its raw state is frequently contaminated with bacteria, great care must be taken to ensure that it is prepared, cooked and stored properly. There are many ways in which poor practice can result in food poisoning; the most common are listed in Box 12.1. Barrie (1996) points out that 'food hygiene is more than cleanliness. It is the use of policies, practices and procedures to protect food from contamination,

---

Box 12.1   The 10 most common causes of food poisoning

1. Food prepared too far in advance
2. Food stored at room temperature
3. Food cooled too slowly before refrigeration
4. Food not reheated to a sufficiently high temperature to destroy food-poisoning bacteria
5. Cooked food contaminated with food-poisoning bacteria
6. Meat and meat products undercooked
7. Frozen meat and poultry not thawed completely
8. Cross-contamination from raw to cooked foods
9. Hot food stored below 63°C
10. Food handlers with gastrointestinal infection

Source: Roberts (1982)

prevent multiplication of bacteria to numbers capable of causing food poisoning or food spoilage and ensure the destruction of disease-producing micro-organisms by thorough cooking'.

The food-handling responsibilities of nurses vary enormously with different healthcare systems and with the type of food delivery. In a large general hospital nurses may be involved only with distribution of pre-prepared meals on trays, although they may be expected to make decisions about storing and reheating meals at ward level. In small hospitals, specialist units or nursing homes, nurses may participate in all stages of food production. As a large proportion of food poisoning occurs in the home, where knowledge of food hygiene may be limited, nurses may be required to advise and educate vulnerable patients on the prevention of gastrointestinal illness in their own homes. An understanding of the principles of food hygiene and infection control is therefore essential if appropriate advice is to be offered.

In the following section, safe handling of food is considered under the headings of 'preparation', 'cooking' and 'storage'.

Food preparation

Raw food is frequently contaminated with pathogens such as campylobacter, *Clostridium perfringens*, salmonella and toxogenic strains of *Escherichia coli* derived from the intestines of animals. Approximately half of raw chicken carcasses have been found to be contaminated with salmonella, and campylobacter is also commonly present (Atabay & Corry 1997, Mackey 1989). Red meat, in particular minced beef, is susceptible to contamination by toxogenic strains of *E. coli* (Centers for Disease Control 1993). *Bacillus cereus* and *C. perfringens* are widely found in the environment and may therefore contaminate a variety of produce including rice and vegetables. Milk and dairy products are readily contaminated during collection or processing.

Most intestinal pathogens must be ingested in very large numbers (at least several hundred in each gram of food) to overcome the acid in the stomach and establish infection in the gut. Thorough cooking will destroy most bacteria in food and the few that remain should be insufficient to cause infection. However, if raw food is brought into contact with cooked food, for example by contact with or dripping on to cold meats in the refrigerator or on equipment such as chopping boards and knives, cross-contamination is likely to occur. The bacteria will then multiply on the cooked

food and will not be killed by further cooking before ingestion. Campylobacter is particularly likely to be transmitted in this way. Although this organism is readily destroyed by cooking, infection can follow the ingestion of only a few hundred organisms as they multiply rapidly in the gut (Eley 1992).

One of the essential principles of safe food handling is to ensure that cooked food is never contaminated by uncooked food. Bacteria can be transferred from raw to cooked food on hands and equipment such as knives and chopping boards. Such equipment must always be washed with hot water and detergent after each use and have smooth surfaces to enable easy cleaning. Cloths used to clean surfaces or equipment will become contaminated rapidly and should be discarded or washed frequently. Raw and cooked food should be covered and stored separately in cold stores or refrigerators because raw food may touch or drip on to other food.

Food that is eaten raw is not decontaminated by heat and must be washed under running water to remove micro-organisms. Salads prepared in hospitals have been found to be contaminated with various **Gram-negative bacilli**, which, although unlikely to cause infection in healthy people, may be harmful to an **immunocompromised** patient (Houang et al 1991). Gastrointestinal viruses, such as small round structured virus, require a very low dose to transmit infection. Outbreaks are frequently associated with salads, sandwiches or desserts prepared by affected food handlers (Luthi et al 1996). It is essential that hands are washed thoroughly before food handling and that those recovering from gastrointestinal illness should not be involved in handling food.

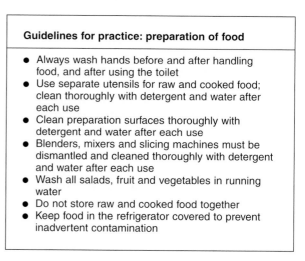

Guidelines for practice: preparation of food

- Always wash hands before and after handling food, and after using the toilet
- Use separate utensils for raw and cooked food; clean thoroughly with detergent and water after each use
- Clean preparation surfaces thoroughly with detergent and water after each use
- Blenders, mixers and slicing machines must be dismantled and cleaned thoroughly with detergent and water after each use
- Wash all salads, fruit and vegetables in running water
- Do not store raw and cooked food together
- Keep food in the refrigerator covered to prevent inadvertent contamination

The important guidelines for practice when preparing food are summarized on page 214.

Cooking food

The destruction of bacteria in food by cooking depends on exposing them to heat for a sufficient period of time. However, there is a balance between eliminating bacteria and spoiling the taste and nutrient value of food by overcooking. Most bacteria are killed at temperatures of around 60°C, but prolonged heating may be required to ensure that these temperatures are achieved throughout the food. It can take some time for heat to penetrate the centre of the food, particularly if the food is dense (e.g. mashed potato, raw meat) or is still frozen in the middle. Standard cooking times are based on the heating of food from room temperature and, if applied to food that is incompletely defrosted, may result in undercooking. This is particularly dangerous with some types of food, such as poultry, because a large proportion are contaminated with salmonella and campylobacter in the raw state (Atabay & Corry 1997). Outbreaks of infection caused by *E. coli* O157 are often associated with the consumption of undercooked mince beef e.g. beefburgers (Centers for Disease Control 1993).

The same principles should be applied to reheating food before consumption. Different foods take different times to reheat and it can therefore be difficult to estimate the reheating time. For example, the gravy in a stew will heat more rapidly than the meat and a bubbling gravy does not mean that the meat has been reheated to the correct temperature. A thermometer should be used to check that the centre of the food is at 70°C before it is safe to serve. The important guidelines for practice when cooking or reheating food are summarized in the Guidelines for practice.

Microwave ovens

Microwave ovens heat food from the inside outwards and vegetative bacteria are unlikely to survive provided that all parts of the food reach 70°C. Unfortunately, heating in microwave ovens tends to be uneven so that some parts of the food may become extremely hot whilst other parts remain cool (Knutson et al 1987). Food should therefore be allowed to stand for 5 min after heating to ensure that the heat is evenly distributed by conduction (Lund et al 1989). Precooked chilled foods should be reheated in the manner specified by the manufacturer. The time necessary to heat other foods is extremely difficult to estimate and a thermometer

---

Guidelines for practice: cooking food safely
• Defrost meat thoroughly before cooking
• Adhere to standard or recommended cooking times
• Use a thermometer to check the temperature in the centre of the food
• Reheat food thoroughly and use a thermometer to check the temperature

should be used to ensure that the food has been heated throughout.

Food storage

Bacteria can multiply in most foods provided there is moisture present and the temperature is between 20 and 40°C (e.g. room temperature). At refrigeration temperatures of 5–10°C multiplication occurs extremely slowly so that food can be stored for a few days without spoiling. Below 0°C food can be stored for prolonged periods as most bacteria are unable to multiply at these temperatures. *Listeria monocytogenes* presents particular problems as it can multiply in the refrigerator. It is transmitted by food and, although rare, may cause serious infection in the immunocompromised, elderly, and unborn child or neonate. It can survive drying, freezing and even cooking. Listeria is frequently isolated from freshly cut salads, paté and soft cheeses (Lund et al 1989). Outbreaks of infection associated with coleslaw, milk and cook–chill chicken have also been reported (Jones 1990). These foods should not be stored in the refrigerator for more than 3 days.

Prolonged storage of food at ambient temperature is responsible for many outbreaks of foodborne infection (Cowden et al 1995). Bacteria may multiply in food eaten raw; for example, salmonella from eggs can contaminate mayonnaise or mousses (Lewis et al 1995) and some bacteria, notably *C. perfringens* and *B. cereus*, may survive the cooking process and multiply during subsequent storage. *C. perfringens* is found in the intestines of animals and in soil, and may contaminate both meat and vegetables. It forms spores when the food is cooked, some of which may survive prolonged boiling. Unless the food is cooled rapidly, the spores will germinate and the bacteria may multiply rapidly in a warm kitchen. If large numbers of the vegetative cells are present in the food when ingested, they release a toxin as they form spores in the intestine. This causes profuse diarrhoea and abdominal pain (Hobbs

& Roberts 1993). *B. cereus* is also able to survive cooking by forming spores. Outbreaks of infection have been associated particularly with prolonged storage of cooked rice at room temperature. Bacteria remaining after cooking multiply in the rice, sporulate and release a heat-resistant toxin that is not destroyed by subsequent reheating (Eley 1992).

To avoid these hazards food should always be stored at temperatures below 8°C or above 63°C. If food is not to be consumed immediately after preparation, it must be cooled quickly and stored in the refrigerator (Food Hygiene Regulations 1995, Food Safety (Temperature Control) Regulations 1995). Meals should not be saved for more than 1 h if a patient is not on the ward at mealtimes. Bacteria may multiply in the food and subsequent reheating may not be sufficient to destroy them. Catering departments must offer a flexible service for patients who have missed meals to avoid the need for reheating at ward level (NHS Executive 1999) (Fig. 12.1).

The method of delivering meals to wards must ensure that the food is kept either hot or cold. Heated trolleys should maintain a temperature of at least 63°C and should incorporate a refrigerated compartment for cold desserts and salads. The meals should be served as rapidly as possible to reduce the risk of bacterial multiplication.

Food stored in the refrigerator should be dated and discarded after it has reached its use-by date. The temperature of the refrigerator must be maintained between 1 and 4°C (Food Hygiene Regulations 1990). Particular care should be taken with the storage and reheating of ready-to-eat chilled foods. Eggs should be stored in the refrigerator to prevent *Salmonella enteritidis*, which has been isolated from a small proportion of eggs, from multiplying to a potentially infectious dose (De Louvois 1993, Humphrey et al 1991). Dishes prepared with raw eggs are a common cause of outbreaks of salmonella poisoning (Ejidokun et al 2000).

Dry foods should be protected from moisture; whilst dry they are unable to support the growth of bacteria.

The standards for temperature control during the storage, processing and distribution of food are

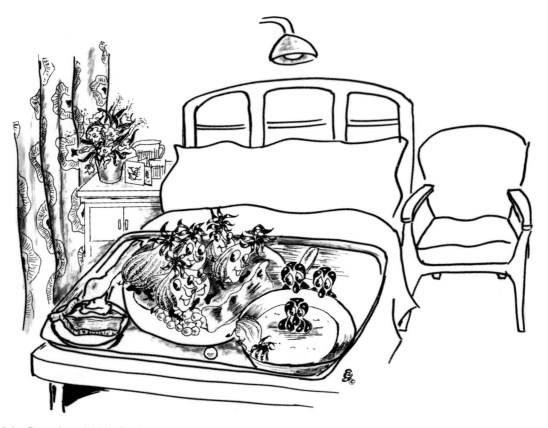

Fig. 12.1 Bacteria multiply in food at room temperature.

Guidelines for practice: storage of food

- Do not keep prepared food at room temperature for more than 1 h
- Plug heated food trolleys in as soon as they arrive on the ward and serve the food immediately
- Do not keep meals in a warm oven
- Do not save and reheat meals for patients absent at mealtimes
- Do not use chilled meals or food beyond its sell-by date
- Ensure the refrigerator is fitted with a thermometer and is maintained between 1 and 4°C
- Date items stored in the fridge and discard after 3 days

Guidelines for practice: ward kitchens

- Check that the ward kitchen is clean
- Ensure the refrigerator is sited out of direct heat or sunlight
- Monitor the refrigerator regularly, discard unlabelled or outdated items and check the temperature
- Ensure soap and handtowels are available
- Use disposable cloths and paper towels when washing and drying dishes

---

described in the Food Safety (Temperature Controls) Regulations 1995. The principles of safe food storage are summarized in the Guidelines for practice above.

Ward kitchens

These are subject to the Food Hygiene Regulations (see p. 213) and may be inspected during visits by the environmental health officer. The ward manager is responsible for ensuring that the regulations are complied with. The fittings should be designed to be cleaned easily, with smooth surfaces to prevent the collection of dirt or grease. A handwash basin with soap and hand towels must be available. The refrigerator must be checked daily to ensure that food is covered, labelled and discarded when appropriate. Drugs, blood or specimens should never be kept in the food refrigerator. The refrigerator should be sited away from a heat source and out of direct sunlight. A thermometer inside the refrigerator should be used to check the temperature regularly. Goldthorpe et al (1991) found that very few ward fridges maintained a temperature of between 5 and 7°C, and recommended the use of commercial larder refrigerators in place of the domestic fridge. Ice-making machines are prone to contamination, especially if ice is removed by hand. They should be cleaned and maintained regularly and a designated receptacle used to remove the ice (Barrie 1996, Medical Devices Directorate 1993).

To minimize the risk of cross-contamination separate colour-coded mops, buckets and cloths should be used to clean kitchen areas and should not be confused with equipment used to clean other areas. Patients and their relatives should be discouraged from bringing food into the hospital because there is no control on how it is prepared.

Crockery and cutlery

Bacteria are easily removed from crockery and cutlery by washing in hot water and detergent. This is best done in a central wash-up area where dishes can be washed in an automatic machine at very high temperature. If items have to be washed at ward level, use clean hot water and detergent, rinse, and leave to drain rather than dry with a cloth which may easily become contaminated with potential pathogens. If dishcloths are necessary, they should be disposable.

Personal hygiene

Food is easily contaminated by bacteria carried on the hands. Pathogens, such as salmonella or campylobacter, may be acquired by handling raw food and transferred to other food or equipment. *Staphylococcus aureus*, a pathogen carried on the skin of many people, can also cause gastrointestinal illness if transferred to food. Particular care should be taken when handling food eaten cold (e.g. sandwiches, desserts) as any contamination will not be removed by subsequent cooking.

People suffering from a gastrointestinal infection may excrete a large number of micro-organisms in their faeces. Some bacteria (e.g. salmonella, *E. coli*) may continue to be excreted in faeces for many months. Infected food handlers may be the primary cause of some outbreaks of food poisoning (Cowden et al 1995, Patterson et al 1997). Staff who develop gastrointestinal infection must be particularly scrupulous about hand hygiene before handling food and should seek advice from the occupational health department before returning to work.

In ward areas, staff should put on a clean apron and wash their hands before distributing food. Cold or cooked food such as salads and cold meats should be handled with gloves or utensils. (See Guidelines for practice.)

Guidelines for practice: personal hygiene

- Wash hands before handling food
- Wash hands after using the toilet, after handling raw meat and vegetables, after cleaning procedures and after handling waste food
- Use a clean plastic apron when handling food
- Keep hair tied back
- Report any gastrointestinal illness to the occupational health department

Meal delivery systems in hospitals

Safe food handling and delivery systems are of paramount importance in hospitals where many vulnerable patients and staff are at risk of food poisoning if the systems break down. In 1984 an outbreak of food poisoning at the Stanley Royd Hospital for the mentally ill affected 355 residents and resulted in the deaths of 19 (Fig. 12.2). The subsequent enquiry found standards in the handling, storage and preparation of food in the hospital kitchens to be very poor. This incident highlighted the vulnerability of hospital patients to food poisoning and resulted in the removal of Crown Immunity, which until 1987 had protected hospitals from prosecution by environmental health officers.

In large hospitals, meals may need to travel considerable distances between the kitchens and ward areas. The delivery system must therefore ensure that hot food is kept above 63°C and that cold food is refrigerated. Many institutions use cook–chill or cook–freeze catering systems, where the meals are prepared in the usual way but are then either rapidly cooled to a temperature of 0–3°C or frozen to –8°C. Cook–chill meals can be kept for up to 5 days, frozen meals for up to 8 weeks. Cook–chill or cook–freeze meals are delivered to wards in chilled cabinets and reheated in the cabinet at a set temperature for a predetermined period of time. These delivery systems are an effective means of large-scale catering and, provided the correct controls are in place, especially in relation to the temperature used during preparation, storage and plating, are safe (Barrie 1996, NHS Executive 1996b). The *Control Assurance Standard: Catering and Food Hygiene* (NHS Executive 1999) requires that all food storage, preparation and handling in NHS premises complies with current food safety legislation as well as providing for the nutritional requirements of patients. There must also be systems in place for monitoring the food safety management system at Trust Board level. Any member of staff involved in handling food must receive training in food handling and as a minimum

PUBLIC INQUIRY INTO SALMONELLA OUTBREAK

SOCIAL SERVICES SECRETARY Norman Fowler has set up a full-scale public inquiry into the outbreak of food poisoning which has killed 27 patients at the Stanley Royd psychiatric hospital in Wakefield.

Announcing his decision last week, Mr Fowler said there was a need to establish 'the full facts surrounding the outbreak', although priority had been to bring it under control. Eight patients were still suffering from salmonella symptoms and three of them were seriously ill as *NT* went to press, but no new cases had been reported for 48 hours.

Investigation into the infection has shown that cold roast beef left out for 10 hours on a warm day had caused the rapid spread of the bacteria, according to Wakefield health authority, although the actual source of the infection is still not known.

District medical officer Dr Geoffrey Ireland said last week that the meat had been taken out of the refrigerator in the morning to be sliced and been left out until it was served later that afternoon. This has been denied by the hospital's kitchen staff. NUPE branch secretary George Rusling told *NT* the meat had been left out of the refrigerator no longer than four hours.

Fig. 12.2 Press report of an outbreak of food poisoning at Stanley Royd Hospital.

must have a basic knowledge of the principles of food hygiene (NHS Executive 1999).

Hazard analysis critical control points (HACCP)

A systematic approach is essential in monitoring standards of food safety and hygiene. A concept called hazard analysis critical control points (HACCP) is now widely used in the food industry and catering establishments, and systematic hazard analysis is also expected in NHS catering services (NHS Executive 1999). HACCP involves the identification of possible hazards in the production process and specification of the critical controls required to ensure safety (critical control points). Each control point is then monitored using defined criteria (e.g. a specific temperature or other check). Microbiological testing of food is usually not necessary, except where an outbreak of food poisoning is suspected.

HACCP can also be applied to other aspects of food provision such as the handling of expressed breast milk and enteral feeding (see below) (Anderton 1994, Hunter 1991).

Enteral feeds

Feeding via a nasogastric or gastrostomy tube is increasingly used as an alternative to parenteral nutrition when patients are unable to feed themselves. However, there are significant microbiological hazards associated with it (Anderton 1985, 1993). Many types of bacteria, including salmonella, klebsiella, enterobacter, E. coli and S. aureus, have been found in high concentrations in enteral feeds. These may cause gastroenteritis and, through **colonization** of the gut, may result in **septicaemia** and **pneumonia** (Thurn et al 1990).

The liquid nutrients provide a favourable medium in which bacteria can grow and are easily contaminated during assembly and manipulation of the administration sets. Once the administration reservoir or tubing is contaminated, the bacteria can multiply rapidly in the feed at room temperature. If feeds are administered over several hours, bacteria may multiply considerably. Contamination of enteral feeds occurs frequently, despite strict protocols for their management. Crocker et al (1986) found that the onset of contamination is delayed if the feed is supplied in prefilled, ready-to-use administration reservoirs. Where feeds were transferred to an administration reservoir, the rate of contamination was much higher and, if the mixture had to be reconstituted before adding to the reservoir, 75% were contaminated after 12 h and 100% after 24 h in use. The standards used in the preparation and handling of enteral feeds must therefore be even higher than with conventional meals.

Currently there are no accepted recommendations concerning the management of enteral feeds but the strong association between infection and contaminated feeds suggests that a rigorous no-touch technique must be used when assembling the administration sets and handling the feed. The risk of contamination may be reduced by the use of clean, disposable gloves (Anderton & Aidoo 1991). Commercially prepared feeds in ready-to-use administration reservoirs are preferable as they are supplied as sterile liquids. However, if the connection between nutrient container and administration set is contaminated during assembly, large numbers of micro-organisms may be recovered from the feed after 24 h (Beattie & Anderton 1999).

Administration reservoirs and tubing should be discarded after a maximum of 24 h in use (Ward et al 1997). Attempts to decontaminate containers with detergent and water or disinfectants may not be successful. Tubing experimentally inoculated with klebsiella could be decontaminated only after flushing with soapy water for 10 min followed by immersion in 125 ppm hypochlorite for 7 h (Anderton & Nwoguh 1991).

There is considerable potential for feeds prepared in a hospital kitchen or ward to become contaminated through contact with equipment such as blenders, mixers or liquidizers. Feeds must be prepared under controlled conditions, preferably in the dietary department, using an extremely high standard of hygiene (Thurn et al 1990). Once a container of feed has been opened, it must be stored in the refrigerator and discarded after 24 h.

Anderton (1994) recommended the application of HACCP to enteral tube feeding. A team of key staff should be involved, such as dietician, representative ward/unit nurses and doctors, pharmacist, infection control nurse and microbiologist. This team should then define the process and identify the key hazards (Box 12.2). Control measures can then be defined for each of the hazards identified, for example selecting well-designed feed administration systems, protocols

---

Box 12.2 Steps in a hazard analysis critical control point

- Assemble a HACCP team
- Define the process
- Identify and assess the hazards and risks
  - characteristics
  - micro-organisms
  - severity and frequency
- Identify the critical control points
  - points where control must be achieved
- Specify monitoring and control procedures
  - when is action taken
  - what action is taken
  - who takes action
  - limits requiring further action
- Implement control at critical points
- Verify HACCP periodically

Adapted from Anderton (1994)

for handling feeds, systems for recording the time feeds are left at ward temperature, and a system to audit the control established.

Enteral feeds prepared by patients at home are also susceptible to contamination and these patients should be prepared with a rigorous education programme before discharge (Anderton et al 1993). In the home, syringes used to check the position of the nasogastric tube or to flush tubing with water between feeds can be used more than once provided they are supplied by the manufacturer for this purpose and are not packaged as single-use disposable items.

The important guidelines for practice for the management of enteral feeding are summarized below. Gastrostomy tubes may be in place for prolonged periods and patients may also be vulnerable to infection at the entry site, and peritonitis (Peters & Westerby 1994).

The potential for contamination during preparation and handling also applies to milk feeds and expressed breast milk. Most milk feeds can be supplied safely in commercial sterile, prefilled bottles. When special milk diets are required, the milk should be prepared using an extremely high standard of hygiene (Burnett et al 1989).

Rowan & Anderson (1998) highlighted the problem of contamination of dietary food supplements such as 'build-up' by *Bacillus cereus*. This spore-forming organism may contaminate pasteurized milk and be present in low numbers in powdered food supplements. When the powdered supplement is reconstituted with the milk and stored above 5°C, the presence of glucose in the milk enables *B. cereus* to multiply and enterotoxin to be produced by toxogenic strains of *B. cereus*.

Guidelines for practice: the management of enteral feeds

- Use commercially prepared feeds in prefilled administration reservoirs where possible
- Pay scrupulous attention to principles of food hygiene if feeds are mixed on the ward
- Blenders used to prepare feed must be dismantled, thoroughly washed with detergent and dried after each use
- Wash hands before handling enteral feeding systems
- Avoid direct contact between the administration set connections and any non-sterile object
- Administer feed over as short a time as possible
- Store opened feeds in the refrigerator and discard after 24 h
- Replace administration sets and reservoirs every 24 h. Do not wash out and re-use
- Flush tubing with plenty of water after administering intermittent feeds

---

Careful controls must also be in place if expressed breast milk is being handled and stored (Hunter 1991). Graham et al (1999) reported a case of Gram-negative bacteraemia in a premature baby that originated from expressed breast milk (EBM) given to the baby via a nasogastric tube. The authors pointed to the need for careful controls and clear guidelines for ensuring that EBM is stored and handled safely (Balmer et al 1997). Hunter (1991) has recommended the use of HACCP in controlling the safe delivery of EBM.

PREVENTING THE SPREAD OF GASTROINTESTINAL INFECTION

Some micro-organisms that cause gastrointestinal infection spread mainly from person to person following contact with excreta (e.g. rotavirus, *Clostridium difficile*).

Micro-organisms transmitted by food can also be spread to others by cross-infection. In outbreaks of foodborne illness, cross-infection may cause what are described as secondary cases of infection, occurring several days after the main outbreak. Joseph & Palmer (1989) reported that 30% of outbreaks of salmonella infection in hospitals affecting two or more patients or staff resulted from cross-infection rather than food poisoning. Person-to-person transmission occurred particularly frequently in elderly care, maternity or paediatric units where contact with faecal material is more likely. Faulty bedpan washers were implicated in four outbreaks and contaminated gastroscopes in a further two. Person-to-person transmission of shigella occurs readily because the ingestion of only a very few organisms may result in infection (Benenson 1995). *E. coli* O157 presents particular problems. A significant proportion of symptomatic patients require hospitalization because they develop thrombocytopenia, purpura or haemolytic uraemic syndrome (Coia 1998). The rate of secondary spread associated with this organism is high, and some people continue to excrete it for prolonged periods, even once symptoms have resolved. Cross-infection of *Clostridium perfringens* amongst the elderly has also been reported (Cooke 1990). Cross-infection by campylobacter is not thought to occur (Skirrow 1990).

Viruses, notably the small round structured viruses, are readily spread from person to person through aerosols and environmental contamination from vomiting and can be either foodborne or introduced by an infected patient or member of staff (Green et al 1998, Owen Caul 1994, Patterson et al 1997). They are also excreted in faeces for several days after the onset of symptoms (Chadwick et al 2000). Outbreaks of infection in hospitals caused by cross-infection of these viruses are frequently reported. Rotavirus is a very common cause of diarrhoea in children and extensive outbreaks of infection amongst susceptible groups of patients such as children and the elderly have been reported although these are rarely foodborne (Lewis et al 1989). During the acute stage of the illness millions of virus particles are excreted in the stools, and virus continues to be shed for several days following recovery. Transmission of the infection on hands following contact with excreta, bedding or nappies can therefore occur extremely easily (Breuer & Jeffries 1990).

C. difficile causes a serious disease of the colon called **pseudomembranous colitis** (PMC). This usually occurs in patients whose normal intestinal flora has been altered by antibiotic therapy, enabling *C. difficile* to multiply and produce toxins (see p. 105). Hospital outbreaks of infection associated with the transmission on the hands of staff and the accumulation of spores in the environment have been reported (Hall 1993).

Spread of gastrointestinal infections occurs particularly easily amongst children or other groups of patients or clients who have a poor understanding of hand hygiene and where staff may have considerable contact with excreta. The routine use of blood and body fluid precautions should prevent the transmission of gastrointestinal illness in most healthcare settings (see Ch. 7). Wearing disposable gloves and aprons for contact with excreta or vomit and scrupulous handwashing after contact with affected patients are particularly important control measures (see Guidelines for practice). Staff may acquire infection from patients with gastrointestinal infection (Reid et al 1990). Gastrointestinal pathogens may be excreted for several days or weeks after the infection, but provided personal hygiene is good (e.g. handwashing after using the toilet) the risk of transmission is minimal once the symptoms have resolved; however, advice should be sought from the occupational health department before affected staff return to clinical duties.

Guidelines for practice: preventing the spread of gastrointestinal infections

- Nurse patient in a single room whilst symptomatic
- Wear gloves and apron for direct contact with faeces/vomit and discard after use
- Wash hands after any contact with the patient
- Remove spills of body fluid promptly and clean the area thoroughly
- Instruct the patient to wash hands thoroughly after using the toilet
- Place bedpans directly into bedpan washer/macerator without emptying the contents first

---

OUTBREAKS OF GASTROINTESTINAL ILLNESS

A sudden increase in diarrhoea or vomiting among patients or staff may indicate an outbreak of infection. Outbreaks may be foodborne or occur as a result of person-to-person transmission. Despite the major improvements in hospital food delivery systems that have been made since the outbreak at the Stanley Royd Hospital, more than 50 outbreaks of food poisoning occur in hospitals or residential homes in England and Wales every year (Cowden et al 1995). Viruses that cause gastroenteritis can be highly infectious and spread extremely rapidly (Mitchell et al 1989).

Control of outbreaks of gastrointestinal illness requires prompt notification of the infection control team, who will then investigate the source and advise on the management of patients to minimize the risk of further spread (Box 12.3). Specimens of faeces should be taken from all symptomatic patients as soon as possible and examined in the laboratory for both bacteria and viral pathogens. The specimens can provide crucial evidence to indicate the source of the infection. Patients whose symptoms have resolved may still

---

Box 12.3 Key steps in the control of suspected outbreaks of gastrointestinal infection

When more than one patient or member of staff is affected by unexplained diarrhoea or vomiting, the following actions should be taken.

In a hospital
- inform the doctor in charge of the patients
- inform the infection control doctor or nurse
- ensure sufficient supplies of gloves and aprons
- collect stool specimens from affected patients for viral and bacterial culture
- wash hands after contact with affected patients
- use protective clothing for handling body fluids
- change gloves and wash hands between patients
- transfer affected patients to single rooms and follow isolation precautions
- ensure affected staff attend the occupational health department

In a nursing home
- inform the general practitioner responsible for affected patients
- inform the consultant for communicable disease control (CCDC)
- ensure sufficient supplies of gloves and aprons
- collect stool specimens from affected patients for viral and bacterial culture
- wash hands after contact with affected patients
- use protective clothing for handling body fluids
- change gloves and wash hands between patients
- ensure affected staff consult their general practitioner

excrete the organism, and specimens should be sent to the laboratory to identify the causative organism.

The infection control team may involve the consultant for communicable disease control or director of public health and local environmental health officers in measures to control outbreaks of gastrointestinal illness.

Outbreaks of infection caused by small round structured virus

Small round structured viruses (SRSVs) are the most common cause of outbreaks of gastroenteritis in hospitals, especially amongst the elderly, and attack rates may be as high as 50%, affecting both patients and staff (Dedman et al 1998). Although person-to-person spread is the most common mode of transmission, outbreaks may be initiated by exposure to contaminated drinking water or shellfish (PHLS Viral Gastroenteritis Subcommittee 1993). Infection is characterized by severe, often projectile, vomiting and this is an important factor in transmission. Environmental contamination has been implicated in the spread of SRSV, which has been found to survive for 12 days on contaminated carpets (Cheeseborough et al 1997). Control measures should be instituted as soon as an outbreak of SRSV is suspected, without waiting for virological confirmation. Gloves and aprons should be worn for contact with affected patients and their body fluids, and rigorous handwashing should be applied. Control measures should be focused on preventing the infection from spreading to other clinical areas. Non-essential staff should be excluded from the affected area, and staff and patients should be prevented from moving to other clinical areas where possible. Comprehensive cleaning of affected areas should be carried out 72 h after resolution of the last case (Chadwick et al 2000).

REFERENCES

Anderton A (1985) Growth of bacteria in enteral feeding solutions. *J. Med. Microbiol.*, **20**: 63–8.

Anderton A (1993) Bacterial contamination of enteral feeds and feeding systems. *Clin. Nutr.*, **12** (Suppl. 1): 16–32.

Anderton A (1994) What is the HACCP (hazard critical control point) approach and how can it be applied to enteral tube feeding? *J. Hum. Nutr. Diet.*, **7**: 53–60.

Anderton A, Aidoo KE (1991) The effect of handling procedures on microbial contamination of enteral feeds – a comparison of the use of sterile vs non-sterile gloves. *J. Hosp. Infect.*, **17**(4): 297–301.

Anderton A, Nwoguh CE (1991) Re-use of enteral feeding tubes – a potential hazard to the patient? A study of the efficacy of a representative range of cleaning and disinfection procedures. *J. Hosp. Infect.*, **18**: 131–8.

Anderton A, Nwoguh CE, McCune I et al (1993) A comparative study of the numbers of bacteria present in enteral feed prepared and administered in hospital and the home. *J. Hosp. Infect.*, **23**: 43–9.

Atabay HI, Corry JEL (1997) The prevalence of campylobacters and arcobacters in broiler chickens. *J. Appl. Microbiol.*, **83**: 619–26.

Balmer SE, Nicoll A, Weaver GA et al (1997) *Guidelines for the Collection, Storage and Handling of Mother's Breast Milk to be Fed to Her Own Baby on a Neonatal Unit.* Queen Charlotte and Chelsea Hospitals, London.

Barrie D (1996) The provision of food and catering services in hospital. *J. Hosp. Infect.*, **33**: 13–33.

Beattie TC, Anderton A (1999) Microbiological evaluation of four enteral feeding systems which have been deliberately subjected to faulty handling procedures. *J. Hosp. Infect.*, **42**(1): 11–20.

Benenson AS (1995) *Control of Communicable Diseases in Man*, 16th edn. American Public Health Association, Washington.

Breuer J, Jeffries DJ (1990) Control of viral infections in hospital. *J. Hosp. Infect.*, **16**: 191–221.

Burnett IA, Wardley BL, Magee GS (1989) The milk kitchen, Sheffield children's hospital, before and after a review. *J. Hosp. Infect.*, **13**: 179–86.

Centers for Disease Control (1993) Multistate outbreak of *Escherichia coli* O157 infections from hamburgers – Western United States 1992–1993. *MMWR*, **42**: 258–63.

Chadwick PR, Beards G, Brown D et al (2000) Management of hospital outbreaks of gastro-enteritis due to small round structured viruses. *J. Hosp. Infect.*, **45**: 1–10.

Cheeseborough JS, Barkess-Jones L, Brown DW (1997) Possible prolonged environmental survival of small round structured viruses. *J. Hosp. Infect.*, **35**: 325–6.

Coia JE (1998) Nosocomial and laboratory acquired infections with *Escherichia coli* O157. *J. Hosp. Infect.*, **40**(2): 107–14.

Cooke EM (1990) Epidemiology of foodborne illness: UK. *Lancet*, **336**: 790–3.

Cowden JM, Wall PG, Adak G et al (1995) Outbreaks of foodborne infectious intestinal disease in England and Wales: 1992–1993. *CDR Rev.*, **5**(8): R109–24.

Crocker KS, Krey SH, Markovic M et al (1986) Microbial growth in clinically used enteral delivery systems. *Am. J. Infect. Control*, **14**: 250–6.

De Louvois J (1993) Salmonella contamination of eggs. *Lancet*, **342**: 366–7.

Dedman D, Laurichesse H, Caul EO et al (1998) Surveillance of small round structured virus (SRSV) infection in England and Wales, 1990–5. *Epidemiol. Infect.*, **121**: 131–49.

Ejidokun OO, Killalea D, Cooper M et al (2000) Four linked outbreaks of *Salmonella enteritidis* phage type 4 infection – the continuing egg threat. *Commun. Dis. Public Health*, **3**(2): 95–100.

Eley AR (ed.) (1992) *Microbial Food Poisoning*. Chapman & Hall, London.

Goldthorpe G, Kerry P, Drabu YJ (1991) Refrigerated food storage in hospital ward areas. *J. Hosp. Infect.*, **18**: 63–6.

Graham JC, Morgan S, Ford M et al (1999) Sepsis and ECMO: beware the breast milk. *J. Hosp. Infect.*, **43**: 75–6.

Green J, Wright PA, Gallimore CI et al (1998) The role of environmental contamination with small round structured virus in a hospital outbreak investigated by reverse transcriptase polymerase chain reaction assay. *J. Hosp. Infect.*, **39**(1): 39–45.

Hall S (1993) *Clostridium difficile* – epidemiological aspects. *PHLS Microbiol. Digest.*, **10**(2): 87–90.

Hobbs BC, Roberts D (1993) *Food Poisoning and Food Hygiene*, 6th edn. Arnold, London.

Houang E, Bodnarak P, Ahmet Z (1991) Hospital green salads and the effects of washing them. *J. Hosp. Infect.*, **17**: 125–31.

Humphrey TJ, Whitehead A, Gawler AHL et al (1991) Numbers of *Salmonella enteritidis* in the contents of naturally contaminated hens' eggs. *Epidemiol. Infect.*, **106**: 489–96.

Hunter PR (1991) Application of Hazard Analysis Critical Control Point (HACCP) to the handling of expressed breast milk on a neonatal unit. *J. Hosp. Infect.*, **17**: 139–46.

Jones D (1990) Foodborne listeriosis. *Lancet*, **336**: 1171–4.

Joseph CA, Palmer SR (1989) Outbreaks of salmonella infection in hospitals in England and Wales 1978–87. *BMJ*, **298**: 1161–4.

Knutson KM, Marth EH, Wagner MK (1987) Microwave heating of food. *Food Sci. Technol.*, **20**: 101–10.

Lewis DA, Paramathasan R, White DE et al (1995) Marshmallows cause an outbreak of infection with *Salmonella enteritidis* phage type 4. *CDR Rev.*, **6**(13): R183–5.

Lewis DC, Lightfoot NF, Cubitt WD et al (1989) Outbreaks of astrovirus type 1 and rotavirus gastroenteritis in geriatric inpatient populations. *J. Hosp. Infect.*, **14**: 9–14.

Lund BM, Knox MR, Cole MB (1989) Destruction of *Listeria monocytogenes* during microwave cooking. *Lancet*, **i**: 218.

Luthi TM, Wall PG, Evans HS et al (1996) Outbreaks of foodborne viral gastroenteritis in England and Wales 1992 to 1994. *CDR Rev.*, **6**(10): R131–5.

Mackey BM (1989) The incidence of food poisoning bacteria in red meat and poultry in the United Kingdom. *Food Sci. Technol. Today*, **3**: 246–9.

Medical Devices Directorate (1993) *Ice Cubes: Infection Caused by* Xanthomonas maltophilia. HN(93)42. Department of Health, Wetherby, UK.

Mitchell E, O'Mahoney M, McKeith I et al (1989) An outbreak of viral gastroenteritis in a psychiatric hospital. *J. Hosp. Infect.*, **14**(1): 1–8.

NHS Executive (1996a) *Hospital Catering: Delivering a Quality Service.* DoH, Wetherby, UK.

NHS Executive (1996b) *Management of Food Hygiene and Food Services in the National Health Service.* HSG(96)20. DoH, Wetherby, UK.

NHS Executive (1999) *Control Assurance Standard: Catering and Food Hygiene.* DoH, Wetherby, UK.

Owen Caul E (1994) Small round structured viruses: airborne transmission and hospital control. *Lancet*, **343**: 1240–2.

Patterson W, Haswell P, Fryers PT et al (1997) Outbreak of small round structured virus gastro-enteritis arose after kitchen assistant vomited. *CDR Rev.*, **7**(7): R101–3.

Peters R, Westerby D (1994) Percutaneous endoscopic gastrostomy. Indications, timing and complications of the technique. *Brit. J. Int. Care*, **4**: 88–94.

Public Health Laboratory Service Viral Gastroenteritis Subcommittee (1993) Outbreaks of gastro-enteritis associated with SRSVs. *PHLS Microbiol. Digest*, **10**(1): 2–8.

Reid JA, Breckon D, Hunter PR (1990) Infection of staff during an outbreak of viral gastroenteritis in an elderly persons' home. *J. Hosp. Infect.*, **16**: 81–6.

Roberts D (1982) Factors contributing to outbreaks of food poisoning in England and Wales 1970–79. *J. Hyg.*, **89**: 491–8.

Rowan NJ, Anderson JG (1998) Growth and enterotoxin production by diarrhoeagenic *Bacillus cereus* in dietary supplements prepared for hospitalised HIV patients. *J. Hosp. Infect.*, **38**: 139–46.

Sharp JMC (1992) Epidemiology. In *Microbial Food Poisoning*, pp. 125–42 (AR Eley, ed.). Chapman & Hall, London.

Skirrow MB (1990) Campylobacter. *Lancet*, **336**: 921–3.

Thurn J, Crossley K, Gerdts A et al (1990) Enteral hyperalimentation as a source of nosocomial infection. *J. Hosp. Infect.*, **15**: 203–18.

Ward V, Wilson J, Taylor L et al (1997) *Preventing Hospital-acquired Infection. Clinical Guidelines.* Public Health Laboratory Service, London.

FURTHER READING

Crawford LM (1998) Bovine spongiform encephalopathy. *Am. J. Infect. Control*, **26**: 5–7.

Department of Health (1990) *Management of Food Services and Food Hygiene in the National Health Service.* National Health Service Management Executive. HMSO, London.

Department of Health (1994) *Management of Outbreaks of Food Borne Illness.* The Stationery Office, London.

Department of Health, Public Health Medicine Environmental Group (1996) *Guidelines on the Control of Infection in Residential and Nursing Homes.* DoH, Wetherby, UK.

DHSS (1986b) *The Report of the Committee of Inquiry into an Outbreak of Food Poisoning at Stanley Royd Hospital.* HMSO, London.

Hobbs BC, Roberts D (1993) *Food Poisoning and Food Hygiene*, 6th edn. Edward Arnold, London.

Lund BM (1990) Foodborne disease due to *Bacillus* and *Clostridium* species. *Lancet*, **336**: 982–6.

Pien ECT, Hume KE, Pien FD (1996) Gastrostomy tube infection in a community hospital. *Am. J. Infect. Control*, **24**: 353–8.

Public Health Laboratory Service (1995) Interim guidelines for the control of infections with verocytotoxin producing *Escherichia coli* (VTEC). *CDR Rev.*, **5**(6): R77–80.

Public Health Laboratory Service Salmonella Committee (1995) The prevention of human transmission of gastrointestinal infections, infestations and bacterial intoxications. *CDR Rev.*, **5**(11): R158–72.

Schlech WF (1991) Listeriosis: epidemiology, virulence, and significance of contaminated foodstuffs. *J. Hosp. Infect.*, **19**: 211–24.

Tranter HS (1990) Foodborne staphylococcal illness. *Lancet*, **336**: 1044–6.

13

Cleaning, disinfection and sterilization

INTRODUCTION

The transmission of infection in association with equipment has been recognized as a problem since micro-organisms were first perceived as the cause of infection. Inadequate decontamination has frequently been responsible for outbreaks of infection in hospital (Cefai et al 1990, Kolmos et al 1993). The emergence of human immunodeficiency virus has focused attention on the potential of medical equipment to transmit infection. Safe decontamination of equipment between patients is an essential part of routine infection control (see Ch. 7). The method of decontamination selected should consider the risk of the item acting as a source or vehicle of infection and the processes that it will tolerate.

The environment is commonly perceived as a more important source of infection than evidence suggests. Microbes cannot multiply in dry environments and most die fairly rapidly on surfaces or in the air. The few that remain are unlikely to be present in sufficient numbers to initiate infection even if they could reach a susceptible site on the patient. The environment does provide a more important microbiological hazard where moisture is present, for example in food, solutions or equipment containing water. Here, bacteria may multiply rapidly to create a source of infection, provided that a suitable vehicle transfers them to a susceptible site on the patient.

LEVELS OF DECONTAMINATION

There are three levels of decontamination which are defined in Table 13.1. Cleaning involves the use of detergent to remove visible contamination from equipment but also removes a large proportion of the micro-organisms. Cleaning alone is an adequate method of decontamination of a wide range of equipment. Cleaning, by removing organic material and reducing the number of micro-organisms present, is an essential preparation for most equipment undergoing

225

Table 13.1   Levels of decontamination

Method	Process
Sterilization	Removes or destroys all micro-organisms, including spores
Disinfection	Reduces the number of micro-organisms to a level at which they are not harmful. Spores are not usually destroyed
Cleaning	Physical removal of contamination (blood, faeces, etc.) and many micro-organisms with detergent

sterilization or disinfection. Disinfection and steriliz-ation can be achieved by physical methods such as heat, or by chemicals. Chemical disinfectants exhibit a wide variation in their effect on different micro-organisms and are susceptible to inactivation by organic material and instability. Decontamination by heat is the preferred method as it is more efficient and easier to regulate.

When equipment is exposed to heat or chemical agents there is a delay in effect on micro-organisms whilst the agent penetrates the cells. The penetration time is extended if organic material is present. Micro-organisms are then steadily destroyed, rapidly by some methods, more slowly by others. If the process destroys all micro-organisms including spores, it is described as *sterilization*. Physical processes, such as steam sterilization, are the most effective method of sterilization, although a few chemicals, used in a specific way, can be used to sterilize. Other processes will not destroy all micro-organisms, particularly bac-terial spores and are described as *disinfection*. The terms sterilization and disinfection are often used incorrectly. For example, it is not correct to refer to the immersion of baby bottles in hypochlorite solution as sterilization. In fact, this is a disinfection procedure which destroys some, but not all, micro-organisms present.

Selecting the level of decontamination

The decision to clean, disinfect or sterilize depends on the risk of the equipment transmitting infection or acting as a source of infection (Table 13.2).

This risk depends on how the item is used. If the skin is penetrated, normally sterile body areas are entered or there is contact with broken mucous membranes, then the risk of introducing infection is high and the items used must be sterile. Items that have contact with less susceptible sites, such as mucous membranes, or that may be contaminated by micro-organisms that are easily transmitted to others are in a medium-risk cate-gory. Disinfection is usually adequate for these items, although sterilization is preferable as it reliably removes contamination. Equipment used on intact skin presents a low risk, is unlikely to transmit infection and may be decontaminated by cleaning.

The level of decontamination selected for routine use must be adequate to destroy any pathogens likely to be present. It should not be necessary to use a higher level of decontamination for a patient known to have an infection, although special procedures are indicated for some instruments used on patients with *Mycobacterium tuberculosis* or Creutzfeldt–Jakob disease (see p. 236).

As a general rule, methods of sterilization or disin-fection employing heat, such as autoclaves and bedpan washers, are more reliable than chemicals and should be used wherever feasible. Quality control is more easily achieved in a central sterile supply depart-

Table 13.2   Categories of decontamination

Category	Indication	Examples	Level of contamination	Methods
High risk	Items that penetrate skin or mucous membranes, or that enter sterile body areas	Surgical instruments, needles, syringes	Sterilize	Autoclave and use sterile Sterile single-use disposable
Medium risk	Items that have contact with mucous membranes or are contaminated by microbes that are easily transmitted	Vaginal speculum, endoscopes, bedpans, crockery	Disinfect or sterilize	Autoclave (not in packs) Chemically disinfect Pasteurize
Low risk	Items used on intact skin	Washbowls, mattresses	Clean	Wash with detergent and hot water and dry

ment (CSSD) and, if possible, equipment should be decontaminated there.

Decontamination policy

Confusion often surrounds the decontamination of equipment used in healthcare. To prevent unsafe or unnecessary decontamination, hospitals should have a decontamination policy. This will provide guidance on the method of decontamination for instruments, equipment and the environment. The policy will be developed by those with expertise in decontamination, including the infection control nurse, consultant microbiologist, pharmacist and sterile supplies department manager. An example of advice contained in a decontamination policy is described in Appendix 1.

Medical equipment is also used in primary care and a range of invasive procedures are now commonly performed in general practice surgeries by practice nurses, general practitioners and other healthcare professionals. These staff also need guidelines on safe decontamination procedures (Finn & Crook 1998, Morgan et al 1990). Useful advice for the primary healthcare team can be found in the British Medical Association's publication *Code of Practice for Sterilisation of Instruments and Control of Cross-infection* (BMA 1984), and can also be obtained from the local infection control team.

Decontamination of equipment before service or repair

Equipment that has been in contact with patients or their body fluids may transmit infection to those required to service or repair it. Such equipment must be thoroughly cleaned and decontaminated before it is inspected and a certificate documenting the method of decontamination should accompany the item (NHS Management Executive 1993). This also applies to equipment that is returned to the manufacturer. An example of a decontamination certificate is shown in Fig. 13.1.

Re-use of single-use equipment

The re-use of equipment intended for single-use is sometimes practised within hospitals in the name of economy. Although it may seem wasteful to discard expensive items, their decontamination and re-use raises a number of issues and requires careful consideration.

First, the decontamination process may cost more in staff time and materials than the item itself. Second,

the decontamination procedure may damage the item and cause it to malfunction on subsequent uses. For example, plastics may lose flexibility or crack. Third, the manufacturer's warranty for the product is likely to be voided by reprocessing and the person who reprocesses it may take on liability should it cause injury to a patient. If it is planned to re-use single-use, disposable items, the method used must be demonstrated to be safe and effective. The exact procedure and number of times an item can be reprocessed must be documented (Medical Devices Agency 1995). A group of people with the relevant expertise, for example the infection control nurse, infection control doctor, purchasing officer, sterile supplies manager and risk manager, should assess whether re-use is both possible and economically viable and determine the quality control checks that would be required to ensure efficacy (Working Party of the Central Sterilising Club 1999).

METHODS OF DECONTAMINATION
Cleaning

Cleaning is important for two reasons: in its own right as a method of decontaminating low-risk items, and as preparation for disinfection or sterilization. Many pieces of equipment classed as low risk can be decontaminated safely between patients by cleaning for example washing bowls, cots, beds and commodes.

Cleaning involves the use of detergent and water to remove organic material and with it micro-organisms. Detergent is essential for effective cleaning. It breaks up grease and dirt and improves the ability of water to remove soil. Approximately 80% of micro-organisms are removed during the cleaning procedure (Ayliffe et al 1967). However, drying the equipment after it has been cleaned is also extremely important to prevent any bacteria that remain from multiplying. The importance of thoroughly drying equipment before storage was demonstrated by Greaves (1985): 34% of washing bowls were not dried completely before storage and more than 50% of these damp bowls were found to be contaminated with large numbers of **Gram-negative bacilli**. These bacteria could be transmitted readily to another patient when the bowl was next used.

Cloths used for cleaning also become heavily contaminated with bacteria, which are readily transferred to hands and equipment (Scott & Bloomfield 1990) and they should be discarded after each use.

Gram-negative bacilli can survive in solutions of detergent and items should not be left to soak for

DECONTAMINATION CERTIFICATE

For issue prior to inspection, service or repair of any medical or laboratory equipment.

TO (Works dept/Manufacturer): ....

Description of equipment ....

Serial No .... Unit .... Date ....

Tick box A if applicable, otherwise complete sections B and C.

A. ☐ **This equipment has not been in contact with blood, body fluid, respired gases or pathological specimens.**

B. **Has this equipment been exposed to hazardous material?**

Blood, body fluids, respired gases
pathological specimens   Yes/No

Chemicals or substances hazardous
to health   Yes/No

Other hazards   Yes/No

Provide details of contamination: ....

C. **Has this equipment been cleaned and decontaminated?**

Yes/No   Method..

If No, state why ....

Note: equipment which has not been decontaminated must not be returned/presented without prior agreement of recipient.

I declare that I have taken all reasonable steps to ensure the accuracy of the above information.

Signature .... Name .... Position ....

Fig. 13.1 Example of a decontamination certificate.

prolonged periods in bowls of detergent (Werry et al 1988).

Blood and body fluids must be completely removed from instruments before they are subjected to a disinfection or sterilization process. Thorough cleaning with detergent and water removes a significant proportion of the micro-organisms and increases the efficiency of disinfection. Organic material such as blood is coagulated by heat or chemicals and consequently difficult to remove after sterilization. Hollow tubing is particularly difficult to clean effectively and requires the use of special brushes or high-powered water jets. Most tubing is single-use and disinfection of this type of item should not be attempted because of the difficulty of ensuring complete decontamination and the risk of subsequent cross-infection (Anderton & Nwoguh 1991).

Automated washing machines provide a highly efficient means of cleaning. They enable contaminated instruments to be decontaminated safely without direct handling by staff. Ultrasonic cleaning machines are also useful for removing body fluids from delicate instruments.

Decontamination by heat

Heat is the best method of decontamination for medical equipment. Its effects are predictable and it is easily controlled. The process is most efficient in the presence of water because the heat will be conducted evenly to all parts of an object.

The number of micro-organisms destroyed depends on the temperature and the period of exposure: the higher the temperature the shorter the period of exposure. Additional time should be allowed for all parts of the item to reach the selected temperature.

There are a number of decontamination methods based on the use of heat; those used most commonly are described below.

Pasteurization

In this process items are heated to temperatures between 65 and 80°C at which many micro-organisms are destroyed provided they are exposed for a sufficient length of time. The higher the temperature, the shorter the exposure period required. Pasteurization is used to disinfect a variety of medium-risk equipment, but cannot be used to sterilize.

Examples of pasteurization used in a clinical setting are: bedpan washers which disinfect at a temperature of 80°C for at least 1 min; the disinfection of linen at 71°C for not less than 3 min during the wash cycle (NHS Executive 1995); and automatic dishwashers.

Washer–disinfectors may be used in operating theatres or sterile supply departments to wash instruments in hot water before sterilization. They enable blood and body fluid to be removed without the need to handle the instruments and will destroy many pathogens.

Boiling

Although not commonly used in hospitals, boiling can be used to disinfect medium-risk equipment. Most bacteria and viruses are destroyed by boiling for a few minutes; however, sterilization by this method is not possible as some bacterial spores will not be destroyed.

Boiling is relatively easily controlled visually. Instruments should be completely immersed in boiling water, and the 5-min disinfection period timed from when the water returns to boiling point. Additional instruments should not be added during this time.

Water boilers are still used in some general practice surgeries for the decontamination of vaginal specula, ear syringes, etc. They must not be used to decontaminate surgical instruments or other equipment used for high-risk procedures. A small autoclave is usually a more practical option and these are widely used in clinics and surgeries (Medical Devices Agency 1997b).

Steam under pressure (autoclave)

This is the most reliable method of sterilizing equipment and used widely in healthcare settings. At atmospheric pressure water boils at 100°C and, while this temperature is sufficient to destroy vegetative bacteria, much higher temperatures are required for the destruction of spores.

If water is heated inside a closed container at increased pressure, it boils at a higher temperature. For example, at a pressure of 1.03 bar (15 lb per inch^2) it boils at 121°C, at 2.2 bar (32 lb per inch^2) it boils at 134°C. The steam produced at these higher temperatures will destroy any micro-organisms present on items inside the container, by condensing on to their surface and releasing energy in the form of heat. The higher the temperature of the steam, the more rapidly spores will be destroyed. At 121°C this takes 15 min, at 134°C 3 min. As a mixture of air and steam inside the chamber reduces the temperature inside and prevents steam from penetrating completely, the efficiency of sterilization is improved if air is removed.

There are two main types of autoclave: porous-load and bench-top.

Porous-load autoclaves These are large industrial machines that use pumps to remove the air from the chamber before steam is introduced. The vacuum created inside the chamber allows steam to penetrate all parts of the load, including porous materials such as paper or linen, enabling prewrapped instruments to be sterilized. The drying cycle, which completes the process, ensures that packs removed from the autoclave are dry. Packed instruments will remain sterile indefinitely provided the wrapping remains intact and does not become wet. Porous-load autoclaves are used in central sterile supply departments (CSSDs) to process surgical instruments and other equipment supplied in packs.

Bench-top autoclaves These simpler autoclaves (Fig. 13.2) do not usually have a prevacuum stage in

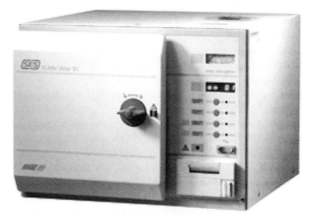

Fig. 13.2 A bench-top autoclave.

the process. They can therefore not be used to sterilize equipment that requires penetration of steam, such as wrapped instruments, porous materials (e.g. dressings) or hollow items. The chamber should not be overloaded so that steam is able to condense easily on all surfaces. Wrapped instruments must not be sterilized in these autoclaves, but they can be protected from recontamination by covering with sterile paper or storing in a sterile container after sterilization.

There are a number of small, relatively inexpensive, autoclaves that are appropriate for processing unwrapped instruments for use in clinics or general practice surgeries. Guidance on their suitability can be found in documents produced by the Medical Devices Agency (1997b) and British Standards Institution (1990).

Staff responsible for processing instruments in autoclaves must be properly trained in their use and in the preparation and loading of instruments (see Guidelines for practice).

Autoclaves are the most common method of sterilization for high- and medium-risk equipment. Instruments used for medium-risk procedures require pathogens from one patient to be removed before use on another and can be used again in a clean, but not necessarily sterile, condition. They should be stored in a clean, covered container after autoclaving (e.g. vaginal specula). Instruments used in high-risk procedures *must* be sterile at the point of use. To prevent contamination of these instruments on removal from the autoclave, they must either be autoclaved inside a sealed packet or autoclaved immediately before use.

Autoclave maintenance An autoclave that is not functioning correctly may not sterilize instruments. Autoclave tape that changes colour on exposure to specific temperatures indicates that an item has been through an autoclave but is not a guarantee of sterility. Internal controls should indicate when the process has failed and these should be closely monitored. For porous-load autoclaves, the temperature and pressures achieved in the chamber must be recorded and checked for each cycle (NHS Estates 1994).

All autoclaves require regular, skilled maintenance to ensure their safety and reliability. There should be a planned and documented testing and maintenance programme carried out by specialist technicians (British Standards Institution 1994, Medical Devices Agency 1998). Advice on installing, testing and maintaining autoclaves should be obtained from a qualified, authorized person, registered with the Institute of Healthcare Engineers and Estates Management.

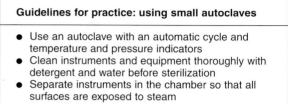

Guidelines for practice: using small autoclaves
• Use an autoclave with an automatic cycle and temperature and pressure indicators
• Clean instruments and equipment thoroughly with detergent and water before sterilization
• Separate instruments in the chamber so that all surfaces are exposed to steam
• Wash cleaning brushes after use and store dry
• Ensure the autoclave is tested and serviced regularly

Hot air ovens

Hot air can also be used to sterilize, but higher temperatures and longer exposure times are necessary because air does not conduct heat as efficiently as steam. Sterilization can be achieved by holding at a temperature of 170°C for 1 h; however, instruments must reach the required temperature before commencing timing and must be allowed to cool before removal. This limits their use to instruments that can withstand high temperatures and to situations where a rapid turnround of equipment is not essential (UK Health Departments 1994).

Instruments must be cleaned thoroughly before sterilization because organic matter will be baked on to the surface and become very difficult to remove.

Ethylene oxide

Equipment easily damaged by heat cannot be sterilized in an autoclave or hot air oven and, for these items, a lower temperature can be used in combination with ethylene oxide gas.

Ethylene oxide is not corrosive, but it is irritant and toxic. It is absorbed into many materials and will then gradually leach out, causing harm to patient and staff in contact with the equipment. Items must therefore be completely aired after the process to remove all traces of the chemical. This can take up to 7 days.

Ethylene oxide is flammable and can be explosive when mixed with air in certain concentrations. It is harmful at far lower concentrations than can be detected by smell, and the gas must be safely vented from the area. Ethylene oxide sterilization requires the use of specialist facilities and the process must be closely controlled by trained operators. Ethylene oxide facilities are not available in most hospitals, but it is used by industry for the sterilization of medical devices and drugs. Gas plasma sterilisation using

---

Guidelines for practice: important principles of chemical disinfection

- Check the disinfection policy to ensure disinfection is necessary and which agent to use
- Check the appropriate COSHH assessment
- Wear protective clothing if indicated
- Clean equipment thoroughly with detergent to remove blood and body fluid
- Make up the correct dilution of the chemical
- Completely immerse equipment for the correct time
- Discard disinfectant after use, clean container and store dry

---

hydrogen peroxide vapour is an alternative to ethylene oxide.

Irradiation

This method is not used in hospitals but is widely employed commercially for the sterilization of plastic disposable items such as syringes and cannulas. The process may alter plastic materials and resterilization of disposable equipment should not be attempted. Ultraviolet light radiation can be used to kill microorganisms, but not spores.

Decontamination by chemicals

A variety of chemicals is used for the decontamination of skin, equipment and the environment. Most can be used only to disinfect, not to sterilize, equipment, as they are mostly not active against spores and have limited antimycobacterial activity. Some viruses with lipid membranes are easily destroyed, whereas those without are more resistant.

Box 13.1   Disadvantages of chemical disinfectants

- Most are not active against all micro-organisms
- Mycobacteria and spores are not easily destroyed
- Variable ability to destroy viruses
- Poor penetration of blood, pus and other organic material
- May be inactivated by organic material, detergent, rubber or plastics
- May be unstable, particularly if diluted, and may support the growth of some micro-organisms
- Often corrosive, toxic or irritant
- Variable exposure time required to achieve disinfection

Chemical disinfection has considerable disadvantages (Box 13.1). Many disinfectants are corrosive and highly irritant, and disposable gloves and aprons should be worn to handle them. After disinfection, equipment usually needs to be rinsed in water to remove traces of the irritant chemical. Disinfectants must be used at the correct dilution: too high a concentration may be corrosive, toxic and irritant, too low a concentration may be ineffective. Diluted disinfectants are often unstable and lose activity, enabling some bacteria, particularly pseudomonas, to grow in the solution.

Effective disinfection cannot be achieved unless the solution is in contact with a surface for a reasonable period of time. Some solutions have a very rapid antimicrobial action, for example alcohols and hypochlorite disinfectants, and on clean surfaces kill microbes within a few minutes. Other disinfectants may take longer, for example immersion in glutaraldehyde for several hours is required to destroy bacterial spores. The important principles for using chemical disinfectants are summarized in the Guidelines for practice. It is important to check with the hospital disinfection policy or infection control team to ensure the correct method of decontamination is selected.

Decontamination by heat is a considerably more reliable process and should be used in preference to chemicals wherever possible. This may mean the purchase of additional instruments to enable processing by CSSD or using single-use equipment.

COSHH regulations and the use of chemical disinfectants

The Control of Substances Hazardous to Health (COSHH) Regulations 1999 require employers to assess the risks presented by the use of hazardous substances in the workplace, and to determine the control measures required to ensure that they are handled safely (Health & Safety Executive 1999a). The COSHH Regulations first came into force in 1989. They incorporate Codes of Practice on general substances hazardous to health, carcinogenic substances and biological agents (see p. 134). Chemical disinfectants may be inflammable, toxic if inhaled or ingested, and irritant to eyes or skin. Even detergent can damage the skin but may be used safely if the proper precautions are followed. Where possible a hazardous chemical should be replaced by a less dangerous chemical or a different process. If this is not possible, equipment should be provided to protect against exposure (e.g. a covered container), and a safe system of work established for handling the chemical. Box 13.2 lists the factors that should be considered when assessing the risk of a chemical disinfectant.

> **Box 13.2** Control of Substances Hazardous to Health: factors to be considered for risk assessment of chemical disinfectants
>
> - Establish how the chemical is used (e.g. how often, what for, in what amounts)
> - Determine potential harmful effects of the chemical
> - Decide how to prevent or control exposure to the chemical
>   - use an alternative
>   - restrict use
>   - use an automated process
>   - use covered containers and/or install ventilation
>   - define a safe system of working with the chemical, including management of spillages
>   - use protective clothing if exposure cannot be prevented by other means
> - Inform and train users
> - Health surveillance (if appropriate)

Information about each chemical used in a department should be provided in the form of a risk assessment and a copy kept in a readily accessible place. This should specify how the chemical should be stored and handled, protective clothing required and how to manage spillages.

The pharmacy or supplies department can often help to draw up risk assessments. The risk of injury from disinfectants can be minimized provided the staff who use the chemicals are properly trained and follow the guidelines for use of the chemical described in the assessment.

Occupational exposure standards

The Health and Safety Executive also publishes occupational exposure limits to certain substances that may have serious effects on health if inhaled (Health & Safety Executive 1999b). The Occupational Exposure Standards (OESs) are levels of exposure that scientific information suggests will not damage the health of workers regularly exposed to the substance. Maximum Exposure Limits (MELs) are applied to more hazardous substances, for which a safe level of exposure does not exist or cannot be practically achieved. This places a duty on the employer to reduce exposure to the substance below the MEL, and to minimize the number of people exposed and the duration of exposure.

The Health and Safety Executive recommends an OES for a number of disinfectants, including chlorine gas, phenol, iodine and alcohol as these chemicals may irritate the eyes, skin or mucous membranes and should not be used in large quantities in poorly ventilated areas. Glutaraldehyde may cause more serious health effects including asthma, and has been assigned a MEL.

Properties of common chemical disinfectants

Alcohol

Examples: 70% industrial methylated spirit (IMS), 70% isopropyl alcohol solution, alcohol handrub, alcohol impregnated wipes.

Alcohol rapidly destroys both bacteria and **fungi**, although it has no effect on bacterial spores. Isopropyl alcohol has poor activity against some **viruses**; IMS at a concentration of 90% is effective against most viruses. Alcohol does not penetrate protein-based organic matter and should be used only on clean surfaces. It damages some materials (e.g. lens cement in fibreoptic scopes) and is inflammable. It is not a suitable disinfectant for most equipment but its rapid action and volatility make it useful for skin disinfection and it is often used for this in combination with other chemicals such as chlorhexidine. Mixed with emollients it is a highly effective hand disinfectant (Rotter et al 1980). Handrub solutions are not suitable for disinfecting equipment (Van den Berg et al 2000).

Alcohol-impregnated wipes are widely used to disinfect surfaces but because of the short contact time are unlikely to have much effect and their use is probably unnecessary (Thompson & Bullock 1992).

Chlorhexidine

Examples: handwash solution (Hibiscrub), chlorhexidine in 70% alcohol (Hibisol), aqueous chlorhexidine (Savlon, Savlodil, Hibidil).

Gram-positive bacteria are more susceptible to chlorhexidine than **Gram-negative** organisms, but this chemical has no effect on tubercle bacilli or spores, and little effect on viruses. Chlorhexidine is recommended mainly as a skin disinfectant, combined either with a detergent in a handwash solution or with alcohol as a preoperative skin disinfectant or handrub. It has the advantage of being highly effective against the resident microbial flora of the skin, with an action persisting for several hours after the initial application. Although not an irritant to intact skin, some studies have suggested that chlorhexidine is toxic to fibroblasts and may interfere with the healing of wounds (Neidner & Schöpf 1986).

Its limited spectrum of activity, inactivation by organic matter and expense make chlorhexidine an unsuitable disinfectant for most equipment. It is sometimes used for the disinfection of low-risk equipment (e.g. thermometer, aural speculum) in combination with alcohol, although the alcohol is the primary disinfectant. Solutions used to immerse equipment may become contaminated by bacteria after time and should be discarded immediately after use (Oie & Kamiya 1996). Savlon, an aqueous chlorhexidine preparation, is often used for cleaning equipment before decontamination. However, general purpose detergent is just as effective and considerably cheaper. The main use of chlorhexidine is in surgical scrubs, but these are not recommended for routine handwashing in most ward areas, where soap is a cheaper and more suitable solution (see p. 135).

Glutaraldehyde

Examples: Cidex, Asep, Totocide.

Glutaraldehyde has a wide range of antimicrobial activity. It kills bacteria, fungi and viruses rapidly, mycobacteria in 20–60 min and bacterial spores in 3–10 h, depending on the product. Glutaraldehyde does not corrode metal and is not seriously inactivated by organic material, although it penetrates such material only slowly. Protein material will be coagulated on to the surface; therefore blood or other organic material must be removed completely before immersion.

Once activated, alkaline solutions of glutaraldehyde remain active for 14–28 days (depending on the product), although they should be replaced if organic matter builds up and if the solution becomes cloudy.

Unfortunately, glutaraldehyde is highly irritant to skin and mucosa and extensive exposure has been associated with sensitization reactions, including dermatitis, running nose and eyes, and asthma (Russell 1994). As a result, most hospitals restrict the use of glutaraldehyde to equipment that cannot be decontaminated by heat or other chemicals and where destruction of a broad spectrum of micro-organisms is essential. The best example of such equipment is fibre-optic endoscopes which would be damaged by heat but need to be disinfected before and after contact with mucous membranes or sterilized before use in surgical procedures.

Where there is no alternative disinfection method to glutaraldehyde, precautions must be used to ensure minimal exposure to the user (Health & Safety Executive 1998). Nitrile gloves (e.g. household gloves) and eye protection must always be worn to handle the solution. It must be kept in a container with a fitted lid and good ventilation provided to remove glutaraldehyde vapour from the atmosphere. After immersion, the equipment must be thoroughly rinsed with water.

Peracetic acid

Examples: Nu-cidex, Steris-System.

This peroxygen compound kills bacteria, fungi and viruses rapidly, and bacterial spores within 10 min, and has better penetration of organic matter than glutaraldehyde (Medical Devices Agency 1997a). In buffered solutions containing corrosion inhibitors peracetic acid causes minimal corrosion, although it may damage rubber and brass after prolonged immersion (Haythorne 1998). It has a strong smell and should be used in an area with exhaust ventilation, but currently there is no evidence of toxicity or adverse health effects.

Hydrogen peroxide

Examples: hydrogen peroxide, Virkon.

These solutions have a wide range of activity against bacteria, viruses and fungi. Hydrogen peroxide has a low toxicity and irritancy but may be corrosive to some metals. Concentrated solutions may irritate the skin, mucous membranes and respiratory tract (Block 1991).

Hypochlorites (and other chlorine-based disinfectants)

Examples: Milton, Chloros, Domestos, sodium dichloroisocyanurate (NaDCC) – Presept, Haz-Tabs.

Hypochlorites are inexpensive and effective disinfectants. They are active against most micro-organisms, including human immunodeficiency virus and hepatitis B, and may also destroy bacterial spores and mycobacteria. Although probably the best general purpose disinfectant, hypochlorites have a number of disadvantages which make them unsuitable for the decontamination of instruments. Particular problems are the corrosive effect on some metals and ready inactivation by organic material.

To prevent corrosion of surfaces, hypochlorite should be washed off with detergent and water, and should not be used on fabric or carpets because it will

Table 13.3 Recommended uses of different strengths of chlorine-releasing agents

Available chlorine (parts per million)	Recommended usage
0.5–1	Drinking water
4–6	Hydrotherapy pools
125	Infant feeding bottles
1000	Contaminated surfaces (e.g. laboratories)
10 000	Treatment of body fluid spills

bleach out the colour. Hypochlorites should not be mixed with large volumes of acidic substances (e.g. urine) in confined spaces because it may result in the release of harmful chlorine gas (Department of Health 1990).

Dilute solutions of hypochlorite lose their activity quite rapidly and fresh solution should be made up daily. The concentration of hypochlorite solutions is often expressed as parts per million of available chlorine (ppm av. Cl). In strong concentrations (e.g. 10 000 ppm av. Cl) the chlorine is less likely to be inactivated by the organic matter and can be used to decontaminate spills of body fluid (Table 13.3). A granular form of NaDCC is useful for decontamination of body fluid spills as the spill is absorbed and can be removed more easily (Coates & Wilson 1989) (see p. 150). Domestos and other brands of thick bleaches contain between 10 000 and 50 000 ppm av. Cl and may need to be diluted before use.

Making the correct dilution of hypochlorite solutions can be difficult but the addition of NaDCC tablets (e.g. Presept, Haz-Tabs) to water, provides the easiest method of making up solutions of the required strength.

Non-abrasive powders that contain hypochlorite are sometimes used to clean baths, although whether these powders have any advantage over detergent is debatable.

Phenolics

Examples: Hycolin, Clearsol, Stericol.

The phenolics are active against most bacteria, including mycobacteria, but have little effect on bacterial spores and a variable activity against viruses, particularly those without lipid envelopes. Although inexpensive, stable and not readily inactivated by organic material, phenolic disinfectants are no longer widely used for environmental disinfection. Their spectrum of activity is not wide enough to enable them to be used to disinfect equipment. In addition, phenolics are absorbed by rubber and plastics, and are irritants. They should therefore not be used to disinfect equipment that is used on skin or mucous membranes.

Hexachlorophane is a phenolic compound which is used on intact skin as a preoperative disinfectant and, as Ster-Zac Powder, for reducing staphylococcal colonization and preventing infection on the umbilicus in the newborn (Teece 1997).

Decontamination of the environment

The complete removal of micro-organisms from the environment is neither practical nor desirable (Collins 1988). The majority of micro-organisms present are not harmful and not readily transferred on to susceptible sites on the patient. In epidemics of infection, contamination of the environment with the epidemic strain is frequently reported; however, in most circumstances it is difficult to demonstrate that the environment is either the source of infection or responsible for transmission (see p. 36). Micro-organisms acquired on hands through direct contact with an infected patient or body fluids is a more likely route of cross-infection in most situations (Barrett et al 1993, Mylotte 1994). The termination of outbreaks of infection is sometimes associated with extensive cleaning programmes, but it is often difficult to establish whether other factors such as the removal of affected patients or staff have had a more important effect (Noone & Griffiths 1997).

None the less, some micro-organisms are particularly adept at surviving in the environment, notably those that withstand desiccation such as staphylococci, enterococci and acinetobacter, and those that form spores such as *Clostridium difficile* and *Bacillus cereus*. In some circumstances, high levels of environmental contamination with these organisms probably contribute to their spread, for example where patients with *C. difficile* or vancomycin-resistant enterococci have diarrhoea (Boyce et al 1994, Kim et al 1981). Outbreaks of infection caused by enteric viruses have also been associated with environmental contamination (Green et al 1998).

While disinfectants may help to reduce environmental contamination, their effect is short lived (Ayliffe et al 1967). Most micro-organisms are present in visible dust and dirt, so that significant reductions are therefore more likely to be achieved by vacuuming up dust and removing dirt by cleaning with detergent. Disinfectants may sometimes have a place in the treatment of high-level environmental contamination where it may be contributing to the spread of infection. Noble et al (1998) reported a case of vancomycin-resistant enterococci

---

Guidelines for practice: Promoting a clean environment

- Ensure clinical areas are tidy and surfaces cleared
- Report faults or damage requiring repair promptly (e.g. broken tiles)
- Find out about the specified cleaning programme and results of audits of the department
- Be aware of own cleaning responsibilities (e.g. commodes)
- Liaise with domestic staff when body fluid spills occur
- Discuss problems with cleaning with the domestic staff
- Report concerns to domestic services manager

transmitted as a result of extensive flooding of a blocked toilet. Decontamination of the environment in this instance required the use of disinfectants in addition to thorough cleaning.

Many authors lament the decline of standards in hospital cleaning. Whilst there is little direct evidence to demonstrate a corresponding increase in hospital-acquired infection, a good standard of cleanliness is likely to minimize the risk of transmission of a range of pathogenic bacteria and viruses (Chadwick & Oppenheim 1996). In addition, cleanliness is important for aesthetic reasons and to maintain the confidence of patients (Dancer 1999). A comprehensive cleaning service with clearly defined routine cleaning programmes, well-trained staff and regularly monitored standards is therefore essential (Infection Control Nurses Association 1999). Effective cleaning requires teamwork. Nursing staff or other managers can make an important contribution in promoting a clean environment (Thompson & Hempshall 1999). See Guidelines for practice.

Furniture, floors and walls

Surfaces in clinical areas should be kept clean and dry to prevent the accumulation and growth of micro-organisms. Most of the micro-organisms found on floors and other horizontal surfaces are from dust particles that have settled (Collins 1988). Dust particles are largely composed of skin scales, respired droplets and fibres from clothing or linen, of which a small proportion carries micro-organisms. The most important component of an effective cleaning programme is the regular removal of dust from these surfaces by using either a vacuum cleaner or a dust control mop. Removal of dust by these methods is more effective than a damp mop which tends to redistribute bacteria in dust rather than remove them.

Mopping with detergent and water is of value for surfaces that are soiled or exposed to spillages. Ayliffe et al (1967) demonstrated that, although disinfectants removed more bacteria from floors than detergent, recontamination of the floor occurred within 1 h of treatment (Fig. 13.3). Disinfectant granules (e.g. sodium dichloroisocyanurate) can be used to remove spills of body fluids and to destroy micro-organisms present, reducing the risk of infection to the person clearing up the spillage (Coates & Wilson 1989, UK Health Departments 1998). These granules should not be used on urine spills, as irritant chlorine vapour may be released (Department of Health 1990). They should also not be used on fabric or carpet, as they will damage these materials.

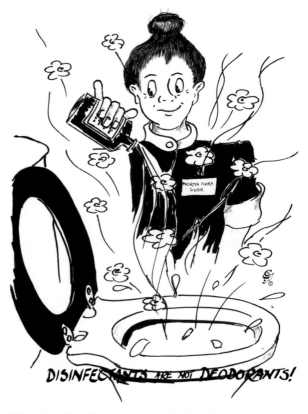

Fig. 13.3 Disinfectants are not deodorants.

There is no evidence that carpets present a greater risk of infection than hard floors. They should be vacuum cleaned daily to remove bacteria in dust, and spillage of body fluid should be removed with detergent and water, preferably using a cleaning machine. For practical reasons, it is probably not advisable to fit carpets to areas where frequent spillage is anticipated. Carpets fitted in clinical areas must be washable and the fibres should be short and water-repellent to enable spills to be dealt with more easily.

Bacteria are rarely found on vertical surfaces such as walls and these require only spot cleaning to remove splashes or stains (Ayliffe et al 1967). Some fixtures and fittings are difficult to clean and if not included in the routine cleaning programme may gather significant amounts of dust. Teare et al (1998) reported a persistent outbreak of *C. difficile* related to the accumulation of dust behind radiators in the affected clinical area.

Mops Wet, dirty mops, stored in buckets of dirty water for long periods, encourage the multiplication of micro-organisms. Such mops are more likely to deposit bacteria on floors than to remove them. The water used for mopping should be changed regularly during cleaning and discarded after use. Mop heads should be decontaminated by laundering daily and stored dry. Disinfection with chemicals should not be attempted as it is unlikely to be effective.

Baths, washbasins and toilets

Bacteria are able to survive more easily in these moist environments; however, the routine use of disinfectants is not justified because they do not present a major source of micro-organisms (Levin et al 1984). Bacteria **colonizing** washbasins and taps are usually environmental organisms and unlikely to cause disease in humans even if transferred to vulnerable sites on patients (Ayliffe et al 1974, Orsi et al 1994). Toilet seats do not usually become heavily contaminated by faecal micro-organisms and are an unlikely route of cross-infection (Newsom 1972). Regular cleaning with detergent will remove pathogens and reduce the risk of cross-infection. Disinfectants are not necessary for routine use but may sometimes be indicated in outbreaks of gastroenteritis (Chadwick et al 2000, Nyström 1981).

Baths may become contaminated with pathogenic bacteria after use by a patient with a large open wound. An outbreak of group A streptococci in episiotomy wounds was associated with two baths that were not properly cleaned between patients. An important factor in this outbreak was the damaged surface on the baths, which prevented effective cleaning (Dowsett & Wilson 1981). Harsh scouring agents should not be used to clean baths as these may damage the enamel. Thorough cleaning with detergent after each patient is sufficient.

Whirlpool baths and birthing pools, which have channels where stagnant water may collect, have been associated with the transmission of infection and require maintenance and the use of disinfectants to prevent the multiplication of pathogenic Gram-negative bacilli (Hollyoak et al 1995, Kingsley et al 1999). Thorough cleaning with detergent between patients is sufficient. Bath hoists may become easily contaminated with bacteria and should be thoroughly cleaned with detergent after each use (Murdoch 1990). Washbowls have been associated with outbreaks of infection by Gram-negative bacilli when not washed and dried properly after use (Joynson 1978).

Beds and mattresses

Bedframes accumulate dust and should be cleaned regularly. Babies' incubators should be cleaned routinely with detergent and water. If disinfection is required, a dilute solution of hypochlorite (125 ppm av. Cl) is suitable but should be rinsed off. Some incubators have an integral humidifier. These should be disinfected by raising the temperature of the water to at least 70°C for 10 min, or removed and autoclaved (Ayliffe et al 1993).

Mattresses with an intact impermeable cover do not support the growth of bacteria if clean and dry. If contaminated with body fluid, they should be cleaned with detergent and water, and the surface thoroughly dried. Some chemical disinfectants (e.g. phenol) can damage mattress covers and their use should be avoided (Loomes 1988). The mattress cover should be inspected carefully for signs of wear or loss of impermeability and should be turned over regularly to prolong its life (Department of Health 1991). Outbreaks of infection caused by *Pseudomonas aeruginosa* and acinetobacter have been associated with damaged mattresses (Fujita et al 1981, Sherertz & Sullivan 1985).

SPECIAL DECONTAMINATION PROBLEMS

Fibreoptic endoscopes

Decontamination of flexible fibreoptic endoscopes presents particular problems as the narrow channels are difficult to clean and they will not withstand the high temperatures in an autoclave. Decontamination must therefore rely on thorough cleaning followed by chemical disinfection or sterilization.

A number of cases of pathogens transmitted between patients on endoscopes have been reported. These have included salmonella, Gram-negative bacilli and *Helicobacter pylori* associated with gastroscopy; hepatitis C associated with colonoscopy; and *Mycobacterium tuberculosis* following bronchoscopy (Bronowicki et al 1997, Earnshaw et al 1985, Langenberg et al 1990, Spach et al 1993). Infections may also be acquired where micro-organisms from tap water, such as pseudomonas and mycobacteria, contaminate the rinse water in automatic washing machines.

The risk of infection, and hence the level of decontamination required, depends on the invasiveness of the procedure. Endoscopes used in normally sterile body areas are invasive and should be sterilized before use. Most of these scopes are rigid and modern designs are usually fully autoclavable. Endoscopes that have contact with mucous membranes, but not sterile body cavities, are considered non-invasive and should undergo high-level disinfection after use (Medical Devices Agency 1997a) (see Table 13.4).

Filters can be used on sigmoidoscopes to prevent contamination of the inflation bulb and tubing. Biopsy

Table 13.4 Decontamination of endoscopes: recommended processes

Procedure	Type of endoscope	Decontamination level	Recommended process
Invasive	Rigid Laparoscope Arthroscope Bronchoscope	Sterilization	Autoclave Ethylene oxide
	Flexible Angioscope Cystoscope Fetoscope	Sterilization	Chemical sterilant Glutaraldehyde (3–6 h)[a] Peracetic acid (10 min)[a]
Non-invasive	Flexible Bronchoscope Gastrointestinal endoscope	High-level disinfection	Chemical sterilant Glutaraldehyde (4–60 min)[a] Peracetic acid (5 min)[a]

[a] Times may vary according to make of chemical and type of scope. Refer to manufacturer's instructions.
Source: Medical Devices Agency (1997a). Crown copyright material is reproduced with the permission of Her Majesty's Stationery Office.

forceps should be sterilized after each patient (Communicable Disease Report 1999).

Thorough cleaning of the external and internal surfaces of the scope with detergent and water is essential to maximize the efficacy of decontamination. All channels should be brushed and flushed with detergent and water. Biopsy forceps and other accessories should be cleaned to ensure that all debris is removed. Automatic washer–disinfectors that clean, disinfect and rinse endoscopes are now widely used. These not only significantly improve the quality of disinfection but also reduce exposure of staff to the disinfectant. These machines must be cleaned and maintained regularly to prevent contamination by micro-organisms. Ultrasonic washers can be used to clean rigid endoscopes but the channels must be flushed after cleaning to remove debris. After cleaning, flexible endoscopes should be fully immersed in the appropriate disinfectant, ensuring that all channels are filled (Medical Devices Agency 1997a, NHS Estates 1995).

Immersion in glutaraldehyde for at least 4 min between each patient is recommended (British Society of Gastroenterology 1988). Longer immersion times of 20 min are recommended at the beginning and end of each list as bacteria may multiply in the damp channels while the endoscope is stored.

The main infection risk associated with flexible bronchoscopes is the transmission of respiratory pathogens, particularly mycobacteria and bloodborne viruses. Decontamination by immersion in glutaraldehyde for 20 min after each patient is recommended (British Thoracic Society 1989). Provided the bronchoscope has first been cleaned thoroughly, this immersion time should be adequate to destroy mycobacteria if the scope is used on patients suspected of having tuberculosis (Ayliffe et al 1993). *Mycobacterium avium intracellulare* is more resistant to chemical disinfectants and an immersion time of 90–120 min is recommended after use on a patient with known or suspected infection (Collins 1986, Russell 1994).

After immersion, endoscopes must be rinsed with water to remove the disinfectant. Glutaraldehyde may irritate mucous membranes, tissues or the operator, and both glutaraldehyde and hydrogen peroxide may damage the gut mucosa if introduced on an inadequately rinsed endoscope (Ryan & Potter 1995). Automatic washing machines leave lower levels of residual glutaraldehyde than manual methods (Farina et al 1999). Sterile or filtered water should be used to rinse the channels as tap water may contain mycobacteria which can contaminate the scope and cause misleading laboratory results from specimens.

The extensive use of glutaraldehyde in endoscopy units may expose staff to serious health risks including contact dermatitis, rhinitis and asthma (Sherwood Burge 1989). Systems that use peracetic acid, which is not associated with the same adverse effects on health as glutaraldehyde, are becoming more popular (Haythorne 1998). Vapour-phase hydrogen peroxide is also being developed as an option for sterilizing endoscopes. Quaternary ammonium compounds and alcohol are sometimes used, but have a poor spectrum of activity (Medical Devices Agency 1997a). Adequate facilities, particularly protective clothing and ventilation, must therefore be available to minimize the number of people exposed and the duration of exposure (Health & Safety Executive 1998). The health of the staff should be monitored by the occupational health department.

> **Box 13.3** High-level decontamination processes required for instruments used on patients at risk of CJD
>
> - Use automated decontamination processes where possible, and do not mix with other instruments
> - Clean instruments thoroughly (at least twice) to remove body fluids
> - Decontaminate using one of the following methods:
>   - immersion in sodium hypochlorite (20 000 ppm av. Cl) for 1 h
>   - immersion in sodium hydroxide 2 mol/l for 1 h[a]
>   - porous-load steam sterilization, 134–137°C for a single 18-min cycle
>   - porous-load steam sterilization, 134–137°C for six cycles of 3 min each[a]
>
> [a] Not known to be completely effective.
>
> Source: Advisory Committee on Dangerous Pathogens (1998). Crown copyright material is reproduced with the permission of the Controller of Her Majesty's Stationery Office

Prions

These proteins, which cause Creutzfeldt–Jakob disease (CJD), bovine spongiform encephalopathy and scrapie, are particularly resistant to conventional methods of decontamination. They cannot be inactivated by most chemicals, including glutaraldehyde and formaldehyde or by autoclaving at 121°C. The main risk of transmission is related to surgery involving nervous tissue where the concentration of the prion proteins is greatest, although lymphoid tissue may also present a risk (Advisory Committee on Dangerous Pathogens 1998).

Instruments and protective clothing used for any invasive procedures on patients known or suspected to have CJD should be destroyed by incineration after use. No attempt should be made to sterilize re-usable instruments and, where possible, single-use items should be used. Instruments and protective clothing used for invasive procedures on the brain, spinal cord or eyes of patients at risk of CJD (see p. 125) should also be destroyed by incineration. For other invasive procedures on these patients, single-use items should be used if possible, but re-usable instruments may be re-used provided they are subjected to high-level decontamination (Box 13.3) (Advisory Committee on Dangerous Pathogens 1998).

Viruses

The fragile structures of most viruses, including blood-borne viruses, results in their destruction at temperatures of 70°C or higher, for example in washing machines, dishwashers and bedpan washers. They are also readily destroyed by autoclaving. Not all chemicals are virucidal, but glutaraldehyde, peracetic acid and hypochlorite are (Bloomfield et al 1990, Hanson et al 1994, Wood & Payne 1998). Alcohol is effective against some viruses, but not those without lipid envelopes (Hanson et al 1989). Phenolics and quaternary ammonium compounds (e.g. Dettol, Savlon) are also not a reliable method of destroying viruses and are not recommended for routine disinfection (Ayliffe et al 1993).

Bacterial spores

Some Gram-positive bacteria are able to enclose their cells in highly resistant casings called spores (see p. 4). Spores are resistant to a wide range of physical processes and chemical agents. They can be reliably destroyed by steam sterilization (e.g. 121°C for 15 min), but not by boiling at 100°C or pasteurization at a lower temperature. The only liquid chemical agents that will destroy spores are glutaraldehyde and peracetic acid.

REFERENCES

Advisory Committee on Dangerous Pathogens, Spongiform Encephalopathy Advisory Committee (1998) *Transmissible Spongiform Encephalopathy Agents, Safe Working and the Prevention of Infection.* The Stationery Office, London.

Anderton A, Nwoguh CE (1991) Re-use of enteral feeding tubes – a potential hazard to the patient? A study of the efficacy of a representative range of cleaning and disinfection procedures. *J. Hosp. Infect.*, **18**: 131–8.

Ayliffe GAJ, Collins BJ, Lowbury EJ (1967) Ward floors and other surfaces as reservoirs of hospital infection. *J. Hyg. (Lond.)*, **2**: 181.

Ayliffe GAJ, Babb JR, Collins BJ et al (1974) *Pseudomonas aeruginosa* in hospital sinks. *Lancet*, **ii**: 578–81.

Ayliffe GAJ, Coates D, Hoffman PN (1993) *Chemical Disinfection in Hospital*. Public Health Laboratory Service, London.

Barrett SP, Teare EL, Sage R (1993) Methicillin-resistant *Staphylococcus aureus* in three adjacent health districts of South East England 1986–91. *J. Hosp. Infect.*, **24**: 313–25.

Block SS (1991) *Disinfection, Sterilisation and Preservation*, 4th edn. Lea & Febiger, Philadelphia.

Bloomfield SF, Smith-Burchnell CA, Dalgleish AG (1990) Evaluation of hypochlorite-releasing disinfectants against the human immunodeficiency virus (HIV). *J. Hosp. Infect.*, **15**: 273–8.

Boyce JM, Opal SM, Chow JW et al (1994) Outbreak of multi-drug resistant *Enterococcus faecium* with transferable VanB class vancomycin resistance. *J. Clin. Microbiol.*, **32**: 1148–53.

British Medical Association (1984) *A Code of Practice for the Sterilisation of Instruments and Control of Cross Infection*. BMA, London.

British Society of Gastroenterology (1988) Cleaning and disinfection of equipment for gastrointestinal flexible endoscopy: interim recommendations of a working party. *Gut*, **29**: 1134–51.

British Standards Institution (1990) *Sterilising and Disinfecting Equipment for Medical Products; Specification for Benchtop Steam Sterilisers for Unwrapped Instruments and Utensils*. BS3970: Part 4. BSI, London.

British Standards Institution (1994) *Bench Top Autoclaves. Specialist technicians*. BS EN 554. BSI, London.

British Thoracic Society Research Committee (1989) Bronchoscope and infection control. *Lancet*, **ii**: 270–1.

Bronowicki J-P, Venard V, Botté C et al (1997) Patient-to-patient transmission of hepatitis C virus during colonoscopy *N. Engl. J. Med.*, **337**: 237–40.

Cefai C, Richards J, Gould FK et al (1990) An outbreak of *Acinetobacter* respiratory tract infection resulting from incomplete disinfection of ventilatory equipment. *J. Hosp. Infect.*, **15**: 177–82.

Chadwick C, Oppenheim BA (1996) Cleaning as a cost-effective method of infection control. *Lancet*, **347**: 1776.

Chadwick PR, Beards G, Brown D et al (2000) Management of hospital outbreaks of gastro-enteritis due to small round structured viruses. *J. Hosp. Infect.*, **45**: 1–10.

Coates D, Wilson M (1989) Use of dichloroisocyanurate granules for spills of body fluids. *J. Hosp. Infect.*, **13**: 241–52.

Collins BJ (1988) The hospital environment: how clean should a hospital be? *J. Hosp. Infect.*, **11** (Suppl. A): 53–6.

Collins FM (1986) Bactericidal activity of alkaline glutaraldehyde solution against a number of atypical mycobacterial species. *J. Appl. Bacteriol.*, **61**: 247–51.

Communicable Disease Report (1999) Sigmoidoscopy and rectal biopsy – failure of infection control. *CDR Weekly*, **9**(16): 139.

Dancer SJ (1999) Mopping up hospital infection. *J. Hosp. Infect.*, **43**: 85–100.

Department of Health (1990) *Spills of Urine: Potential Misuse of Chlorine-releasing Disinfecting Agents*. SAB59(90) 41. Medical Devices Agency, DoH, London.

Department of Health (1991) *Hospital Mattress Assemblies: Care and Cleaning*. Safety Action Bulletin SAB(91)65. DoH, Wetherby, UK.

Dowsett EG, Wilson PA (1981) An outbreak of *Streptococcus pyogenes* infection in a maternity unit. *CDR*, **81**(17): 3.

Earnshaw JJ, Clark AW, Thom BT (1985) Outbreak of *Pseudomonas aeruginosa* following endoscopic retrograde cholangiopancreatography. *J. Hosp. Infect.*, **6**: 95–7.

Farina A, Fievet M-H, Plassart F et al (1999) Residual glutaraldehyde levels in fiberoptic endoscopes: measurement and implications for patient toxicity. *J. Hosp. Infect.*, **43**: 293–7.

Finn L, Crook S (1998) Minor surgery in general practice – setting standards. *J. Public Health Med.*, **20**(2): 169–74.

Fujita K, Lilly HA, Kidson A et al (1981) Gentamicin-resistant *Pseudomonas aeruginosa* infection from mattresses in a burns unit. *BMJ*, **283**: 219–20.

Greaves A (1985) We'll just freshen you up, dear. *Nursing Times*, **March 6** (Suppl.): 3–8.

Green J, Wright PA, Gallimore CI et al (1998) The role of environmental contamination with small round structured viruses in a hospital outbreak investigated by reverse-transcriptase polymerase chain reaction assay. *J. Hosp. Infect.*, **39**: 39–45.

Hanson PJV, Gor D, Jeffries DJ et al (1989) Chemical inactivation of HIV on surfaces. *BMJ*, **298**: 862–4.

Hanson PJV, Bennett J, Jeffries DJ et al (1994) Enteroviruses, endoscopy and infection control: an applied study. *J. Hosp. Infect.*, **27**: 61–7.

Haythorne A (1998) Alert to alternatives. *Nursing Times*, **94**(37): 76.

Health & Safety Executive (1998) *Glutaraldehyde*. Chemical Hazard Alert Notice 7 (revised). HSE, London.

Health & Safety Executive (1999a) *Control of Substances Hazardous to Health Regulations. Approved Codes of Practice for General COSHH, Carcinogens and Biological Agents*. HSE Books, Sudbury, UK. Available: http://www.hsebooks.co.uk

Health & Safety Executive (1999b) *Occupational Exposure Limits*, EH 40/99. HSE Books, Sudbury, UK. Available: http://www.hsebooks.co.uk

Hollyoak V, Boyd P, Freeman R (1995) Whirlpool baths in nursing homes: use, maintenance and contamination with *Pseudomonas aeruginosa*. *CDR Rev.*, **5**(7): R102–4.

Infection Control Nurses Association/Association of Domestic Management (1999) *Standards for Environmental Cleanliness in Hospitals*. ICNA, Bathgate, West Lothian.

Joynson DHM (1978) Bowls and bacteria. *J. Hyg.*, **80**: 423–4.

Kim KH, Fekety R, Batts DH et al (1981) Isolation of *Clostridium difficile* from the environment and contacts of patients with antibiotic-associated colitis. *J. Infect. Dis.*, **143**: 42–50.

Kingsley A, Hutter S, Green N et al (1999) Waterbirths: regional audit of infection control practices. *J. Hosp. Infect.*, **41**: 155–7.

Kolmos HJ, Thuesen B, Nielsen SV et al (1993) Outbreak of infection in a burns unit due to *Pseudomonas aeruginosa* originating from contaminated tubing used for irrigation of patients. *J. Hosp. Infect.*, **24**: 11–22.

Langenberg W, Rauws EAJ, Oudbier JH et al (1990) Patient-to-patient transmission of *Campylobacter pylori* infection by fibreoptic gastroduodenoscopy and biopsy. *J. Infect. Dis.*, **161**: 507–11.

Levin MH, Olsen B, Nathan C et al (1984) Pseudomonas in the sinks of an intensive care unit: relation to patients. *J. Clin. Pathol.*, **37**: 424–7.

Loomes S (1988) Is it safe to lie down in hospital? *Nursing Times*, **84**(49): 63–5.

Medical Devices Agency (1995) *The Re-use of Medical Devices for Single Use Only*. MDA DB 9501. DoH, London.

Medical Devices Agency (1997a) *Decontamination of Endoscopes*. DB 9607. DoH, Wetherby, UK.

Medical Devices Agency (1997b) *Purchase, Operation and Maintenance of Bench-top Steam Sterilisers*. DB 6905. DoH, Wetherby, UK.

Medical Devices Agency (1998) *Validation and Periodic Testing of Bench-top Vacuum Steam Sterilisers*. DB 9804. DoH, Wetherby, UK.

Morgan DR, Lamont TJ, Dawson JD et al (1990) Decontamination of instruments and control of cross-infection in general practice. *BMJ*, **300**: 1379–80.

Murdoch S (1990) Hazards in hoists. *Nursing Times*, **86**(49): 68–70.

Mylotte JM (1994) Control of methicillin-resistant *Staphylococcus aureus*: the ambivalence persists. *Infect. Control Hosp. Epidemiol.*, **15**: 73–7.

Neidner R, Schöpf R (1986) Inhibition of wound healing by antiseptics. *Br. J. Dermatol.*, **115**(S31): 41–4.

Newsom SWB (1972) Microbiology of hospital toilets. *Lancet*, **ii**: 700–3.

NHS Estates (1994) *Sterilisation*. Health Technical Memorandum 2010. DoH, Wetherby, UK.

NHS Estates (1995) *Washer–disinfectors*. Health Technical Memorandum 2030. DoH, Wetherby, UK.

NHS Executive (1995) *Hospital Laundry Arrangements for Used and Infected Linen*. HSG(95)18. DoH, Wetherby, UK.

NHS Management Executive (1993) *Decontamination of Equipment Prior to Inspection, Service or Repair*. HSG(93)26. HMSO, London.

Noble MA, Issac-Renton JL, Boyce DL et al (1998) The toilet as a transmission vector of vancomycin-resistant enterococci. *J. Hosp. Infect.*, 40: 237–41.

Noone P, Griffiths RJ (1997) The effect on sepsis rates of closing and cleaning hospital wards. *J. Clin. Pathol.*, 24: 721–5.

Nyström B (1981) The disinfection of baths and shower trolleys in hospitals. *J. Hosp. Infect.*, 2: 93–5.

Oie S, Kamiya A (1996) Microbial contamination of antiseptics and disinfectants. *Am. J. Infect. Control*, 24: 389–95.

Orsi GB, Mansi A, Tomao P et al (1994) Lack of association between clinical and environmental isolates of *Pseudomonas aeruginosa* in hospital wards. *J. Hosp. Infect.*, 27: 49–60.

Rotter M, Koller W, Wewalka G (1980) Povidone–iodine and chlorhexidine gluconate-containing detergents for disinfection of hands. *J. Hosp. Infect.*, 1: 149–58.

Russell AD (1994) Glutaraldehyde: current status and uses. *Infect. Control Hosp. Epidemiol.*, 15: 724–33.

Ryan CK, Potter GD (1995) Disinfectant colitis. Rinse as well as you wash. *J. Clin. Microbiol.*, 21(1): 6–9.

Scott E, Bloomfield SF (1990) The survival and transfer of microbial contamination via cloths, hands and utensils. *J. Appl. Bacteriol.*, 68: 271–8.

Sherertz R, Sullivan M (1985) An outbreak of infections with *Acinetobacter calcoaceticus* in burn patients: contamination of patients' mattresses. *J. Infect. Dis.*, 151: 252–8.

Sherwood Burge P (1989) Occupational risks of glutaraldehyde. *BMJ*, 299: 342.

Spach DH, Silverstein FE, Stamm WE (1993) Transmission of infection by gastrointestinal endoscopy and bronchoscopy. *Ann. Intern. Med.*, 118: 117–28.

Teare EL, Corless D, Peacock A (1998) *Clostridium difficile* in district general hospitals. *J. Hosp. Infect.*, 39: 241–2.

Teece J (1997) Ster-Zac powder in the care of the umbilical cord following childbirth *Br. J. Midwifery*, 5(4): 200–2.

Thompson G, Bullock D (1992) To clean or not to clean? *Nursing Times*, 88(34): 66–8.

Thompson M, Hempshall P (1999) Dirt alert. *Nursing Times*, 94(28): 63–4.

UK Health Departments (1994) *Dry Heat Sterilisers: Purchase, Maintenance and Use*. SAB (94)23. HMSO, London.

UK Health Departments (1998) *Guidance for Clinical Health Care Workers: Protection Against Infection with Blood-borne Viruses. Recommendations of the Expert Advisory Group on AIDS and the Advisory Group on Hepatitis*. DoH, Wetherby, UK.

Van den Berg RW, Claahsen HL, Niessen M et al (2000) *Enterobacter cloacae* outbreak in the NICU related to disinfected thermometers. *J. Hosp. Infect.*, 45: 29–34.

Werry C, Lawrence JM, Sanderson PJ (1988) Contamination of detergent cleaning solutions during hospital cleaning. *J. Hosp. Infect.*, 11: 44–9.

Wood A, Payne D (1998) The action of three antiseptics/disinfectants against enveloped and non-enveloped viruses. *J. Hosp. Infect.*, 38(4): 283–96.

Working Party of the Central Sterilising Club (1999) Reprocessing of single use medical devices in hospitals. *Zentralbl. Steril.*, 7: 37–47.

FURTHER READING

Association of Practitioners in Infection Control & Epidemiology (1996) Guideline for selection and use of disinfectants. *Am. J. Infect. Control*, 24(4): 313–42.

Atwell C (1990) Control of substances hazardous to health. *Surg. Nurse*, 3(6): 10–13.

Castille K (1999) To re-use or not to re-use – that is the question. *Nursing Times*, 13(34): 48–52.

Coates D (1988) Household bleaches and HIV. *J. Hosp. Infect.*, 11: 95–6.

Cowan T (1997) Sterilising solutions for heat-sensitive instruments. *Prof. Nurse*, 13(1): 55–8.

Department of Health (1987) *Decontamination of Equipment, Linen or Other Surfaces Contaminated with Hepatitis B or Human Immunodeficiency Virus*. Health Notice HN (87)1. HMSO, London.

Department of Health (1994) *Instruments and Appliances Used in the Vagina and Cervix; Recommended Methods for Decontamination*. Safety Action Bulletin SAB(94)22. DoH, London.

Department of Health (1998) *Sterilisation, Disinfection and Cleaning of Medical Equipment*. Guidance from the Microbiological Advisory Committee to the Medical Devices Directorate. HMSO, London. Online. Available: http://www.doh.nhsweb.nhs.uk/health/decontamination-guidance.htm

East J (1992) Implementing the COSHH regulations. *Nursing Standard*, 6(26): 33–5.

Hoffman PN (1987) Decontamination of equipment in general practice. *The Practitioner*, 231: 1411–15.

Morgan DR, Lamont TJ, Dawson JD et al (1990) Decontamination of instruments and control of cross-infection in general practice. *BMJ*, 300: 1379–80.

Nyström B (1981) The disinfection of baths and showers trolleys in hospitals. *J. Hosp. Infect.*, 2: 93–5.

Parker LJ (1999) Managing and maintaining a safe environment in the hospital setting. *Br. J. Nurs.*, 8(16): 1053–66.

Russell AD (1986) Bacterial resistance to antiseptics and disinfectants. *J. Hosp. Infect.*, 7: 213–25.

Russell AD, Hugo WB, Ayliffe GAJ (eds) (1992) *Principles and Practice of Disinfection, Preservation and Sterilisation*, 2nd edn. Blackwell Scientific, Oxford.

Talon D (1999) The role of the hospital environment in the epidemiology of multiresistant bacteria. *J. Hosp. Infect.*, 43: 13–18.

Weber DJ, Rutala WA (1997) Role of environmental contamination in the transmission of vancomycin-resistant enterococci. *Infect. Control Hosp. Epidemiol.*, 18: 306–9.

Appendix 1: A policy for the decontamination of equipment

Item	Method	Frequency
Ambu-bags	Protect with filter Autoclave	Change filter after each patient After each patient
Anaesthetic masks	Clean	After each patient
Auriscopes	Clean	After each use
Baby bottles	Use presterilized feeds if possible Clean, immerse in hypochlorite (125 ppm av. Cl) for 1 h or boil for 5 min	After each use
Baby scales	Clean	After each use
Baths	Clean If patient has large open wounds or bathwater contaminated by body fluid, wipe with hypochlorite (1000 ppm av. Cl) after cleaning	After each use
Bath hoists	Clean	After each use
Bedpans	Washer–disinfector Disposables – macerate, clean bedpan carriers	After each use
Bowls (washing)	Clean, dry and store inverted	After each use
Commodes	Clean	When visibly soiled

Duvets
  PVC covered
  Fabric
  Duvet cover
	
	Clean
	Launder
	Launder
		
		After each patient
		Every three months
		After each patient and when soiled

Humidifiers	Clean	Every 48 h Refill with sterile water Maintain at at least 50°C while in use
Incubators	Clean	After each patient
Instruments	Autoclave or hot air oven	After each use
Jugs	Washer–disinfector, or clean and dry, or CSSD	After each use

Laryngoscopes
  Blades
  Handles
	
	Clean and autoclave or washer–disinfector
	Clean
		
		After each use
		After each use

Mattresses	Clean, allow to dry before turning Ensure cover intact	After each patient and when visibly soiled
Mops	Launder	Daily
Nailbrushes (operating department)	Use sterile, send to CSSD or discard	After each use
Nebulizers (medicine)	Clean and dry Discard	After each use After each patient
Ophthalmic prisms	Clean, immerse in hydrogen peroxide for 10 min, or hypochlorite (500 ppm av. Cl), rinse and dry	After each use

cont.

Appendix 1 (*cont.*)

Item	Method	Frequency
Pillows	Clean Ensure cover intact	After each patient and when visibly contaminated
Razors Electric	Brush out hairs; immerse head in alcohol for 10 min	After each use
Specula Vaginal	Autoclave Use sterile speculum for IUD insertion	After each use
Spirometer	Change mouthpiece	After each patient
Suction Bottles Tubing Filter	Clean or autoclave if possible Single-use	After each use Change between patients Change when discoloured and every three months
Temperature probes	Use a plastic sleeve Clean, wipe with alcohol, store dry	For each use or after each patient
Thermometers	Wipe with alcohol or use a plastic sleeve Clean, immerse in alcohol for 10 min and store dry	After each use, for each use After each patient
Thermometer holders	Clean	After each patient
Toys Hard Soft	Clean Launder	When soiled
Tracheostomy tubes (silver)	Autoclave	After each patient
Trolleys Dressing	Clean	Daily
Urinals	Washer–disinfector Macerate disposables	After each use
Ventilators Machine Tubing	Protect with filter on expiratory circuit Protect with filter at patient end of circuit or change regularly	Change every 48 h Change filter (or tubing) every 48 h

Clean = wash with detergent and water, then dry.

14

Management of the infectious patient

INTRODUCTION

Micro-organisms cause a wide variety of human infections, some of which are described in Chapter 6. For many of these pathogens, the simple precautions outlined in Chapter 7 are sufficient to prevent their spread from person to person. However, there are a few for which additional precautions are considered necessary to minimize the risk of transmission. Although such precautions are most relevant in hospitals where the fre-quency of contact with staff and the presence of other vulnerable patients may facilitate their spread, they may also be required in residential or nursing homes, where they should be adapted to local circumstances. In the past these precautions were referred to as 'barrier nursing', but are now more commonly known as isolation precautions. Some hospitals use the term 'source isolation' to indicate that the patient is the source of infection and to distinguish them from 'protective isolation', which may be required for patients at risk of infection.

The assessment of whether such measures are necessary is influenced by a number of factors including the ease with which the micro-organism is transmitted, the route of transmission, the epidemiological significance of the organism in the local setting, and the extent to which other susceptible individuals may be exposed (Box 14.1). For example, isolation in a single room is recommended for a patient admitted to hospital with open tuberculosis to minimize the risk of the infection spreading by an airborne route to other susceptible patients in the same ward. After a short period of treatment the patient is no longer likely to transmit infection and the precautions can be discontinued.

Many isolation procedures in use today are based on tradition and there is a lack of empirical evidence regarding their efficacy in preventing the transmission of infectious diseases (Jackson & Lynch 1985, 1996). Examples of such practices include the use of separate cleaning equipment for isolation rooms and the use of masks.

Box 14.1 Factors that influence the requirement for isolation precautions

Ease of transmission
Some micro-organisms cause diseases that spread easily from person to person and are known as infectious or communicable diseases (e.g. rotavirus, diphtheria).

Route of transmission
Routine infection control precautions are sufficient to minimize the risk of transmission of most micro-organisms spread by direct contact with blood or body fluid (e.g. bloodborne viruses). Additional precautions are required to prevent the spread of micro-organisms transmitted by airborne particles (e.g. tuberculosis) or contact with skin (e.g. impetigo).

Epidemiological significance
Special infection control measures may be necessary to limit the spread of strains of micro-organisms resistant to the antibiotics conventionally used to treat the infections they cause. These measures are often necessary only in hospitals, where extensive use of antibiotics encourages the emergence of resistant strains and aspects of care facilitate their spread.

Presence of susceptible individuals
People who are immunosuppressed as a result of therapy or underlying disease are at increased risk of acquiring a wide range of infections, including infectious diseases, and precautions may be required to protect them, such as the use of negative pressure isolation rooms for patients with tuberculosis admitted to HIV units. Hospital patients, who have invasive devices or procedures, are also more vulnerable to some infections and the precautions recommended in hospital may therefore be different to those in a community setting.

Systems used to apply isolation precautions have evolved in response to changes in healthcare provision and hospital pathogens. Most recently, the widespread adoption of routine precautions for contact with blood and body fluids has enabled many infections to be managed without additional isolation precautions.

HISTORICAL PERSPECTIVE

The fear of infectious disease was recorded long before microbes were identified as the cause of infection in the late nineteenth century. Isolation was an early remedy for infection, and segregation of infected individuals has been practised for at least 4000 years. The oldest comprehensive isolation system is set out in the Bible, in the book of Leviticus, and these principles applied throughout the Middle Ages, particularly for leprosy and plague (Selwyn 1991).

Isolation procedures were first introduced in hospitals in the early twentieth century. To cope with the lack of single rooms or cubicles two approaches were employed: barrier nursing and 'bed isolation'. Barrier nursing involved the use of special procedures to prevent the spread of micro-organisms, for example gloves and gowns as a barrier for patient contact. Bed isolation involved the segregation of the infected patient to one part of the ward. Frequently the bed was surrounded by a partition, wire screen or curtain soaked in disinfectant (Glenister 1991). The purpose of the screen was to keep the patient away from other patients and to remind the staff to take barrier precautions. Many workers, including Florence Nightingale in her concept of 'fever nursing' for the care of patients with infection, realized that infection was rarely transmitted by the air or from the environment but that contact with body fluids was usually responsible and transmission could be prevented by the use of barrier precautions. This was an early recognition of the importance of basing isolation precautions on the **epidemiology** of the infecting micro-organism; that is, how it spreads from person to person.

In the early twentieth century patients with infectious diseases were commonly segregated in 'fever hospitals'. As the century progressed, improvements in public health and the introduction of antimicrobial agents had a marked effect on the incidence of infectious disease. Most patients could be treated in the community or as outpatients, and the demand for fever hospitals declined. By the 1960s most fever hospitals had closed and patients with infectious diseases were admitted to general hospitals instead.

Categories of isolation

In the 1950s categories of isolation precautions were developed; these aimed to simplify the application of precautions in these general hospital settings (Bagshawe et al 1978). Infections were allocated to a particular category according to their principal route of transmission and a specific set of precautions was defined for each category. Commonly used categories were strict isolation for highly infectious disease such as viral haemorrhagic fevers; respiratory isolation for tuberculosis and viral respiratory infections; wound and skin isolation for infected or colonized wounds; and enteric isolation for gastrointestinal pathogens such as salmonella (Control of Infection Group 1974, Garner & Simmons 1983).

The advantage of this type of system was that staff needed to learn a few procedures and were less likely to make mistakes. The disadvantage was that it could not be tailored to particular patients or types of infection. As not all infections allocated to a category would be spread in exactly the same way, in some cases more precautions would be applied than necessary.

Disease-specific isolation precautions

Categories of isolation were particularly difficult to apply to multidrug-resistant micro-organisms that could be spread by a variety of routes depending on the micro-organisms and the site of infection. As the problems with these organisms increased in the 1980s the need for isolation precautions tailored to individual infections incorporating an element of local decision-making was recognized and disease-specific isolation precautions were introduced (Garner & Simmons 1983). In this system only the precautions needed to prevent transmission of a particular infection were used. For example, hepatitis A is a gastrointestinal infection that spreads by contact with faeces. The precautions necessary to prevent the spread of infection would be the use of protective clothing for direct contact with faeces and handwashing after contact with the patient. This system had the advantage of eliminating unnecessary practices and could be adapted for individual patients. However, as staff were expected to make more decisions about what precautions were necessary, mistakes were likely to occur. In addition the procedures were diagnosis driven, that is they would be implemented only when a particular infection or disease was diagnosed. Frequently a patient may have been infectious for several days before the clinical illness had become apparent or the micro-organisms detected. For example, a patient may carry methicillin-resistant *Staphylococcus aureus* (MRSA) for many days before a swab result indicates its presence.

Integrating routine and isolation precautions

By the end of the 1980s the routine use of precautions to minimize the transmission of bloodborne viruses in all healthcare settings, commonly known as 'universal precautions', was advocated. These precautions were first recommended by the Centers for Disease Control in Atlanta, USA, in 1985 in response to growing concerns about the risk to healthcare workers from human immunodeficiency virus (HIV) (CDC 1987). Until then, special precautions had been taken only with body fluids from patients known or suspected to be infected with bloodborne viruses. HIV had highlighted the difficulty of identifying people who were incubating a disease and who were infectious, but who had no outward signs of the infection. Universal precautions

recognized that there were a few simple practices that could be used in the care of all patients that would minimize the risk of bloodborne viruses being transmitted to healthcare workers, for example the safe management of sharps and the use of protective clothing in situations where blood or body fluid was likely (see Ch. 7).

The change in emphasis towards regarding blood and body fluids from all patients as a major source of infection had important implications for isolation precautions. As body fluids are involved in the transmission of a wide range of other pathogens, universal precautions could be used in routine care to prevent the transmission of other pathogens (Lynch et al 1987, 1990, Wilson & Breedon 1990). The routine precautions could adequately contain many infectious diseases without the need for isolation. For example, if gloves were worn routinely for contact with excreta, patients with infections spread through contact with excreta would not require additional isolation precautions.

However, if universal precautions were to be effective in preventing cross-infection between patients, as well as protecting staff from bloodborne viruses, it was important to ensure that protective clothing was both used and changed appropriately. By changing protective clothing after each procedure, micro-organisms acquired on gloves used for contact with body fluid were not introduced to a susceptible site on the same or another patient. In 1987, Lynch et al introduced a new system called 'body substance isolation' which recommended the use of universal precautions with all moist body substances as a means of preventing the transmission of hospital pathogens. Healthcare workers were required to use clean gloves for contact with moist body substances, mucous membranes and non-intact skin, and to change them after each procedure. By ensuring that basic precautions were taken to prevent transmission from patients who are unknowingly incubating infection or colonized with pathogens, isolation procedures for patients known to have infectious disease could be simplified and focused on a smaller number of pathogens. Additional precautions (e.g. the use of masks) were recommended only for a few infections transmitted by airborne respiratory droplets (e.g. varicella, tuberculosis) (Jackson & Lynch 1985). The approach also helped to address the problem of preventing transmission of micro-organisms before a diagnosis being made.

Although the integration of routine and isolation precautions has caused some controversy, particularly in relation to the cost of protective clothing and the effect of lapses in routine use of precautions, it has now been incorporated into the latest advice on isolation precautions (Garner 1996, Garner & Hierholzer 1993). This adopts a simplified approach to isolation recommending the routine use of standard precautions and three categories of additional isolation precautions. Isolation is recommended for infections, such as MRSA, which can be transmitted through direct contact with patients or their environment (contact precautions); infections spread by coughs and sneezes, such as meningococcal meningitis (respiratory droplet precautions); and infections such as tuberculosis that are transmitted via inhaled droplet nuclei (airborne precautions) (Box 14.2).

THE PRINCIPLES OF ISOLATION PRECAUTIONS

The objective of isolation is to minimize the risk of micro-organisms from the affected person being transferred to others. It is important to recognize that it is the micro-organisms rather than the person that requires isolation, and precautions should be specifically directed at the usual route of transmission of the micro-organisms concerned. Care should be planned for individual patients, avoiding the use of unnecessary precautions and taking his or her needs into account.

The advice contained in the following section is intended to provide some general principles of isolation precautions, when they may be required and the rationale behind their use. If standard infection control precautions are used routinely for contact with blood and body fluid from all patients (Box 7.2), additional precautions will be necessary only for a limited number of infections (Box 14.2). A guide to routes of transmission and recommended precautions for infections commonly encountered in hospitals in the UK can be found in **Appendix 1** of this chapter. The precautions should be used for patients who are either known or suspected to have an infectious disease or when a patient presents with significant signs or symptoms, such as vomiting or diarrhoea, skin rash or pyrexia of unknown origin.

Local policies should be consulted before placing a patient in isolation. The application of precautions may vary according to the type of ward or unit and the presence of other patients at particular risk of infection. The infection control nurse (ICN) will be able to advise on appropriate precautions and identify unnecessary practices. A simple set of isolation procedures suitable for minimizing the risk of transmission of micro-organisms spread by direct contact or exposure to respiratory droplets is illustrated in **Appendix 2**.

Box 14.2 Indications for the use of isolation precautions in hospitals

If standard infection control precautions are used routinely for contact with blood and body fluid from all patients, additional precautions will be necessary only for infections or micro-organisms transmitted by the following routes.

Airborne
Infections transmitted by the inhalation of micro-organisms on droplet nuclei. These minute particles are expelled from the respiratory tract and may remain suspended in air for a long time.

Examples: tuberculosis, varicella, measles

Isolation precautions: single room (preferably with air-handling system); limit patient movement; masks recommended for some procedures; use gloves and plastic aprons for handling respiratory secretions; wash hands on leaving the room

Respiratory droplets
Infections transmitted by contact with respiratory secretions, including particles produced during coughing and sneezing. These particles do not travel far or remain airborne. Many of these infections are also spread by direct contact with infective material.

Examples: meningococcal meningitis, mumps, pertussis, diphtheria, some respiratory viruses

Isolation precautions: single room; limit patient movement; use gloves and plastic aprons for contact with infective material; wash hands on leaving the room

Contact with patients or their environment
Infections transmitted by direct contact with patients (e.g. by touching their skin, lesions or nasal secretions). Some micro-organisms may also be able to survive in the immediate environment and be transferred by contact with surfaces or equipment.

Examples:
- Enteric infection where prolonged survival in the environment may contribute to the transmission of infection (e.g. *Clostridium difficile*, enteroviruses)
- Some respiratory viral infections such as respiratory syncytial virus, influenza
- Skin infections such as impetigo, group A streptococcus
- Antibiotic-resistant micro-organisms infecting or colonizing skin or other body sites (e.g. MRSA, vancomycin-resistant enterococcus)

Isolation precautions: single room preferable; limit patient movement; use gloves and plastic aprons for contact with infective material from patients or their immediate environment; wash hands on leaving the room

Adapted from Garner J (1996)

Single room accommodation

Physical separation from other patients is indicated where an infection is transmitted by airborne particles. This is particularly important for micro-organisms carried on droplet nuclei (e.g. measles, chickenpox, pulmonary tuberculosis). Droplet nuclei are minute particles expelled from the respiratory tract that may remain airborne for long periods, travel long distances in air currents and, if inhaled, may penetrate deep into the lung (see p. 36). As a minimum, patients with these infections must be placed in a well-ventilated single room with the door kept closed. Ideally, specially ventilated isolation rooms should be used to ensure that droplet nuclei are diluted by extracting room air outside the building (Fig. 14.1). This negative pressure isolation is required for the management of patients with tuberculosis who are being cared for in areas where immunocompromised patients are present as they are particularly vulnerable to acquiring the infection, even after brief exposure (Breathnach et al 1998). Procedures that induce the patient to cough (e.g. bronchoscopy, sputum collection, administration of nebulized medication) should always take place in a room with adequate exhaust ventilation. The recommended minimum level of infection control precautions required for patients in hospital with pulmonary tuberculosis are summarized in Table 14.1 (Interdepartmental Working Group on Tuberculosis 1998).

Some infections are transmitted by larger respiratory droplets (e.g. pertussis, meningococcal meningitis). Unlike droplet nuclei, these will not travel a great distance or remain airborne for prolonged periods; however, a single room is recommended to minimize the risk of transmission to other patients likely to be in close proximity in an open ward.

Single rooms are not essential to prevent the transmission of infections spread by direct contact, although they may be preferred as a means of ensuring that infection control procedures are observed. Notices at the entrance of the room or displayed by the patient's bed can indicate to visitors and staff, particularly those who may not work regularly on the ward, that special precautions are being observed (Fig. 14.2). Sometimes a private room is advisable because the patient's illness is particularly likely to result in contamination of the environment (e.g. profuse diarrhoea, vomiting or bleeding) or because the patient is unable to follow infection control measures, for instance young children or the psychologically disturbed. Some micro-organisms, notably *Clostridium difficile* and antibiotic-resistant bacteria such as glycopeptide-resistant enterococci, are able to survive in the environment for prolonged periods and environmental contamination has been implicated in their spread (Teare et al 1998, Weber and Rutala 1997). A single room may therefore be required to limit the extent of environmental contamination and facilitate cleaning once the patient has been discharged or the isolation discontinued.

Usually patients with infections that are transmitted only by direct contact can be allowed to leave their rooms for treatment. This is particularly important for those who require physiotherapy or other forms of rehabilitation.

If more than one patient is infected or colonized with the same organism, they can be nursed together in the same ward or area rather than individual rooms. This is called cohorting and can be a useful approach for managing outbreaks of infection, as demonstrated in the study by Doherty et al (1998) on the management of respiratory syncytial virus amongst children. A few hospitals have specialist isolation facilities for the management of patients with infectious diseases. Regional infectious diseases units in London and Newcastle have high-level facilities with air-handling systems and bed isolators. Patients with viral haemorrhagic fevers must be transferred to these units (Advisory Committee on Dangerous Pathogens 1996).

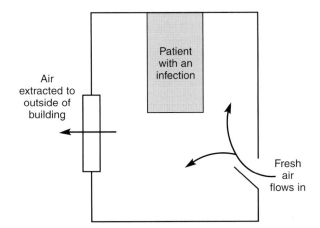

Fig. 14.1 Negative pressure room ventilation. The aim is to reduce the risk for those entering the room of acquiring the infection by diluting the number of infectious airborne particles and ensuring that air flows from the room to the outside of the building, not to other patient areas. Air is extracted to create a lower pressure inside the room. Air from adjacent rooms will be drawn in through vents and around doors. The rate at which air is extracted must exceed the rate of supply, and doors and windows must be kept shut to ensure that the pressure differential and direction of airflow are maintained. The ventilation system should be checked regularly by a trained engineer.

Table 14.1 Summary of isolation precautions recommended for patients with *Mycobacterium tuberculosis*

Status of patient	Recommended infection control precautions	
	Patient in ward area with no immunocompromised patients	Patient in ward area with significantly immunocompromised patients
TB suspected	Isolate in a single room	Isolate in single room with automatically monitored negative air pressure[a]
	Encourage patient to cover mouth and nose when coughing	
TB confirmed and sputum smear positive	Isolate in single room	Isolate in single room with automatically monitored negative air pressure[a]
	Encourage patient to cover mouth and nose when coughing	
	Staff who have regular or prolonged contact with the patient should wear a mask	
	Discontinue isolation after 2 weeks of chemotherapy, provided there is clinical improvement, the patient can adhere to therapy and there is no multidrug-resistant mycobacterium in sputum	
TB confirmed or suspected but sputum smear negative	Isolation not necessary	Isolate in a single room
Multidrug-resistant TB suspected or confirmed	Isolate in a single room with negative air pressure	Isolate in single room with automatically monitored negative air pressure[a]
	Patient to wear a mask when being transported to other clinical areas	
	Encourage patient to cover mouth and nose when coughing	
	All persons entering the room should wear a high-efficiency filtration mask	
	If multidrug-resistant TB is confirmed, isolation may need to be continued indefinitely while the patient is in hospital	

[a]Air flows into the room and is extracted to the outside, not into other patient areas.
Source: Interdepartmental Working Party on Tuberculosis (1998).

STANDARD ISOLATION

Visitors please check with nurse before entering

- Remove white coats before entering

- **Wash hands before leaving**

For further information refer to Isolation Policy

Fig. 14.2 Example of an isolation notice.

In nursing or residential homes, the most commonly encountered infectious diseases are viral respiratory infections and gastroenteritis. These can often spread rapidly amongst the residents, and the isolation of affected residents either in a single room or by sharing with others who are affected may be necessary to prevent spread. The room should have a handwash basin to ensure that staff can easily wash their hands after contact and a designated toilet is helpful where a resident has gastroenteritis (Public Health Medicine Environmental Group 1996).

Protective clothing

Protective clothing should be used to minimize the risk of acquiring pathogens on hands or clothing and worn when contact with material likely to transmit the infection is anticipated. It is not usually necessary to wear protective clothing every time the room is entered, as some activities are unlikely to result in contact with infective material, but it should be readily available both inside and outside the room (Fig. 14.3).

The infective material varies according to the type of infection (see Appendix 1). For example, if a patient has cellulitis the micro-organisms will be present on the affected area of skin. Gloves and plastic apron should be used for direct contact with the skin and for handling bed linen. If a patient has shigella, the pathogen will be excreted in faeces. Gloves and apron should be worn for any direct contact with faeces or items contaminated with faeces. If protective clothing is worn routinely for contact with blood and body fluid, in many instances additional protective clothing will not be required for isolated patients because body fluids are the main source of infectious material.

The important principle is to ensure that protective clothing is discarded before contact with another patient. Usually this means removing protective clothing before leaving the room; however, it may sometimes be necessary to take equipment out of the room (e.g. to place a bedpan in the washer–disinfector). In this situation the gloves and apron should be removed and hands washed once the procedure has been completed. *It may also be necessary to change protective clothing several times during a particular episode of care to ensure that bacteria from an infected or colonized site on the patient are not transferred to a susceptible site such as a wound or urinary catheter.*

Gloves

Disposable gloves are worn to reduce the contamination of hands with micro-organisms. They should be worn for direct contact with infectious material and changed between procedures to ensure that bacteria from an infected or colonized site on the patient are not transferred to a susceptible site such as a wound or urinary catheter. Gloves should be discarded before leaving the room or before initiating care on another patient. Hands are easily contaminated during the removal of gloves and should therefore be washed after gloves have been discarded (Olsen et al 1993).

Gowns and aprons

Clothing may become contaminated while caring for patients, particularly during procedures involving heavily contaminated sites such as infected wounds and burns (Hambraeus 1973, Speers et al 1969). The number of organisms actually transferred to the

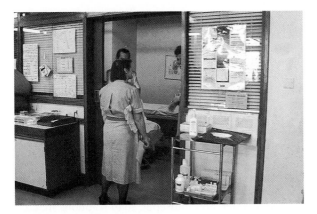

Fig. 14.3 An isolation room.

> **Example in practice**
>
> *Mrs Jones has been admitted with gastroenteritis caused by salmonella. She has frequent diarrhoea and is receiving intravenous fluids, but is mostly able to care for herself.*
>
> To prevent the transmission of salmonella to other patients on the ward, gloves and a plastic apron should be worn by staff who have direct contact with faeces, commodes or bedpans. These should be removed, and hands washed, afterwards. For any other care, such as adjusting Mrs Jones' intravenous therapy or assisting her with daily hygiene, gloves and apron are not necessary. Staff should always wash their hands before leaving the room, although an alcohol handrub can be used if the hands are not soiled. Mrs Jones' visitors need not wear protective clothing, but should be asked to wash their hands before leaving.

clothing is quite small and most will not survive there for very long periods. The front, the part that has most direct contact with patients and their immediate environment, is most likely to become contaminated (Babb et al 1983).

Micro-organisms can pass through fabric gowns, particularly when they are wet (Hoborn 1990). Plastic aprons are impermeable and therefore provide the most practical form of protection for the parts of the clothing most likely to become contaminated (Babb et al 1983). They should be worn when contact with infectious material is anticipated and changed between procedures and before leaving the room. The re-use or **disinfection** of aprons is impractical and not cost-effective.

Masks

Masks may be of value as a means of protection against airborne infection spread by droplet nuclei, although there is no scientific evidence to demonstrate their efficacy. To protect the wearer they must fit closely around the mouth and nose, otherwise air will be drawn in around the sides (Belken 1997). The mask should filter particles of 1 μm in diameter with at least 95% efficiency. The European Standard (1991) EN 149 describes the filtering standards for respiratory protection. The Control of Substances Hazardous to Health Regulations 1999 require that all other control measures, such as room ventilation, should be taken before considering the use of personal protective clothing such as masks. In a well-ventilated isolation room, masks are probably of limited value (Fennelly & Nardell 1998). They are recommended for aspects of care of patients with open tuberculosis that increase the exposure to infectious airborne particles, for example cough-inducing procedures and prolonged periods of care for high-dependency patients. Patients should be educated to minimize the release of tubercle bacilli into the air by coughing and sneezing into tissues, keeping their mouth covered. Provided the patient is able to cooperate with this practice, it is not usually necessary for them to wear a mask while being transported through other patient areas (Interdepartmental Working Group on Tuberculosis 1998).

Another more effective means of protecting staff from infections transmitted by an airborne route is immunization. The BCG vaccine for tuberculosis confers 70–80% immunity lasting at least 15 years. Although it does not completely eliminate the risk of acquiring the infection, it does reduce it considerably (Interdepartmental Working Group on Tuberculosis 1996).

Immunity is also the most reliable factor protecting staff against acquiring chickenpox (varicella zoster virus) and measles. Varicella zoster virus (VZV) is highly transmissible. Most adults born in the UK acquire and develop immunity to the virus during childhood, although people born in some other countries, such as the West Indies and Hong Kong, are less likely to have been exposed. Staff who have no immunity to VZV are unlikely to be protected by the use of masks and should therefore avoid contact with the infected patient. VZV is a particular problem in wards or units that care for immunocompromised patients (e.g. haematology, renal or HIV units), as these patients are vulnerable to developing serious disease. Staff who work in these areas should have their immunity checked so that, if non-immune, they can be managed appropriately should they be exposed to the infection or an outbreak occur (Jones et al 1997). Measles usually occurs in children and vaccination is now offered routinely in the UK (UK Health Departments 1996).

Other respiratory infections expelled in larger respiratory droplets are more likely to be transmitted on hands than inhaled (Ansari et al 1991). However, masks may help to reduce the risk of transmission during some procedures where there is close contact with respiratory secretions (e.g. bronchial suction, intubation) and they should be worn to protect staff when there is a risk of blood or body fluid splashing into the mouth.

Handwashing

Hands are probably the most important route by which micro-organisms are transmitted from patient to patient. Handwashing is therefore an essential component of preventing the spread of infection (Garner & Hierholzer 1993).

Micro-organisms may be acquired on the hands by contact with the patient, equipment or the patient's immediate environment. Although the use of gloves to handle infective material will reduce the extent of contamination, gloves may become punctured during use and micro-organisms may be transferred to the skin as gloves are removed (Olsen et al 1993). Hands should therefore always be washed when protective clothing is removed and before leaving the room. As the micro-organisms are acquired transiently on the skin, most are easily removed by washing with soap and water. However, some antibiotic-resistant Gram-negative bacilli appear to be particularly resistant to removal by soap and water, and antiseptic soap solutions may be recommended to prevent their spread (Wade et al 1991).

Alcohol handrubs provide a quicker alternative to soap and water for hands that are physically clean, for example for decontaminating hands after gloves have been removed (Mackintosh & Hoffman 1984).

Excreta

Safe disposal of excreta from patients with infections transmitted by the faecal–oral route is particularly important, although excreta from all patients should be treated as potentially infectious and disposed of in the same way. Excreta may be discarded into a toilet, a bedpan washer or a macerator. Bedpans can be taken out of an isolation room wearing gloves and plastic apron, and emptied directly into the bedpan washer. Protective clothing can then be discarded into a yellow waste bag and hands washed. There is no risk of cross-infection if the nurse has no direct contact with other patients until gloves and aprons have been removed and hands washed. The practice of attempting to remove intestinal **pathogens** from excreta with **disinfectants** is unnecessary because more pathogens enter the sewage system in domestic waste than from hospitals.

Pathogens on re-usable bedpans are destroyed provided the bedpan washer achieves a temperature of 80°C for at least 1 min during the wash cycle. Most modern bedpan washers have a temperature display to enable the temperature to be checked.

Spillage of excreta should be cleaned up promptly, preferably with disposable wipes and using gloves and a plastic apron. Decontamination with disinfectants may be indicated where contamination affects a large area (see p. 150). Toilets splashed with excreta from patients with intestinal infections may in theory present a risk to others. This risk can be eliminated by regular cleaning of the toilet with detergent and ensuring that patients have access to handwashing facilities after using the toilet. Particular care must be taken to ensure that commodes are cleaned thoroughly after use by a patient with an enteric infection.

Waste material and linen

Waste generated during the care of an infected patient may be contaminated with infectious material and must be disposed of safely. In the UK all waste contaminated with blood or body fluid should be destroyed by incineration (Health & Safety Executive 1999). Waste from an infectious patient does not require any special labelling, but should be discarded into yellow waste bags. A national colour-coding system dictates that yellow bags are incinerated (see p. 147). The outer surfaces of waste bags do not become significantly contaminated and there is no reason to enclose them inside a second bag before disposal (Maki et al 1986).

Linen may transmit infection to laundry workers who sort it before washing. To minimize this risk, it is recommended that linen used by patients with certain infectious diseases should not be sorted until it has been disinfected by washing. Linen used by patients with enteric infection, open tuberculosis and some other infections specified by the infection control team should be segregated by placing in a water-soluble bag with water-soluble stitching. This should then be sent to the laundry in a red outer bag. The alginate bag is placed directly into a washing machine and splits open when in contact with water. Micro-organisms on linen are removed by detergent and the dilution of the water, and destroyed by the water temperature of at least 71°C during the wash cycle (NHS Executive 1995).

Equipment

In most situations routine decontamination procedures are sufficient to prevent cross-infection on equipment used by patients in isolation. These are discussed in Chapter 13.

Items that are likely to become contaminated by infectious material, such as a commode used by a patient with an enteric infection, should be cleaned with detergent after each use. It may, however, be more practical to allocate such equipment for sole use by the patient and to clean thoroughly when no longer required.

Items that do not become contaminated with infectious material do not require special cleaning and it is not usually necessary to discard unused disposable items in the room after the patient has been discharged or taken out of isolation.

Disposable crockery and cutlery for infectious patients is not necessary. Crockery and cutlery are unlikely to become contaminated with significant numbers of pathogens and bacteria will not be able to survive and multiply on the surface of clean, dry plates or cutlery. After use they should be washed in hot water and detergent, preferably in a dishwasher that has a rinse temperature of approximately 80°C, and allowed to dry before storage or re-use (Barrie 1996).

Cleaning

The environment is not a significant factor in the transmission of most infections because most micro-organisms cannot survive for long on clean, dry surfaces. Some bacteria are able to survive for prolonged periods in dust as they form spores or are extremely resistant to desiccation. The spores of *C. difficile* have been found to persist in the environment for 5 months and large numbers are dispersed from patients with diarrhoea (Hoffman 1993). The contamination of the environment has been associated with outbreaks of infection caused by this micro-organism (Cartmill et al 1994, Department of Health/Public Health Laboratory Service 1994). Although the **spores** are difficult to remove, disinfectants do not appear to be more effective than detergents for cleaning (Hoffman 1993). Similarly Boyce et al (1994) reported widespread contamination of the environment when patients with glycopeptide-resistant enterococcus had diarrhoea. In some cases disinfectants may be necessary to eliminate the contamination (Noble et al 1998). Contamination of the environment is not implicated in the spread of mycobacteria, as infection can be acquired only through the inhalation of droplet nuclei (British Thoracic Society 1990).

Equipment and surfaces should be kept free of dust and spills of body fluid to prevent micro-organisms accumulating. The room or bed area of the infected patient should be cleaned routinely in the same way as other areas. Disposable cleaning cloths should be used and discarded. Some hospitals designate a separate mop and bucket to clean the room.

Domestic staff do not usually have direct contact with the patient and the risk of their acquiring infection from a patient is even less than that of nursing or medical staff. To reduce the risk to a minimum they should be instructed to wear protective clothing to clean the room and to remove it and wash their hands before leaving. Careful reassurance is essential as they may be extremely concerned about acquiring infection from the isolated patient and the standard of cleaning may suffer as a result.

After an isolated patient has been discharged the room should be cleaned before the next patient is admitted. A thorough clean to remove all dirt and dust is usually sufficient using normal detergent-based cleaning agents. Afterwards the next patient can be admitted. Leaving isolation rooms for a period of time to air is unnecessary, as most infections are not spread by an airborne route and most harmful micro-organisms will have been removed by cleaning.

Transport of infected patients

Limiting visits to other departments reduces the opportunities for transmission. If transport to another department is necessary, infected lesions should be covered with a dressing and the patient asked to cover the mouth if coughing or sneezing. The personnel involved with the transport are unlikely to have contact with the infectious material and therefore do not need to wear protective clothing; however, they should be instructed to wash their hands afterwards. The receiving department should be informed in advance and advised of the precautions required.

Some infections present particular risk to mortuary staff (e.g. Creutzfeldt–Jakob disease, bloodborne viruses, tuberculosis, gastrointestinal infections). They should therefore be informed when a patient who has died had an infection so that the appropriate precautions can be taken when the body is handled. In some instances the body may need to be placed inside a plastic body bag (e.g. viral haemorrhagic fever, rabies, yellow fever) (Cutter 1999, Department of Health 1991, Healing et al 1995).

Visitors

Visitors are unlikely to have contact with infectious material, such as faeces or respiratory secretions, and unlike staff they will not usually be able to transmit infection through contact with other patients on the ward. Visitors should be advised to wash their hands before leaving the patient's room but there is usually no reason for them to wear protective clothing. Where appropriate, children and elderly visitors, who may be more susceptible to the infection, should be advised of the risks of visiting whilst the patient remains infectious (e.g. if the patient has chickenpox, RSV, etc.).

For patients with tuberculosis, visiting should be restricted to close relatives for the first few days of treatment. They will already have been exposed to the infection before the patient's admission and will be followed up by the Public Health Department to establish whether they have acquired the infection.

Psychological effects of isolation

Isolation affects individual patients in different ways and, as social beings, humans generally do not like being isolated from others (Fig. 14.4). The combination of isolation and fear of being infectious can be particularly stressful for some patients. Gammon (1998) measured four psychological constructs in a group of isolated patients and a control group of patients in hospital but not isolated. He found that the stressor of hospitalization was made worse by isolation. The isolated patients had significantly higher levels of anxiety and depression and lower

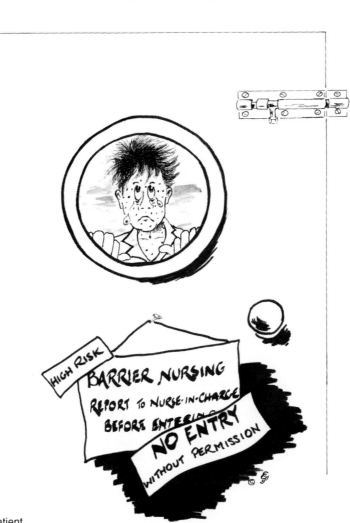

Fig. 14.4   The isolated patient.

self-esteem and sense of control. Anxiety may alter symptoms or induce secondary unrelated symptoms, affect the ability to listen and reduce the ability to cope. Carers must be sensitive to actions that increase anxiety, such as lack of communication, the use of excessive protective clothing or an inconsistency in the use of protective clothing, which can be confusing. A nurse who understands how the infection is transmitted can reassure and explain things to the patient. The value of providing information to isolated patients was demonstrated in a second study by Lewis et al (1999). This showed that providing patients in isolation with information about their disease, its symptoms and treatment, the control measures and their rationale, together with advice about their responsibilities, significantly reduced their levels of anxiety and depression and increased their self-esteem and sense of control.

Psychological disorders have been reported in patients who have been isolated (e.g. anxiety, time disturbance, hallucinations) (Denton 1986). Some become extremely demanding, fussy or irritable, and the nurse should recognize this behaviour as a response to isolation rather than that of a 'difficult' patient. Knowles (1993) studied eight patients in isolation. Many expressed feelings of loneliness, abandonment, inferiority and boredom (Table 14.2). Although the nurses often understood the patient's response to isolation, they did not take account of these problems and change the nursing care that they gave.

Table 14.2   Patient's response to isolation and nurses' perception of the situation. From Knowles (1993) with permission.

Patient	Patient's response to isolation	Nurses' perception of patient's response
A	Feels 'browned off' and isolated Feels confined and frustrated by lack of progress Feels lonely, misses company of others No meaningful activities when alone	Is depressed, feels isolated Is neglected and stigmatized Dislikes being alone
B	Feels neglected and imprisoned Feels inferior, stigmatized	Gets forgotten by staff Feels cut off
C	Feels isolated and abandoned Feels physically separate from the ward Makes sleeping and pastimes easier	Feels isolated Appreciates quiet
D	Feels enclosed Makes pastimes more pleasurable Values own company, not lonely	Gets forgotten by staff Values quiet, facilitates pastimes
E	Feels neglected, shunned, inferior Feels shut in Lack of meaningful activity when alone Misses company of others	Feels neglected, isolated, lonely Feels shut in Easier access to television
F	Is bored Values privacy Feels isolated, enclosed, imprisoned, stigmatized, punished Lacks information and control, feels anxious as a result	Is bored Values privacy

Patients with an infectious disease are often isolated for far longer than is necessary. The recommended period of isolation varies for each infection but usually precautions can be stopped once the symptoms have resolved, for example when diarrhoea has stopped, or for some infections after a short course of appropriate antimicrobial therapy (see Appendix 1).

For many infections, where transmission occurs only through direct contact with the infectious material, the stress of isolation can be relieved by allowing the patient out of the room. Isolation procedures should not interfere with rehabilitation, for example physiotherapy or occupational therapy.

Implementing isolation precautions and information for patients

At a clinical level isolation precautions can be difficult to implement; often there is confusion about how to apply the precautions and uncertainty about their effectiveness (Box 14.3). Prieto & Clark (1999) point to the conflicting advice given in a variety of national guidelines in relation to the use of gloves and how the importance of changing gloves between procedures is frequently overlooked. They go on to describe how, in practice, staff tend to put on gloves when they enter an isolation room and remove them only on leaving the room. As a result they observed occasions when soiled gloves continued to be used for clean activities where cross-infection could have occurred. This highlights the importance of clear, simple and consistent policies that address the issues that most commonly lead to confusion and explain the rationale behind them. The infection control nurse has a major role to play in explaining isolation precautions and should be called upon for advice whenever necessary. The precautions must be applicable to all members of the healthcare team. In general, they tend to be regarded as the sole responsibility of nurses, are often not addressed in medical textbooks, and have little place in doctors' training.

Consistency is also important for the patient. Patients need to understand the rationale for the pre-

---

Box 14.3   Nurses' concerns about isolation precautions

- Confusion about the correct way to implement precautions, leading to inconsistencies in practice
- Lack of information at ward level
- Uncertainty about effectiveness of precautions
- Lack of adherence to precautions
- Inadequate isolation facilities
- Detrimental effects of isolation on patients

Source: Prieto & Clark (1999)

cautions themselves and be reassured that all staff with whom they have contact apply them similarly. When a patient is discharged, the same precautions may not be necessary in their home or if they are transferred to residential care. The reasons for this may require careful explanation and good communication between hospital, nursing home and community staff.

The nurse must also play an important role as health educator. For example, patients with *Salmonella typhi* may continue to excrete the organisms in their stool for several weeks after the symptoms have resolved. To ensure that the infection is not transmitted to other members of the patient's family the importance of handwashing after using the toilet and before preparing any food should be discussed (see Ch. 12).

REFERENCES

Advisory Committee on Dangerous Pathogens (1996) *Management and Control of Viral Haemorrhagic Fevers*. The Stationery Office, London.

Ansari SA, Springthorpe S, Sattar SA et al (1991) Potential role of hands in the spread of respiratory infections: studies with human parainfluenza virus 3 and rhinovirus 14. *J. Clin. Microbiol.*, **29**: 2115–19.

Babb JR, Davies JG, Ayliffe GAJ (1983) Contamination of protective clothing and nurses' uniforms in an isolation ward. *J. Hosp. Infect.*, **4**: 49–57.

Bagshawe KD, Blowers R, Lidwell OM (1978) Isolating patients in hospital to control infection. Part IV: nursing procedures. *BMJ*, **ii**: 808–11.

Barrie (1996) The provision of food and catering services in hospital. *J. Hosp. Infect.*, **33**: 13–33.

Belken NL (1997) The evolution of the surgical mask; filtering efficiency versus effectiveness. *Infect. Control Hosp. Epidemiol.*, **18**: 48–57.

Boyce JM, Opal SM, Chow JW et al (1994) Outbreak of multidrug resistant *Enterococcus faecium* with transferable vanB class vancomycin resistance. *J. Clin. Microbiol.*, **32**: 1148–53.

Breathnach AS, de Ruiter A, Holdsworth GMC et al (1998) An outbreak of multidrug resistant tuberculosis in a London teaching hospital. *J. Hosp. Infect.*, **39**(2): 111–18.

British Thoracic Society, Joint Tuberculosis Committee (1990) An updated code of practice. *BMJ*, **30**: 995–1000.

Cartmill TDI, Panigrahi H, Worsley MA et al (1994) Management and control of a large outbreak of diarrhoea due to *Clostridium difficile*. *J. Hosp. Infect.*, **27**: 1–16.

Centers for Disease Control (1987) Recommendations for the prevention of transmission of HIV transmission in health care settings. *MMWR*, (Aug 21) **36**: (2S).

Control of Infection Group, Northwick Park Hospital and Clinical Research Centre (1974) Isolation system for general hospitals. *BMJ*, **2**: 41–6.

Cutter M (1999) In the bag? *Nursing Times*, **95**(20): 55–6.

Denton P (1986) Psychological and physiological affects of isolation. *Nursing*, **3**(3): 88–91.

Department of Health (1991) *Safe Working and Prevention of Infection in Clinical Laboratories*, HMSO, London.

Department of Health/Public Health Laboratory Service (1994) Clostridium difficile *Infection. Prevention and Management*. Report by a Joint Working Group. PHLS, London.

Doherty JA, Brookfield DS, Gray J et al (1998) Cohorting of infants with respiratory syncytial virus. *J. Hosp. Infect.*, **38**: 203–6.

European Standard (1991) *Specification for Filtering Half Masks to Protect Against Particles*. BS EN149, British Standards Institution, London.

Fennelly KP, Nardell EA (1998) The relative efficacy of respirators and room ventilation in preventing occupational tuberculosis. *Infect. Control Hosp. Epidemiol.*, **19**(10): 754–9.

Gammon J (1998) Analysis of the stressful effects of hospitalisation and source isolation on coping and psychological constructs. *Int. J. Nurs. Pract.*, **4**: 84–96.

Garner JS (1996) Guideline for isolation precautions in hospital. *Infect. Control Hosp. Epidemiol.*, **17**: 53–80.

Garner JS, Simmons BP (1983) Guideline for isolation precautions in hospitals. *Infect. Control*, **4**: 245–325.

Garner JS, Hierholzer WJ (1993) Controversies in isolation policies and practice. In *Prevention and Control of Nosocomial Infections*, 2nd edn, pp. 70–81 (RP Wenzel, ed.). Williams & Wilkins, Baltimore, MD.

Glenister H (1991) *Surveillance Methods for Hospital Infection*. PhD thesis, Surrey University.

Hambraeus A (1973) Transfer of *Staphylococcus aureus* via nurses' uniforms. *J. Hyg. (Camb.)*, **71**: 799–814.

Healing TD, Hoffman PN, Young SEJ (1995) The infection hazards of human cadavers. *CDR Rev.*, **5**(5): R61–8.

Health & Safety Executive (1999) *Safe Disposal of Clinical Waste*. The Stationery Office, London.

Hoborn J (1990) Wet strike through and transfer of bacteria through operating barrier fabrics. *Hyg. Med.*, **15**: 15–20.

Hoffman PN (1993) *Clostridium difficile* and the hospital environment. *PHLS Microbiol. Dig.*, **10**(2): 91–2.

Interdepartmental Working Group on Tuberculosis (1996) *The Prevention and Control of Tuberculosis in the United Kingdom: Recommendations for the Prevention and Control of Tuberculosis at a Local Level*. Department of Health, London.

Interdepartmental Working Group on Tuberculosis (1998) *The Prevention and Control of Tuberculosis in the United Kingdom: UK Guidance on the Prevention and Control of Transmission of 1. HIV Related Tuberculosis and 2. Drug-resistant, Including Multiple Drug-resistant, Tuberculosis*. Department of Health, London.

Jackson MM, Lynch P (1985) Isolation practices: a historical perspective. *Am. J. Infect. Control*, **13**(1): 21–31.

Jackson MM, Lynch PL (1996) Invited commentary: guideline for isolation precautions in hospitals, 1996. *Am J. Infect. Control*, **24**: 203–6.

Jones EM, Barnett J, Perry C et al (1997) Control of varicella-zoster infection on renal and other specialist units. *J. Hosp. Infect.*, **36**(2): 133–40.

Knowles HE (1993) The experience of infectious patients in isolation. *Nursing Times*, **89**(30): 53–6.

Lewis AM, Gammon J, Hosein I (1999) The pros and cons of isolation and containment. *J. Hosp. Infect.*, **43**: 19–23.

Lynch P, Jackson MM, Cummings MJ et al (1987) Rethinking the role of isolation practices in the prevention of nosocomial infections. *Ann. Intern. Med.*, **107**: 243–6.

Lynch P, Cummings MJ, Roberts PL et al (1990) Implementing and evaluating a system of generic infection precautions: body substance isolation. *Am. J. Infect. Control*, **18**: 1–12.

Mackintosh CA, Hoffman PN (1984) An extended model for transfer of micro-organisms via the hands: differences between organisms and the effect of alcohol disinfection. *J. Hyg.*, **92**: 345–55.

Maki DG, Alvarado C, Hassemer C (1986) Double bagging of items from isolation rooms is unnecessary as an infection control measure: a comparative study of surface contamination with single and double bagging. *Infect. Control*, **7**: 535–7.

NHS Executive (1995) *Hospital Laundry Arrangements for Used and Infected Linen.* HSG(95) 18. Department of Health, Wetherby, UK.

Noble MA, Issac-Renton JL, Boyce DL et al (1998) The toilet as a transmission vector of vancomycin-resistant enterococci. *J. Hosp. Infect.*, **40**: 237–41.

Olsen RJ, Lynch P, Coyle MB et al (1993) Examination gloves as barriers to hand contamination in clinical practice. *JAMA*, **270**(3): 350–3.

Prieto J, Clark J (1999) Dazed and confused. *Nursing Times*, **95**(28): 49–53.

Public Health Medicine Environmental Group (1996) *Guidelines on the Control of Infection in Residential and Nursing Homes.* Department of Health, Wetherby, UK.

Selwyn S (1991) Hospital infection – the first 2500 years. *J. Hosp. Infect.*, **18** (Suppl. A): 5–65.

Speers R, Shooter RA, Gaya H et al (1969) Contamination of nurses' uniforms with *Staphylococcus aureus. Lancet*, **ii**: 233–5.

Teare EL, Corless D, Peacock A (1998) *Clostridium difficile* in district general hospitals. *J. Hosp. Infect.*, **39**: 241–2.

UK Health Departments (1996) *Immunization Against Infectious Disease.* The Stationery Office, London.

Wade JJ, Desai N, Casewell MW (1991) Hygienic hand disinfection for the removal of epidemic vancomycin-resistant *Enterococcus faecium* and gentamicin-resistant *Enterobacter cloacae. J. Hosp. Infect.*, **18**: 211–18.

Weber DJ, Rutala WA (1997) Role of environmental contamination in the transmission of vancomycin-resistant enterococci. *Infect. Control Hosp. Epidemiol.*, **18**: 306–9.

Wilson J, Breedon P (1990) Universal precautions. *Nursing Times*, **86**(37): 67–70.

FURTHER READING

Bowell B (1992) A risk to others. *Nursing Times*, **88**(4): 38–40.

Bowell E (1986) Nursing the isolated patient: lassa fever. *Nursing Times*, **33** (17 Sept): 72–81.

Crummey V (1997) Major undertaking. Funeral directors' knowledge of infection risks. *Nursing Times*, **93**(11): 72–6.

Curran ET (1993) Taking down the barriers; a new approach to barrier nursing. *Prof. Nurse*, **9**(7): 472–8.

Edmund M (1997) Isolation. *Infect. Control Hosp. Epidemiol.*, **18**: 5–64.

Gammon J (1998) A review of the development of isolation precautions. *Br. J. Nurs.*, **7**(6): 307–10.

Gaskill D, Henderson A, Fraser M (1997) Exploring the everyday world of the patient in isolation. *Oncol. Nurs. Forum*, **24**(4): 695–700.

Grazier S (1988) The loneliness barrier. *Nursing Times*, **84**(41): 44–5.

Oldman T (1998) Isolated cases. *Nursing Times*, **94**(11): 67–9.

Van Rijn RR, Kuijper EC, Kreis RW (1997) Seven-year experience with a 'quarantine and isolation unit' for patients with burns. A retrospective analysis. *Burns*, **23**(4): 345–8.

Vesley D (1995) Respiratory protective devices. *Am. J. Infect. Control*, **23**: 165–8.

Webster O, Bowell E (1986) Thinking prevention. *Nursing Times*, **82**(23): 68–74.

Appendix 1: Routes of transmission and isolation precautions for common infections

This table provides a guide to the routes of transmission for infections that may be encountered in hospital patients and whether isolation precautions are indicated. Routine infection control precautions should be used in the care of all patients. ICT, infection control team; IDU, infectious diseases unit; NA, not applicable.

Infection or disease	Route of transmission	Period of infectivity to others	Isolation precautions	Comments
AIDS: *see* Human immunodeficiency virus				
Amoebic dysentery: *Entamoeba histolytica*	Ingestion of faecally contaminated food or water	While cysts being excreted (may be years)	No	
Bronchiolitis (infants)	Respiratory droplets and direct contact with secretions	While symptomatic (5 days or longer)	Yes	Commonly caused by respiratory viruses (e.g. RSV, parainfluenza)
Campylobacter	Usually foodborne, also contact with contaminated animals or meat. Person-to-person transmission unlikely	Excreted in faeces for several weeks	No	
Candidiasis	Contact with lesions and secretions	Duration of illness	No	Can be spread by hands or equipment
Cellulitis (e.g. group A streptococci)	Direct contact with lesion	Until culture negative or after completion of course of antibiotics	Yes	Organism may be difficult to eradicate from chronic wounds
Chickenpox: Varicella zoster virus	Inhalation or direct contact with vesicle fluid or respiratory secretions	1–2 days before rash and 5 days after lesions first appear (longer in immunosuppressed)	Yes (single room essential)	Staff attending patient must be immune
Chlamydia trachomatis		May be carried on mucous membranes for months		
Conjunctivitis	Sexual contact, contact with discharge from eye		No	
Genital	Sexual contact		No	
Respiratory	Infected mother to baby during birth		No	
Chlamydia pneumoniae	Not defined but probably airborne respiratory droplets and direct contact with secretions		No	Spread may occur among families
Cholera	Ingestion of faecally contaminated food or water	During illness (although persistent, asymptomatic carriage may occur)	Yes	Case-to-case transmission can occur so diligence is required
Clostridium perfringens				
Food poisoning	Contaminated food (usually inadequately heated meat)	NA	No	Heavy bacterial contamination required for transmission to occur
Gas gangrene	Traumatic wounds contaminated by soil; endogenous infection of surgical wounds	NA	No	Poorly perfused, necrotic wounds required for gangrene to develop

cont.

Appendix 1 (*cont.*)

Infection or disease	Route of transmission	Period of infectivity to others	Isolation precautions	Comments
Clostridium difficile – toxigenic strains (pseudomembranous colitis)	Direct or indirect contact with faeces	Duration of diarrhoea	Yes (if symptomatic)	Spores may survive in the environment for prolonged periods. Infection commonly associated with disruption of gut flora as a result of antibiotic activity
Creutzfeldt–Jakob disease (CJD)	Unknown. Can be transmitted by grafts of human brain tissue, instruments, corneas or growth hormone derived from pituitary glands	Duration of illness	No	Variant CJD probably acquired through ingestion of meat contaminated with bovine spongiform encephalopathy agent
Crytococcosis: *Cryptococcus neoformans*	Found in pigeon faeces and soil	Not transmitted from person to person	No	Usually affects immunocompromised. Causes chronic meningitis but can also infect lungs, kidneys and bone
Cytomegalovirus (CMV)	Intimate contact with mucous membranes. Fetus may be infected in utero, during delivery or by breast milk	Virus excreted in urine and saliva for months. May persist episodically for years	No	Severe disease more likely in immunosuppressed
Diphtheria: *Corynebacterium diphtheriae* (toxigenic strains)	Direct contact with oral or nasal secretions of infected person	Until throat swabs negative (usually 2 weeks)	Yes	Immunization in infancy protects against systemic disease; local nasopharyngeal infection may occur
Escherichia coli gastroenteritis				
Enterohaemorrhagic (O157, verotoxin)	Usually foodborne or waterborne, may be transmitted by contact with animals and from person to person	Excreted in faeces for 1 week (longer in children)	Assess risk of transmission for individual patients	Associated with haemolytic–uraemic syndrome, usually in under-5yr
Enterotoxigenic	Foodborne (developing countries)	Prolonged excretion in faeces	No	Major cause of traveller's diarrhoea
Enteropathogenic	Foodborne (baby milk and weaning foods). Transmission via hands, especially in nurseries	Prolonged excretion in faeces	No	Causes severe prolonged diarrhoea in infants, especially in developing countries

Ebola virus: *see* Viral haemorrhagic fever

Erysipelas: *see* Streptococci

Giardiasis: *Giardia intestinalis*	Ingestion of contaminated drinking water; contact with faeces	Duration of infection (may be months)	Assess risk of transmission for individual patients	Often acquired abroad. Can be transmitted from person to person, especially among children

Appendix 1 (*cont.*)

Infection or disease	Route of transmission	Period of infectivity to others	Isolation precautions	Comments
Glandular fever (infectious mononucleosis): Epstein–Barr virus	Contact with saliva	Oropharyngeal carriage may persist for months or years	No	Infection may be transmitted on hands of staff if contaminated with saliva
Gonorrhoea: *Neisseria gonorrhoeae*				
Genital infection	Sexual contact with infected mucous membranes of genital tract	Until organism eradicated by appropriate therapy	No	
Ophthalmia neonatorum	Infection acquired from infected birth canal during delivery	While discharge persists	Yes	Can be spread by contact with conjunctival discharge
Hepatitis A	Faecal–oral route; food contaminated by infected handler; contaminated water	Maximum infectivity immediately before and for a few days after onset of jaundice	Assess risk of transmission for individual patients	Hepatitis A vaccine or immunoglobulin may be used to protect family contacts from infection
Hepatitis B	Sexually transmitted; blood inoculation through skin or on to mucous membranes; acquired transplacentally or intrapartum from infected mother	May persist indefinitely as carrier state	No (unless uncontrolled bleeding)	Main risk to healthcare workers is from contaminated sharps. All healthcare workers should be protected by vaccination – specific immunoglobulin available
Hepatitis C	As hepatitis B	May persist indefinitely	No	
Hepatitis E	Contaminated water; probably transmitted from person to person by faecal–oral route (not commonly)	Probably similar to hepatitis A	No	
Herpes simplex				
Cold sores, herpetic whitlow	Direct contact with lesion, exudate or saliva	Virus may be shed into saliva for several weeks after symptoms resolve	No	Staff may develop herpetic whitlow through contact with active cold sores. Staff with active lesions should avoid contact with immunosuppressed patients
Genital herpes	Sexually transmitted	Active lesions infectious for 7–12 days. Transient asymptomatic viral shedding common	No	
Neonatal herpes	Via infected birth canal; can be transmitted congenitally if mother acquires primary infection during pregnancy	Duration of illness	Yes	Separate infant from other neonates. Handle secretions from mother and baby using gloves and aprons

cont.

Appendix 1 (*cont.*)

Infection or disease	Route of transmission	Period of infectivity to others	Isolation precautions	Comments
Herpes zoster virus: *see* Shingles				
Human immunodeficiency virus (HIV)	Sexually transmitted; inoculation of blood or body fluid through skin or on to mucous membranes; transmitted from mother to baby in utero during delivery, or in breast milk shortly after birth	Indefinitely	No	Main risk to healthcare workers is from contaminated sharps
Impetigo: *Staphylococcus aureus*, group A streptococcus	Direct contact with lesion	Duration of lesion (until culture negative or after completion of course of antibiotics)	Yes	Young children often highly susceptible
Lassa fever: *see* Viral haemorrhagic fever				
Legionnaires' disease: *Legionella pneumophila*	Inhalation of contaminated aerosols. Not spread from person to person	NA	No	
Leptospirosis (Weil's disease)	Contact of abraded skin or mucous membranes with water, soil or vegetation contaminated by urine of animals	NA	No	Hazard to farmers, sewer workers, etc., watersports participants, bathers
Listeriosis: *Listeria monocytogenes*	Ingestion of contaminated food; from mother to baby in utero or during delivery	Shed in faeces for several months; shed in vaginal discharge for 7–10 days	Neonates	Outbreaks of infection in nurseries have been reported. Elderly, neonates and immunocompromised particularly susceptible
Lyme disease: *Borrelia burgdorferi*	Transmitted by tick bite	NA	No	Not spread from person to person
Malaria	Transmitted by mosquito bite; transfusion of blood from infected person	NA	No	No person-to-person spread except (rarely) by transfusion of blood
Marburg virus: *see* Viral haemorrhagic fever				
Measles	Airborne by respiratory droplets; direct contact with nose or throat secretions	From just before rash appears until 4 days after	Yes	Highly infectious. May cause severe illness in immunosuppressed children. Immunoglobulin available for susceptible patients
Meningitis				
Neisseria meningitidis (meningococcal meningitis)	Direct contact with respiratory droplets, nasal or oral secretions	Until organism no longer present in nasal or oral secretions	Yes (first 24 h of antibiotic therapy)	Most infections subclinical. Rifampicin prophylaxis offered to close *family* contacts
Haemophilus influenzae	Direct contact with respiratory droplets, nasal or oral secretions	Until organism no longer present in nasal or oral secretions (after 48 h of antibiotics)	Not usually	Most common in children aged between 2 months and 5 years

Appendix 1 (*cont.*)

Infection or disease	Route of transmission	Period of infectivity to others	Isolation precautions	Comments
Viral (e.g. enteroviruses, mumps)	Faecal–oral or respiratory spread (depends on agent)	Before and during acute illness	No	
MRSA: *see Staphylococcus aureus*				
Mumps	Transmitted by respiratory droplets and direct contact with saliva	7 days before symptoms appear and up to 9 days afterwards	Yes	Highly infectious. Previous infection confers lifelong immunity
Pneumonia (pneumococcal): *Streptococcus Pneumoniae*	Respiratory droplets; direct contact with nasal or oral secretions		No (unless antibiotic-resistant strain)	Susceptibility increased by underlying lung disease, aspiration, immunosuppression, very young, elderly
Poliomyelitis	Mainly by the faecal–oral route but transmission through direct contact with nasal or oral secretions also occurs	Most infectious for the few days before and after onset of symptoms. Virus persists in faeces for several weeks	Yes (IDU)	Vaccine strain of virus shed in faeces following immunization: non-immune contacts may be at risk of infection with vaccine virus
Psittacosis: *Chlamydia psittaci*	Inhalation of dust contaminated by bird droppings, secretions or feathers	Birds may shed organisms for weeks	No	Person-to-person transmission by contact with respiratory secretions is unlikely but has been reported. Laboratory staff may acquire infection by handling cultures
Rotavirus	Mainly by faecal–oral route but possibly also through contact with respiratory secretions	Virus shed in faeces for up to 8 days after onset of symptoms (longer in immunocompromised)	Yes	Outbreaks in elderly care and paediatric units reported
Respiratory syncytial virus (RSV)	By direct contact with respiratory secretions or droplets	While symptomatic	Yes	Highly transmissible on paediatric wards
Rubella	Direct contact with respiratory secretions or droplets. Also shed in urine of infants with congenital infection	7 days before and at least 4 days after onset of rash	Yes	Carers should be rubella-immune. In congenital rubella, babies excrete virus for months
Salmonella Enteric fever (*S. typhi* or *S. paratyphi*) Other species	Usually foodborne but may be transmitted from person to person via hands	Excreted in faeces for several weeks (especially infants)	Assess risk of transmission for individual patients	Carriers may inadvertently infect food
Scabies	Prolonged skin-to-skin contact	Until mite destroyed by treatment	No (unless Norwegian scabies)	Norwegian scabies occurs only in immunocompromised, but is highly contagious

cont.

Appendix 1 (*cont.*)

Infection or disease	Route of transmission	Period of infectivity to others	Isolation precautions	Comments
Scarlet fever: *see* Streptococci				
Shigella	Direct or indirect contact with faeces; can also be water- or foodborne	Infectious while organism present in faeces	Yes (until symptom-free and normal stool)	Highly infectious. Outbreaks in nurseries caused by transmission on hands
Shingles (herpes zoster)	Contact with lesion exudate	7 days after lesions first appear	Yes	Seronegative contacts develop chickenpox and should be excluded while patient is infectious
Staphylococcus aureus, methicillin-resistant (MRSA)	Direct contact with infected or colonized lesions or skin	While organism present in lesions, in nose or on skin	Yes (seek advice from ICT)	Epidemic strains may cause outbreaks of infection
Streptococci (groups A, C and G)	Direct contact with lesions	Until culture negative (or after course of antibiotics completed)	Yes	
Syphilis: *Treponema pallidum*	Direct contact with lesions during sexual contact; from infected mother to baby	During primary and secondary stages	No	Infectivity rapidly reduced by treatment. Wear gloves for contact with lesions
Tetanus: *Clostridium tetani*	Direct inoculation from contaminated source. Not transmitted from person to person	NA	No	Booster immunization not required after five doses in childhood or as adult
Toxoplasmosis: *Toxoplasma gondii*	Ingestion of infective oocysts in dirt or tissue cysts in undercooked meat. Primary infection in early pregnancy may result in transplacental infection of fetus	NA	No	Most infections asymptomatic; immunity develops readily
Tuberculosis (pulmonary) *Mycobacterium tuberculosis*	Inhalation of airborne droplet nuclei	While viable bacilli in sputum	Yes	Prolonged exposure usually required to transmit infection. Infectivity reduced after first 14 days of treatment. Patients with multidrug-resistant strains should be transferred to IDU
Viral haemorrhagic fever Lassa Ebola–Marburg Crimean–Congo (tickborne)	Person-to-person transmission by direct contact with blood, pharyngeal secretions or urine, and by sexual intercourse	Variable; depends on virus	Yes – transfer to regional IDU	Crimean–Congo fever is tickborne; Lassa fever transmitted by direct contact with rat urine. Source of Ebola–Marburg unknown
Whooping cough: *Bordetella pertussis*	Direct contact with respiratory secretions and probably airborne droplets	Highly infectious in early stages; non-infectious 3 weeks after onset of paroxysms	Yes	Children under 5 years most susceptible

From Wilson J (2000) *Clinical Microbiology: A Guide for Healthcare Professionals*, 8th edn. Baillière Tindall, London.

Appendix 2: An isolation policy

Indication

Isolation is necessary when a patient has or is suspected to have a communicable infection.

Check the list of communicable infections to find out whether isolation is necessary and what material from the patient is infectious.

Remember: Standard precautions must be used with all patients including those in isolation.

Aims

- To prevent the transmission of micro-organisms from an infected patient to others
- To provide psychological support and reassurance to the patient while in isolation
- To ensure that all staff are aware of the correct precautions to take and that unnecessary precautions are avoided

Equipment

- Single room with a washbasin
- Remove excess equipment from the room before patient is isolated
  Hand soap
  Disposable gloves
  Paper towels
  Yellow waste bag
  Plastic aprons
  Alcohol handrub

Practice	Rationale
Patient: explain reason for isolation and provide reassurance	To reduce anxiety and gain patient's cooperation
Aprons: wear plastic apron for contact with body fluid and infectious material, discard between procedures and before leaving the room	To protect clothing from contamination and prevent cross-infection
Gloves: wear for contact with body fluids and infectious material. Discard between procedures and before leaving the room	To prevent contamination of hands and prevent cross-infection
Masks: not usually necessary	There is no evidence that they protect from respiratory infection
Hands: always wash hands and forearms when gloves are removed and before leaving the room	To prevent transfer of micro-organisms to other patients
Faeces/urine/vomit: discard directly into bedpan washer/macerator or toilet	Prompt disposal essential to prevent transmission of micro-organisms
Linen: place in an alginate bag, then into a red nylon outer bag	To prevent dissemination of micro-organisms and protect laundry staff
Disposable items: discard used or soiled items into a yellow plastic bag	To ensure waste is incinerated
Equipment: clean/disinfect before removing from the room (see disinfection policy/contact ICN)	To prevent the spread of micro-organisms
Crockery: use normal utensils and return to main kitchens in usual way	Risk of cross-infection from crockery is minimal. Washing in hot water and detergent is sufficient
Visitors: instruct to wash their hands before leaving the room. Children and susceptible visitors should be discouraged from visiting	For most infections the risk to visitors is minimal as they do not have contact with body fluids
Other departments: avoid visits to other departments. If necessary, the department should be notified in advance and the patient seen at the end of the list. Porters need not wear protective clothing but should be instructed to wash their hands on completion of the journey	To keep contact with other patients to a minimum and enable the department to take appropriate precautions
Cleaning: inform domestic supervisor that the patient is being isolated. Use designated cleaning equipment for the room. Ask the domestic to wear gloves and apron to clean, and discard them on leaving the room	To maintain a clean environment and minimize risk of spread

cont.

Appendix 2 (*cont.*)

Practice	Rationale

In case of death: follow the usual last offices procedure. Body bags may be required for some infections

Body fluids leaking after death may present a risk to mortuary staff

Duration of isolation: refer to list of communicable infections or contact ICN

Isolation can be distressing for the patient and should not be continued for longer than necessary

Termination of isolation

See above for treatment of bed linen, disposable items and equipment. It is not necessary to discard unused packets of disposable equipment.

Cleaning: all furniture and surfaces, including the mattress and bed frame, should be cleaned with detergent and water. Once cleaned the room may be re-used immediately.

Special points

Chickenpox, shingles (herpes zoster), measles
Patients with these infections must not be looked after by staff unable to give a definite history of the infection or appropriate vaccination.
Pulmonary tuberculosis (smear positive)
Visitors, apart from immediate family, should be discouraged from visiting for the first week of antituberculosis treatment.

15

Ectoparasitic infections and environmental infestations

INTRODUCTION

This chapter examines the problem of infections and infestations by arthropods and other animals. It begins with a review of **parasites** that can infect the human skin and then looks at the variety of pests that may infest the healthcare environment.

ECTOPARASITIC INFECTIONS

The prospect of a close encounter with lice or scabies usually induces alarm in most people. In reality, most of these infections can be eradicated easily and the risk of staff or other patients acquiring the parasite is slight. An understanding of how they are transmitted is essential if the treatment is to be carried out effectively and the affected individual approached sensitively. It is also important to consider education and treatment of other members of the family.

Lice (pediculosis)

Lice can be caught only by close contact; they cannot jump or fly but need to be close enough to walk on to another host. They feed from the host, usually taking blood about five times a day. An allergic reaction develops to the bites, causing them to itch. This allergic reaction can take up to 3 months to develop and carriers easily become desensitized and therefore no longer notice the bites. Lice found off the body on bedding, chairs, floors, etc. are either dead, dying or injured and are unable to crawl on to another host.

There are about 500 different species of lice but only three of these use humans as their host and each lives on a specific part of the body.

*The head louse (*Pediculus humanus capitis*)*

This species lives on head and eyebrow hair. It mostly affects children, although adults may also acquire the infection. A study in southern England suggested that 10% of schoolchildren acquire lice in a year (Ibarra 1989, Maunder 1993). The adult head louse is between 1 and 4 mm long (Plate 15.1). The female louse can produce over 50 eggs, laying about six each day and sticking them close to the base of hairs where it is warmest. The eggs hatch after 7–10 days, leaving the egg cases or nits so firmly stuck to the hair that they can remain attached until the hair falls out (Plate 15.2). The louse nymphs then moult three times, reaching adulthood after 6–12 days. Some 11–18 h after the last moult they are ready to mate. Transmission to another host occurs when two heads are in direct contact and the louse moves on to a new head. They are able to climb rapidly in dry hair, although they move to a new head only when adult. They are sensitive to cold, preferring temperatures of at least 31°C. This keeps them close to the scalp and their source of food. Consequently lice are not easily passed to others unless heads are in contact for a minute or more, allowing time for the hair to warm up and the lice to pass across (Maunder, 1993). Lice prefer a clean head of hair where they can move around easily. They are able to cling on tightly to hairs and are not removed by washing.

Head lice are invariably acquired from family members or close friends. The infection is difficult to detect in its early stages. Lice use a local anaesthetic to make the feeding process painless. Itching, although a common symptom, may not develop for weeks. A pruritic rash may appear at the back of the neck. They are best detected by using a fine-toothed comb in wet hair. The eggs are only the size of a grain of sugar and are difficult to see as their colour is matched to that of the skin.

Treatment and control Several chemical insecticides are available for the treatment of lice, most of which can be obtained from the pharmacist without a prescription. The conventional treatments are based on the insecticides malathion, an organophosphate (e.g. Prioderm, Suleo-M and Derbac-M), carbaryl (e.g. Carylderm, Derbac-C and Suleo-C) and pyrethroid compounds (e.g. Lyclear, Full Marks). Two applications of lotion applied 7 days apart are recommended for effective treatment (British National Formulary 1999), although for most products the manufacturers recommend only a single application. The lotion should be applied to dry hair and left on the scalp for 12 h. A hair-dryer should not be used for alcohol-based products. After 12 h the hair should be washed.

Shampoos are also available but, although they contain a higher concentration of insecticide, they are not as effective because they are not in contact with the hair for long enough and are unlikely to destroy eggs. Three separate treatments with shampoo are therefore required to eradicate the lice. Lyclear cream rinse leaves a residual pesticide in the hair and, although this may continue to kill nymphs as they hatch from eggs, the reducing concentration of pesticide is likely to encourage resistance to emerge.

Although single, or infrequent, applications of these pesticides is considered safe, some chemicals, especially carbaryl and to a lesser extent malathion, are readily absorbed through the skin and repeated use may be harmful (Communicable Disease Report 1997). Carbaryl and pyrethroids are considered to be potential carcinogens (Calman et al 1995). Alcohol-based solutions are contraindicated in small children or asthmatics. Both local skin irritation and systemic effects such as headache, dizziness and general malaise have been reported (Antony et al 1997).

Resistance to pediculicides is thought to be common, although disputed by some (Burgess et al 1995, Communicable Disease Report 1997, Vander Stichele et al 1995) and high failure rates have been reported (Downs et al 1999). Attempts to prevent resistance emerging by rotating insecticide groups within health authorities have not been effective and are no longer recommended (Lowe 2000).

Unconventional treatments for head lice are available (e.g. essential oils), but their efficacy is unproven and they may also exhibit toxicity (Figueroa et al 1998).

Eradication of head lice by systematic combing In recent years, concerns about the inadequacy and toxicity of pediculicides has led to the development of a mechanical method of eradicating infection. This method, called 'Bug Busting', involves combing the hair with a fine-tooth comb after shampooing and while it is still wet. Lice stop moving when hair is wet and the addition of conditioner lubricates the hair, enabling the lice to be removed easily with the comb. Once the hair has been thoroughly combed, the conditioner should be rinsed out of the hair. The process should then be repeated three more times at intervals of 4 days (Fig. 15.1). This will ensure that any nymphs hatching from eggs in the hair will be removed before they are fully grown and able to lay more eggs. Provided all adult lice are removed on the initial combing and new lice are not acquired, the affected person will not transmit lice. Eggs are not easily removed by a fine-tooth comb, but as they hatch during the Bug Busting period the nymphs will be removed by combing (Figueroa et al 1998). This technique has been reported to be highly

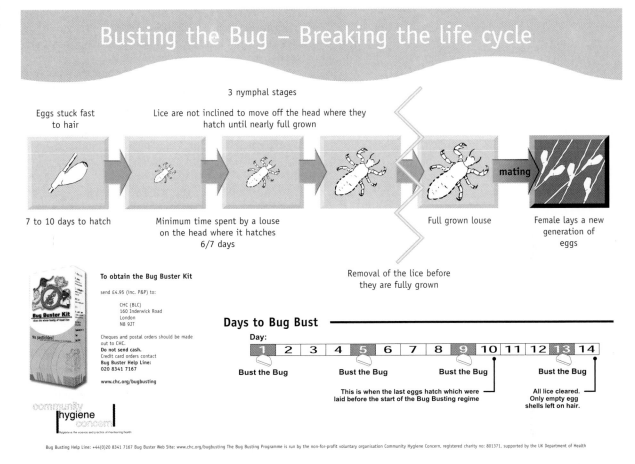

Busting the Bug – Breaking the life cycle

3 nymphal stages

Eggs stuck fast to hair

Lice are not inclined to move off the head where they hatch until nearly full grown

7 to 10 days to hatch

Minimum time spent by a louse on the head where it hatches 6/7 days

Full grown louse

mating

Female lays a new generation of eggs

Removal of the lice before they are fully grown

To obtain the Bug Buster Kit

send £4.95 (inc. P&P) to:

CHC (BLC)
160 Inderwick Road
London
N8 9JT

Cheques and postal orders should be made out to CHC.
Do not send cash.
Credit card orders contact
Bug Buster Help Line:
020 8341 7167

www.chc.org/bugbusting

community hygiene concern

Days to Bug Bust

Day:

| 1 | 2 | 3 | 4 | 5 | 6 | 7 | 8 | 9 | 10 | 11 | 12 | 13 | 14 |

Bust the Bug   Bust the Bug   Bust the Bug   Bust the Bug

This is when the last eggs hatch which were laid before the start of the Bug Busting regime

All lice cleared. Only empty egg shells left on hair.

Bug Busting Help Line: +44(0)20 8341 7167 Bug Buster Web Site: www.chc.org/bugbusting The Bug Busting Programme is run by the non-for-profit voluntary organisation Community Hygiene Concern, registered charity no: 801371, supported by the UK Department of Health

Fig. 15.1 Bug Busting: the eradication of head lice by systematic combing. From the poster 'Busting the bug – breaking the life cycle' 1999. Produced by the charity Community Hygiene Concern.

effective at eradicating infection and is particularly useful for treating children (Figueroa 2000, Ibarra & Hall 1996). However, there is controversy about the practicability of a mechanical method of lice eradication. A randomized controlled trial currently in progress should help to establish the efficacy of this treatment method (Bingham et al 2000).

Close family or friends who have had sufficient contact to enable transmission of lice should also be checked for infection. Head lice cannot be transmitted to others on clothing or linen and therefore no special precautions are necessary. Patients with head lice need not be **isolated**, except on paediatric wards where close contact between children may transmit the lice.

Crab (pubic) lice (Phthirus pubis)

The prevalence of infection with crab lice (phthiriasis) is unknown but probably common. These lice are

much broader and flatter than head lice and have large claws on the second and third pairs of legs (Fig. 15.2) which enable them to move around in the less dense

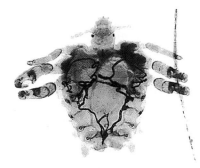

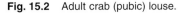
PHTHIRUS PUBIS (pubic, or crab louse)
female

Fig. 15.2 Adult crab (pubic) louse.

coarse body hair. Pubic and perianal hair is most frequently affected, but crab lice can infect all coarse body hair including hair on the axilla, chest, arms, beard, eyebrows and eyelashes, and may also affect head hair. Although frequently considered a sexually transmitted disease, phthiriasis is transmitted by other close physical contact, particularly within families. Children may acquire crab lice through contact with axillary, chest and arm hair. Crab lice are not transmitted on clothing, bed linen or other inanimate objects as, once off the body, they die rapidly.

The female louse lays several eggs on a single hair. These incubate for between 6 and 8 days, and after hatching the lice take 17 days to mature. It can take a minimum of 4–6 weeks for the host to react to the bite of the lice during which time they usually remain undetected, but once sensitized the itching around the affected area is severe.

Treatment and control Crab lice can be treated with the same formulations to those recommended for head lice but aqueous-based solutions are recommended for use on genital hair and phenothrin is not recommended as it causes irritation of the genitalia. The solution should be applied to all hairy parts of the body; a second treatment 7 days later is usually necessary to ensure eradication. A single application of shampoo or cream rinse formulation is unlikely to be effective.

If eyelashes or eyebrows are affected the lice can be eradicated by applying petroleum jelly twice a day for 10 days. This will kill the nymphs as they hatch (Figueroa et al 1998). The Bug Busting method described for the treatment of head lice can also be used to eradicate crab lice, but is unlikely to be effective unless carried out with assistance.

Crab lice on clothing or bedding are not transmitted to other people and can be removed by washing. **Isolation precautions** are not necessary.

Body louse (Pediculus humanus humanus)

The body louse is very similar to, but slightly larger than, the head louse. It causes pediculosis corporis, or infestation of clothing or bedding from where the lice visit the body to feed. It only affects people who are unable to change their clothes at regular intervals and nowadays is confined mostly to vagrants and people living on the streets. The louse lives in the clothing, laying its eggs in clusters on the fibres, especially the seams of underwear. Provided the clothing is worn continuously, nymphs hatch from the eggs after about eight days, but this will take longer if they are exposed to lower temperatures by removal of the clothing. The progress through nymphal moults varies according to the time in contact with the body. If worn continuously, the nymphs reach adulthood in approximately 8 days. If worn for only a few hours a day, this may take 3 weeks. Adult lice live for up to 30 days but will die of starvation after a few days if the clothes are removed and they are unable to feed. Although heavy infestation sometimes occurs, usually only 10 to 20 lice are present (Figueroa et al 1998). Bite marks usually occur along the seams of clothing, particularly underwear. They are often extremely itchy and may be accompanied by evidence of an inflammatory wheal around the bite.

Transmission occurs in overcrowded conditions by contact with infested clothing and bedding.

To survive, body lice depend on the same clothes being worn for prolonged periods, that are washed in cool water and then reworn immediately. They are therefore easy to eradicate as they will die if the clothing is not worn for 3 days and, provided the clothes are changed once a week, the young lice will not be able to feed when they hatch out of the eggs. Lice are also destroyed by washing clothes in hot water, and hot tumble-drying destroys both lice and eggs.

The human body louse is responsible for the transmission of a number of serious **infectious** diseases. Trench fever (Bartonella quintana) can be transmitted by lice. Borrelia recurrentis causes relapsing fever which is characterized by bouts of fever lasting for several weeks. It is a spirochaete which multiplies in the body of the louse and is transmitted to human hosts when the lice feeds. Although not seen in Europe now, cases do occur in Africa and South America. Typhus, caused by Rickettsia prowazeki, is a severe fever associated with a death rate of 10–20% and is transmitted by louse faeces entering a cut on the skin. Epidemics of typhus and relapsing fever are associated with cold, lack of fuel, overcrowding, famine and war – conditions that are conducive to louse infestation.

Treatment and control Clothing should be washed in hot water (60°C or more) and be changed at least once a week. Fifteen minutes in a hot tumble-dryer is sufficient to destroy both lice and eggs. No treatment of the skin or isolation precautions are necessary.

Scabies

Scabies is caused by a small mite, Sarcoptes scabiei (Fig. 15.3). It is a common infection and endemic in many developing countries. Epidemics are cyclical, with the prevalence of infection peaking every 10–30 years. In the UK reported cases of scabies have increased in the 1990s with outbreaks affecting schools, residential homes and hospitals, especially units for

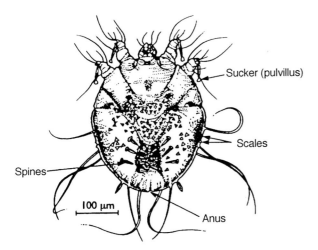

Fig. 15.3 The scabies mite *Sarcoptes scabiei* (dorsal view of female).

patients with acquired immune deficiency syndrome (AIDS) or the elderly (Barrett & Morse 1993).

The mites live in the deeper layers of the epidermis. The female burrows through the stratum corneum, tunnelling up to 5 mm a day. The male mite moves between burrows searching for a mate. A fertilized female lives for approximately 4–6 weeks during which time she lays between 40 and 50 eggs. Eggs hatch after 3–4 days and the larvae establish a new tunnel off the maternal burrow. They moult several times before becoming adults, 10–15 days later. On average an affected person will harbour between 15 and 20 female adult mites.

Despite the conventional view of scabies as a highly infectious disease, it is not easily transmitted from person to person and is not easily spread by social contact. The mite moves extremely slowly and therefore prolonged contact is required for it to move on to another host. It can be transmitted between family members and sexual partners and in hospital is often seen in care of the elderly and psychiatric settings where holding hands may be more common.

The majority of mites are found on the hands and wrists, especially where the skin is thin (e.g. between the fingers). However, they may also occur on the elbows, axillae and nipple areas, groins, buttocks and genitalia. They do not commonly spread to the head and neck except in the elderly or immune-deficient patients, and are unusual on the soles of the feet and palms of the hands, except in children (Taplin 1986).

The main symptoms of scabies infection are caused by an allergic response to the presence of the mite. Sever itching, especially at night, develops 2–6 weeks after the first infection. An allergic rash with erythematous papules, vesicles or itchy nodules appears, characteris-

tically affecting the body symmetrically on the arms, trunk, waist, inner thighs and calves. The rash and itching are not necessarily related to the site of the mites (Maunder 1983). Sarcoptes also affect animals, for example causing mange in dogs. Whilst these mites are usually unable to establish on a human host, exposure to the mite faeces on the animal may cause sensitized individuals to develop a scabies-like allergic rash.

If the person has had a previous infection with the scabies mite, the immune response is rapid and itching develops within hours. The mite may then be killed before it can re-establish an infection.

The appearance of a generalized rash or itch may be diagnosed as scabies, but because of the implications of contact tracing and treatment of contacts it is important to make a definite diagnosis. Burrows are not easily seen but may be visible as tiny white lines, 15–30 cm long and with a (0.5 mm) brown spot, the female mite, at one end. To an experienced eye these are diagnostic of scabies. However, the diagnosis can be confirmed by the examination of skin scrapings from a suspected burrow under the microscope to detect parasites, their eggs or faecal pellets. These are more easily obtained from the skin if a drop of mineral oil is applied before gently collecting scrapings with a needle or scalpel blade.

Norwegian (crusted) scabies

This form of scabies occurs when the scabies mite infects a person with a deficiency of their immune system, caused by either disease or **immunosuppressive** therapy. In the absence of a normal immune system the body cannot control the mite infection, and the mite multiplies rapidly, causing many thousands of mites to spread all over the body, including the head. This widespread infection usually results in hyperkeratotic (crusted) lesions, particularly on the nailbeds, palms, soles, wrists, buttocks and penis, and is known as Norwegian scabies. Sometimes the presentation may be atypical, with no crusted lesions or itching, despite widespread infections with large numbers of mites. Skin scales and crusts are heavily contaminated with mites and affected individuals are highly infectious.

Outbreaks of scabies, from an unrecognized index case of Norwegian scabies, commonly spread through nursing homes or elderly care units and may result in many patients and staff becoming infected (Anderson et al 2000). Particular problems are associated with wards caring for a high proportion of patients with AIDS, where rapid spread may occur and several cases of Norwegian scabies may develop as a result (Sirera et al 1990). Contacts with a normal immune system may develop conventional scabies.

Treatment and control There are two main forms of treatment for scabies: malathion (lotion) and permethrin (cream). These should be applied to the whole body except the head and neck, and left on for up to 24 h. The lotion should be reapplied to the hands when they are washed. Benzylbenzoate can also be used but is not recommended for initial treatment as it does not destroy the mite eggs. In cases of Norwegian scabies or where children or the elderly are infected, treatment should include the neck, face, scalp and ears (*British National Formulary* 1999). A single treatment is usually sufficient but if the infestation is severe a second application one week later may be required. Treatment of pregnant women, nursing mothers or children should be under medical supervision. Recently an oral drug, ivermectin, has been shown to be effective against scabies and may be useful for the treatment of severe infections and for controlling outbreaks (Anderson et al 2000, Griffin et al 1999).

Patients should be a warned that itching persists for some time after treatment because it takes a few days for the allergic response to subside even though the mites have been killed. Retreatment is not indicated unless itching persists for longer than 1 week.

All close contacts of the affected person should be treated at the same time even if they are asymptomatic because of the long delay between infection and the development of symptoms.

Scabies mites are not readily transmitted by clothes or bed linen, and these items should be laundered normally using hot water and a dryer (Barrett & Morse 1993, Maunder 1992, Robinson 1986).

Patients with scabies do not require isolation as actual skin-to-skin contact is required to transmit infection. However, patients with Norwegian scabies are highly **contagious** and isolation precautions are recommended until treatment has been completed. No special treatment of clothing, bedding or the environment is required (Maunder 1992).

Early identification of cases is essential to control spread and ensure effective treatment of affected patients and their contacts. Staff should be vigilant for cases of scabies in nursing and residential homes for the elderly or in units caring for immunocompromised patients. These should have established procedures for diagnosing and managing cases of scabies, and for the identification and simultaneous treatment of contacts.

INFESTATION OF THE ENVIRONMENT

Healthcare premises provide an ideal environment in which pests can flourish. They are warm and full of people whose habits inevitably provide a constant source of food. Pests can be described as animals or insects that cause damage, annoyance or, in some cases, present a risk of infection.

Pests that most commonly infest hospitals are cockroaches, Pharaoh's ants, fleas, birds, rodents and cats. Although it is unlikely that all pests could be totally eradicated from hospitals or other centres of healthcare, an effective and continuous strategy to control their numbers is essential. Healthcare staff have a crucial role to play in the reporting of pests or signs of infestation and should be aware of the system of reporting and treating infestations that occur in their place of work. Pests frequently appear only at night and are not easily observed. Even small signs should be reported. The sighting of a single cockroach, egg case or mouse dropping is probably indicative of an infestation problem.

The Department of Health recommends that each hospital or unit of management should nominate a pest control officer (PCO) with responsibility for all aspects of pest control (NHS Management Executive 1992). These individuals should be trained in the recognition of pests and methods of controlling them, keep a record of pest sightings, investigate reports and ensure that appropriate action is taken. Most hospitals have a contract with a pest control servicing company that will treat infestations and inspect the site regularly for pests. The PCO is responsible for liaison with the contractor and monitoring the contract. This may involve periodic inspections of the site at night when the activity of many pests is at its greatest. In large complex buildings, information on pest sightings from staff is particularly valuable.

Cockroaches

Cockroaches have existed for millions of years and there are over 3000 different species. The two most common species in the UK are the German (*Blattella germanica*) and oriental (*Blatta orientalis*) cockroach; American (*Periplaneta americana*) and brown banded cockroaches are only rarely seen. Any large building that is warm is prone to infestation.

Cockroaches feed on an enormous variety of meat and vegetable matter including sewage and organic waste. They also need a supply of water and cavities in which to hide. They can live in tiny cracks and crevices and behind wall and floor tiles and, because they are strongly nocturnal, infestation often goes unnoticed until the population is very large. The life cycle of the cockroach includes three stages: the eggs are enclosed within a capsule; they hatch out as nymphs – smaller, wingless versions of the adult insect which after several moults mature into adults. Some species hide their eggs in cracks; German cockroaches carry them until nearly ready to hatch; whereas Oriental cockroaches abandon them. Both German and oriental adult cockroaches have wings but do not fly.

The German cockroach is the smallest, about 12 mm long, and accounts for about 10% of cockroach infestations. Its common name is the 'steamfly' as it prefers warm and humid conditions and is therefore most commonly found in kitchens. It is good at climbing and may be found in heated trolleys, vending machines, refrigerator motors and behind false ceilings. The oriental cockroach is larger, about 25 mm long, and accounts for about 90% of all cockroach infestations in heated buildings (Fig. 15.4a). However, it can tolerate cooler conditions and so may be found outside, around the perimeter of buildings and in drains and underground ducting. The American cockroach is the largest species found in the UK, about 35 mm long. It needs access to water and warm conditions of between 24 and 33°C, and is usually found in large heated greenhouses and in ports and airports where it is introduced from abroad on ships or aeroplanes.

Many hundreds of cockroaches can live in gaps behind tiles, gaining access through breaks or cracks (Fig. 15.4b). Nursing staff can help to discourage infestation in ward areas by employing simple preventive measures: storing food in tight-fitting containers and secure cupboards, not leaving out prepared food, discarding waste food and refuse promptly, and ensuring that leaking pipes and damaged surfaces are repaired (DHSS 1984, Smith 1988).

Many bacteria have been isolated from the bodies and faecal droppings of cockroaches, which they probably acquire through feeding on food, decaying matter and faeces. The microbes they carry reflect the microbial flora of the environment in which they live (Bennett 1993, Fotedar et al 1991). Although it is difficult to prove that cockroaches are responsible for particular cases of infection, they could in theory transmit infection if allowed to crawl over working surfaces or prepared food. Circumstantial evidence for transmission of infection by cockroaches was provided by Graffar & Mertens (1950) who reported an outbreak of *Salmonella typhimurium* in a Brussels children's ward. Cockroaches were observed running over the children and their bedclothing by a night nurse. *S. typhimurium* was isolated from one of the captured insects and the outbreak came to an end once the infestation had been eradicated. Cotton et al (2000) reported an outbreak of antibiotic-resistant *Klebsiella pneumoniae* in a neonatal unit infested with cockroaches. Although the outbreak micro-organism was

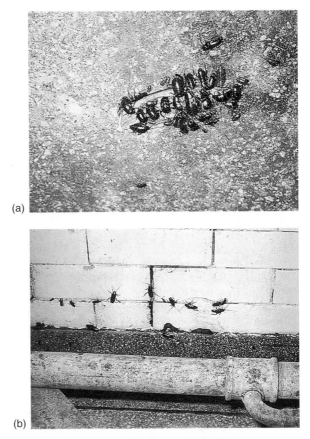

(a)

(b)

Fig. 15.4 (a) Adults and nymphs of the oriental cockroach feeding on a courgette discarded in a kitchen yard. (b) Mixture of oriental and German cockroaches on a kitchen wall. Notice also the slugs!

found on cockroaches, there was no direct evidence that these were responsible for the transmission of infection; other factors such as overcrowding and understaffing were probably of greater significance.

Ants

Garden ants, attracted by food debris, may occasionally cause a minor problem in buildings but are easily controlled by treatment with insecticide. Far more serious problems can be caused by Pharaoh's ants, tiny insects 1–2 mm long which can invade equipment and contaminate food (Fig. 15.5). Originally introduced from tropical countries, they can survive easily in centrally heated buildings in temperate climates. Nest colonies each containing several thousand worker ants are sited in almost any concealed area, for example behind tiles, light fittings and in brickwork. Nests have been found in heated food trolleys, drink-vending

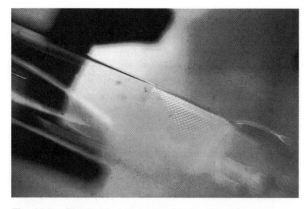

Fig. 15.5 Pharoah's ants trapped in the filter of an administration set.

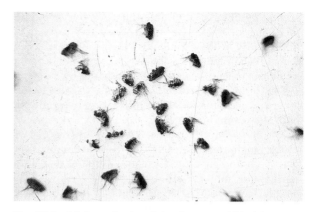

Fig. 15.6 Mixture of cat and dog fleas caught in 1 h on sticky tape in a radiography department.

machines and **autoclave** units. They eat both meat and vegetable matter but prefer meat and sweet substances. They can chew through plastic and have been found in intravenous fluid administration sets and sterile packs (Beatson 1973). They will also search out suppurative lesions and feed on the discharge from the wound.

Infestation in operating theatres or central sterile supply departments enables ants to invade sterile packs. Infestation in the laundry or other service departments results in ants being transferred throughout the hospital. They can also spread through ducting.

There is some evidence that these ants can transmit infection and indeed they are more likely to be found in contact with patients and their equipment than more shy insects, such as cockroaches. A large range of bacteria, including pseudomonas, staphylococci and enterobacter, have been isolated from the surface of their bodies (Beatson 1972). Their affinity for moist areas such as sinks, toilets and sluices means they could acquire **pathogenic** bacteria on their bodies and transfer them on to food, into sterile packs or on to patients' wounds.

Suspected infestation with Pharoah's ants should be reported promptly to the PCO so that extensive treatment by a professional pest control company can be carried out without delay.

Fleas

There are more than 1000 species of flea and, although they feed on any warm-blooded animal, they require a specific host on which to breed. Human fleas are now rarely encountered. They dislike the warm, dry environment of modern homes and are usually found only in association with vagrants or homeless people. They live in the environment, feeding infrequently from their hosts, and should be treated by washing infested clothing and applying insecticide to the environment.

Cat and dog fleas (Fig. 15.6) are responsible for most flea bites on humans (Watkins & Wyatt 1989). They thrive in the warm, dry environment of the domestic home and live in furniture and carpets, jumping on to passing animals and humans for food. The bites are commonly seen on the ankles and lower legs, although many people become desensitized to them and do not develop an immune response to the bite. Infestations in hospitals may originate from colonies of feral cats or animals kept as pets and can be very troublesome. Feral cats living in ducting or basements may support a large population of fleas which may then gain access to the building. Cat flea infestations have even been responsible for the closure of an operating department and a laundry (Baker 1981). If infestation with fleas is suspected in a hospital department, the pest control officer should be contacted who will arrange for the source of the infestation to be identified and treated with insecticides.

Preventing flea infestations depends on control of feral cat populations by neutering. Pet animals should be sprayed regularly with insecticide and bedding should also be treated. The environmental health department of the local authority or a company specializing in pest control can be called in to treat severe infestation with fleas in the home.

Birds

Birds, particularly pigeons and house sparrows, become pests when their population is large enough to cause a nuisance, either by fouling, noise or secondary pests such as mites and fleas. Roosting can be deterred by nets, wires, spikes, etc. and they should be prevented from gaining access to buildings. To avoid attracting birds refuse must be carefully sited, spillages cleared up promptly and deliberate feeding discouraged.

Rodents

The main rodent pests are rats and mice. They can cause damage to furnishings, spoil food and may also carry pathogenic bacteria. They are often detected by evidence of damage or droppings. Rodents can be discouraged by storing food in tightly closing containers or secure cupboards, and discarding waste promptly. Waste for disposal should not be stored for prolonged periods and the storage area should be kept clean and tidy.

REFERENCES

Anderson BM, Haugen H, Rasch M et al (2000) Outbreak of scabies in Norwegian nursing homes and home care patients: control and prevention. *J. Hosp. Infect.*, **45**: 160–4.

Antony H, Birtwhistle S, Eaton K et al (1997) *Environmental Medicine in Clinical Practice*. British Society for Allergy Environmental and Nutritional Medicine, Southampton.

Baker LF (1981) Pests in hospital. *J. Hosp. Infect.*, **2**: 5–9.

Barrett NJ, Morse DL (1993) The resurgence of scabies. *CDR*, **3**(2): R32–3.

Beatson SH (1972) Pharaoh's ants as pathogen vectors in hospitals. *Lancet*, i: 425–7.

Beatson SH (1973) Pharoah's ants enter giving sets. *Lancet*, i: 606.

Bennett G (1993) Cockroaches as carriers of bacteria. *Lancet*, i: 732.

Bingham P, Kirk S, Hill N et al (2000) The methodology and operation of a pilot randomised control trial of the effectiveness of the Bug Busting method against a single application insecticide product for head louse treatment. *Public Health*, **114**: 265–8.

British National Formulary (1999) British Medical Association & Royal Pharmaceutical Society of Great Britain, London.

Burgess IF, Peock S, Brown CM et al (1995) Head lice resistant to pyrethroid insecticides in Britain. *BMJ*, **311**: 752.

Calman KC, Moores Y, Hartley BH (1995) *Carbaryl*. PL CMO (95)4. Department of Health, London.

Communicable Disease Report (1997) Head lice. *CDR Weekly* **7**(41): 365.

Cotton MF, Wasserman E, Pieper CH et al (2000) Invasive disease due to extended spectrum beta-lactamase-producing *Klebsiella pneumonia* in a neonatal unit: the possible role of cockroaches. *J. Hosp. Infect.*, **44**: 13–17.

Department of Health and Social Security (1984) *An Introduction to Pest Control in Hospitals*, Domestic Services Management Advice Notes. HMSO, London.

Downs AMR, Stafford KA, Harvey I et al (1999) Evidence for double resistance to permethrin and malathion in head lice. *Br. J. Dermatol.*, **141**: 508–11.

Figueroa JI (2000) Head lice: is there a solution? *Curr. Opin. Infect. Dis.*, **13**: 135–9.

Figueroa J, Hall S, Ibarra J (eds) (1998) *Primary Health Care Guide to Common UK Parasitic Disease*, 1st edn. Community Hygiene Concern, London.

Fotedar R, Shrinivas U, Banerjee U et al (1991) Nosocomial infections: cockroaches as possible vectors of drug-resistant klebsiella. *J. Hosp. Infect.*, **18**: 155–9.

Graffar M, Mertens S (1950) Le role des blattes dans la transmission des salmonelloses. *Ann. Inst. Pasteur*, **79**: 654–60.

Griffin GE et al (1999) Disease due to infection. In *Davidson's Principles and Practice of Medicine* (C Haslett et al, eds). Churchill Livingstone, Edinburgh.

Ibarra J (1989) Headlice in schools. *Health at School*, **4**: 147–51.

Ibarra J, Hall DMB (1996) Headlice in school children. *Arch. Dis. Child.*, **75**: 471–3.

Lowe J (2000) Are you up to scratch? *Nursing Times*, **96**(3): 51–2.

Maunder J (1983) The increase in scabies. *Postgrad. Doctor*, **6**: 198–202.

Maunder J (1992) The scourge of scabies. *Chemist and Druggist*, **Jan 11**: 54–5.

Maunder J (1993) An update on headlice. *Health Visitor*, **66**(9): 317–18.

NHS Management Executive (1992) *Pest Control Management for the Health Service*, HSG(92)35. Department of Health, Wetherby, UK.

Robinson R (1986) Scratching the surface. *Nursing Times*, **34** (Dec 3): 71–2.

Sirera G, Ruis F, Romeu J et al (1990) Hospital outbreak of scabies stemming from two AIDS patients with Norwegian scabies. *Lancet*, **335**: 1227.

Smith P (1988) An unpleasant case of cracked tiles. *Health Services Journal*, **26 May** (S): 6.

Taplin D (1986) Cutaneous infestations. In *Modern Management of Skin Diseases*, pp. 18–25 (CFH Vickers, ed.). Churchill Livingstone, Edinburgh.

Vander Stichele RH, Dezere EM, Bogaert MG (1995) Systematic review of clinical efficacy of topical treatments for head lice. *BMJ*, **311**: 604–8.

Watkins M, Wyatt T (1989) A ticklish problem; pest infestation in hospitals. *Prof. Nurse*, **May**: 369–92.

FURTHER READING

Commens CA (1994) We can get rid of scabies: new treatment available soon. *Med. J. Aust.*, **160**: 317–18.

Community Hygiene Concern (2000) *Bug Buster Teaching Pack.*, CHC, 160 Inderwick Road, London N8 9JT (Tel: 020 8421 7167). Available: http://www.chc.org/bugbusting

Department of Health (1998) The prevention and treatment of head lice. Online. Available: http://www.doh.gov.uk/headlice/index.htm

Health Service Pest Control (1988) *Health Services Journal* (Suppl.) **26 May**.

Henderson C (1991) Community control of scabies. *Lancet*, **337**: 1548.

Lane RP, Crossley RW (1993) *Medical Insects and Arachnids*, pp. 517–28. Chapman & Hall, London.

Public Health Laboratory Service (1998) Working document combs out guidance on head lice. *CDR*, **8**(46).

Public Health Medicine Environmental Group (1996) *Guidelines on the Control of Infection in Residential and Nursing Homes*. Department of Health, London.

Glossary

Abscess A localized collection of pus.

Active immunity Immunity that develops in response to a stimulus (e.g. infection or vaccine) and is dependent on the production of B and T lymphocytic memory cells.

Acute infection An infection that runs its course in a relatively short period.

Adenosine triphosphate A chemical compound that contains energy-rich bonds and serves as the main 'energy currency' of the cell. It breaks down into adenosine diphosphate and a phosphate ion, releasing energy.

Aerobe A microbe that grows in the presence of oxygen. A strict aerobe requires oxygen. *See* anaerobe.

Agar A polysaccharide made from seaweed and used to solidify bacteriological media.

Agglutinate To stick to one another, clump (of particles, red cells, etc.); the result is agglutination.

Algae Photosynthetic microbes; the blue-green algae are procaryotes and the others are eucaryotes.

Allergic response An exaggerated immune response to an antigen resulting in histamine release, inflammation and tissue damage. The effects may be localized (e.g. hay fever, asthma) or systemic (e.g. anaphylactic shock).

Allergy An undesirable immune response due to hypersensitivity to an antigen.

Amino acid An organic acid, constituent of proteins. It has the structure $R-C-COOH$
$$| $$
$$NH_2$$

Amoeba A eucaryotic organism that lacks a rigid cell wall and moves by means of pseudopods.

Anaerobe A microbe that grows in the absence of oxygen. A strict anaerobe will not grow in the presence of oxygen; a facultative anaerobe can grow in the presence or absence of oxygen.

Anaphylaxis A hypersensitivity reaction.

Antagonism One drug interferes with another so that the sum of the effect is less than if either were given alone (e.g. penicillin and tetracycline).

Antibiotic A substance that is toxic to micro-organisms; the first antibiotics to be used were derived from other micro-organisms, but many are now partly or wholly synthesized (= antimicrobial agent).

Antibody A protein produced by B lymphocytes which appears in the body fluids after contact with a foreign molecule ('antigen') and which combines specifically with that antigen.

Antigen *See* antibody.

Antimicrobial agent *See* antibiotic.

Antiseptic A chemical used to kill microbes on body surfaces.

Antiserum A serum that contains antibodies to a particular antigen.

Antitoxin A serum containing antibodies to a toxin, either as a result of natural infection or, more often, in response to injection of toxoid.

Arthropod An animal that has a hard outer 'skeleton' and jointed legs; examples are insects, ticks and lice.

Aseptic Free of micro-organisms.

ATP See adenosine triphosphate.

Attenuated A microbe that has lost its virulence and can be safely used as a vaccine.

Autoclave A machine in which materials are exposed to steam under pressure and therefore at a temperature higher than that of boiling water.

Autogenous From within the individual.

Bacillus Any rod-shaped bacterium; also the name of a genus of Gram-positive bacteria, often found in soil and dust.

Bacteraemia The presence of bacteria in the blood without clinical signs or symptoms of infection.

Bactericidal Capable of killing bacteria (e.g. penicillins).

Bacteriophage A virus that infects bacterial cells.

Bacteriostatic A drug that prevents bacteria from replicating; if the drug is withdrawn, bacteria can multiply again (e.g. tetracycline). (A drug that is bacteriostatic may in high concentration or in certain circumstances become bactericidal, e.g. fusidic acid.)

Bacteriuria The presence of micro-organisms in the bladder with no signs or symptoms of infection.

Basophil A white cell of the blood. It attracts lymphocytes to the site of an infection by releasing vasoactive chemicals that increase blood flow to the area.

BCG An attenuated strain of tubercle bacilli that is used as a vaccine against tuberculosis.

Binary fission Division of one cell into two daughter cells; the usual method of reproduction in bacteria.

Biofilm A film of proteins and micro-organisms that forms over the surface of foreign material when it is in contact with tissue.

B lymphocyte One of the two main cell types of the immune system, chiefly involved in the production of antibodies.

Broad spectrum Agents that work against many types of bacteria. Often used for initial treatment when the cause of an infection is unknown.

Capsid Protein coat of a virus made from polypeptide subunits.

Capsule A slimy substance, usually polysaccharides, that forms a protective layer around some bacterial cells.

Carbohydrate A compound of carbon, hydrogen and oxygen in a ratio of two hydrogen molecules to each oxygen and carbon molecules (e.g. glucose = $C_6H_{12}O_6$).

Carrier An individual who has a body surface colonized by a pathogen, but without being affected by disease.

Catalyst A substance that increases the rate of a chemical reaction, but is itself unchanged by the reaction.

Cell-mediated immunity The part of the immune response mediated by T lymphocytes and directed against intracellular pathogens, (e.g. viruses, malignant cells).

Cell wall The rigid outer layer of most procaryotic cells and of some eucaryotic cells.

Cellulose A carbohydrate composed of glucose molecules; an important constituent of plant cell walls.

Centrifuge An instrument that can spin liquids in containers at high speed, thus depositing particles on the bottom of the tube. It is often used to concentrate bacteria from body fluids for examination.

Chemotaxis Movement of a cell in response to the presence of a chemical.

Chlorophyll A green pigment found in plants and some bacteria that absorbs light to provide energy for the synthesis of carbohydrates from water and carbon dioxide (photosynthesis).

Chromosome Contains the genetic information of the cell and is composed of long threads of DNA and associated proteins.

Clone A group of organisms descended from a single parent by asexual reproduction and therefore exact copies of it.

Coccobacillus A short oval rod, i.e. between a coccus and a bacillus in shape.

Coccus A spherical bacterium.

Colonization A microbe that establishes itself in a particular environment such as a body surface without producing disease is said to 'colonize' the site.

Colony When a bacterial cell (or a few cells) multiplies on a solid medium until the group is visible to the naked eye, the group is called a colony. A typical colony contains 10–100 million cells.

Commensal A commensal organism lives in association with another, without benefiting or harming it. Many members of the gut flora appear to be commensals. Commensals may be pathogenic if the host is immunocompromised.

Communicable A disease that can be transmitted from one person to another is communicable (*syn.* contagious, infectious).

Community-acquired infection An infection acquired in the community, not as a result of treatment in hospital.

Complement A complex of proteins in the blood that promote the activity of phagocytic cells; the sequential reactions between the component proteins are triggered by micro-organisms or an antigen–antibody complex.

Conjugation The transfer of genetic material from one bacterial cell to another by the formation of a small tube between them (sex pilus).

Conjugative plasmid A plasmid that carries the genes required to form a sex pilus and transfer plasmid DNA into another cell.

Contagious *See* communicable.

Counterstain A stain used to enhance contrast in a differential stain.

Culture A culture of microbes is the result of inoculating a medium with them and incubating it until large numbers are present.

Cystitis Infection of the bladder.

Cytoplasm In a procaryote, everything inside the cytoplasmic membrane; in a eucaryote, everything inside the cytoplasmic membrane, except the nucleus.

Cytoplasmic membrane The membrane that surrounds the cell and retains the cytoplasm.

Delayed(-type) hypersensitivity A hypersensitivity reaction that develops 24 h or more after exposure to an antigen.

Denaturation (a) Of proteins: the loss of folding brought about by heat or chemicals; associated with the loss of normal biological activity. (b) Of DNA: breaking the hydrogen bonds that hold two DNA strands together, resulting in their separation.

Deoxyribonucleic acid (DNA) The large molecule in which genetic information is encoded, the genetic material. The component nucleotides contain the sugar deoxyribose.

Dermatophyte A fungus that infects the skin, hair and nails without invading the deeper tissues.

Diffusion The process whereby random movement of molecules tends to equalize their concentration across areas of higher and lower concentration.

Diploid A diploid cell contains two copies of each chromosome. The body cells of most eucaryotic organisms are diploid.

Disinfection A process that reduces the number of micro-organisms to a level at which they are not harmful, but which does not usually destroy spores.

DNA See deoxyribonucleic acid.

Dysentery A severe form of infectious diarrhoea, characterized by blood and mucus in the stools.

Ectoparasite A parasite that lives on the outer surface of the host (e.g. a tick or louse).

Electron A negatively charged particle.

Electron microscope A microscope in which a beam of electrons is used instead of light rays to produce an image.

Electrophoresis The separation of molecules by subjecting them to an electric field in which they move at different rates.

ELISA (enzyme-linked immunosorbent assay) A technique for detecting antigens and antibodies, in which a coloured compound is formed by an enzyme linked to the detector antibody.

Encephalitis Inflammation of the brain.

Endemic If a disease is endemic, cases regularly occur in the population with little variation in incidence. *See* epidemic.

Endocarditis An inflammation, especially one due to infection, of the lining of the heart, including its valves.

Endogenous From within the body; an endogenous infection is caused by micro-organisms that are part of the normal flora.

Endoplasmic reticulum A complicated membrane system extending throughout the cytoplasm of the eucaryotic cell.

Endotoxin Lipopolysaccharides in outer membrane of Gram-negative cells. When cells are lysed these are released and may cause severe systemic symptoms (endotoxic shock).

Envelope An outer membrane that surrounds the capsid of some viruses and may be derived partly or wholly from the host cell.

Enzyme A protein that catalyses a biochemical reaction.

Eosinophil A white cell of the blood whose main role is to attack large micro-organisms (e.g. protozoa).

Epidemic When the incidence of an endemic infection increases to an unusually high level or infections not usually seen in that population occur.

Epidemiology The study of the occurrence of diseases, how and when they occur, how and why they are transmitted.

Erythema A reddening of the skin caused by dilatation of capillary blood vessels; often a sign of inflammation or infection.

Eucaryotic cell One of two types of living cells, in which the nucleus is delimited from the cytoplasm by a membrane.

Exogenous From outside the body; compare with 'endogenous'. Exogenous infections are caused by micro-organisms acquired from another person, animal or the environment.

Exotoxin Proteins secreted by bacteria that damage host tissues.

Facultative An organism that can adapt its metabolism; thus a facultative anaerobe can live in the absence or presence of oxygen.

Fermentation Production of energy from carbohydrates in the absence of oxygen. The electrons generated are passed to organic molecules.

Fibrin The final product of blood coagulation, formed by the action of the enzyme thrombin on the precursor fibrinogen. Makes a mesh that seals off damaged blood vessels (i.e. a clot).

Flagellum A hair-like appendage on the surface of the cell and used for locomotion.

Fluorescent antibody technique A technique for detecting microbes in which the antibody is tagged with fluorescent dyes and thus rendered visible when viewed with a special microscope (fluorescence microscope) in which ultraviolet light is used.

Fomites Inanimate objects or material on which disease-producing agents may be conveyed (e.g. patients' personal possessions such as bedding, clothes).

Gangrene Death of tissue or part of the body due to deficiency or cessation of the blood supply.

Gas gangrene Death of tissue or part of the body due to infection by *Clostridium perfringens*.

Gene A 'unit of heredity'; a segment of DNA that encodes the structure of a protein.

Genome The complete set of genes contained in the chromosomes.

Genus In biological nomenclature, the genus is the larger grouping and is written with a capital; the species is the smaller grouping. Both words are modern Latin and are printed in italics when the species name is given.

Glycocalyx A more or less diffuse layer outside the cell wall of procaryotes; it consists of polysaccharide, polypeptide, or both.

Glycogen A polysaccharide stored by animals and some bacteria.

Golgi complex An organelle present in the cytoplasm of eucaryotic cells; it is involved in the secretion of proteins from the cell.

Gram stain A staining procedure that distinguishes two types of prokaryote: Gram-positive and Gram-negative.

Granulocytes Phagocytic cells of the immune system that circulate in the blood. There are three types: neutrophils (the largest proportion), basophils and eosinophils.

Haemolysin An enzyme that lyses red cells. Many bacteria produce haemolysins.

Haploid A haploid cell contains only one copy of each chromosome. The cells of procaryotic organisms are haploid. Compare with 'diploid'.

Heat labile Easily destroyed by heat.

Helix, helical Spiral.

Herd immunity Protection of an entire population against a particular infection, through the induction of immunity in at least 60% of individuals.

Histamine A molecule released by mast cells; it causes increased permeability of blood vessels, and is responsible for the signs of inflammation; excess is associated with hay fever, asthma, etc.

Histocompatibility antigens Cell surface antigens involved in many aspects of immunological recognition; they are the main antigens recognized in the rejection of grafts. In humans the chief group of such antigens is called the HLA system.

Hospital-acquired infection An infection acquired as a result of treatment in hospital.

Humoral immune system Antibody production by B lymphocytes.

Hypersensitivity An exaggerated or inappropriate immune response, leading to inflammation or tissue damage.

Icosahedron A solid figure with 12 (vertices) corners and 20 triangular faces.

Immunity Protection against infection by a particular microbe. Results from infection by or immunization against that microbe.

Immunization The process of artificially inducing immunity to infection by a microbe.

Immunocompromised Impaired immune response that renders the host particularly susceptible to infection.

Immunoglobulin An antibody.

Incidence The number of new cases occurring in a population over time.

Incubation period The interval between contact with the microbe and the development of the symptoms and signs of infection.

Infection Entry of a harmful microbe into the body and its multiplication in the tissues.

Inflammation A response to infection or other injury characterized by swelling, heat, redness and pain.

Inoculum Material (containing bacteria) added to a growth medium to initiate a culture; hence 'inoculate'.

Interferons A group of immunological proteins that carry signals between cells.

Interleukins Immunological proteins, messenger molecules released by cells of the immune system.

In vitro 'In glass', i.e. carried out in the test-tube, in the laboratory.

In vivo 'In the living', i.e. in the animal (or patient).

Latent infection A condition in which the clinical signs of infection are absent and the causative organism may be temporarily undetectable; under certain conditions the infection may again become obvious.

Leucocyte *See* granulocytes.

Lipid A fat; a molecule made up of glycerol and fatty acids.

Lipopolysaccharide A constituent of the Gram-negative bacterial cell wall, in which chains of various sugars are linked to lipid A.

Lymphocytes Cells involved in the specific immune response. B lymphocytes produce antibodies; T lymphocytes attack intracellular pathogens and malignant cells and coordinate the activity of other immune system cells.

Lysis Destruction or decomposition of a cell under the influence of a specific agent.

Lysosome An intracellular organelle; contains enzymes that digest unwanted molecules.

Lysozyme An enzyme that can dissolve the cell walls of certain bacteria.

Macrophage A type of phagocyte mainly found in the tissues.

Malaise A general feeling of being unwell.

Mantoux test A tuberculin skin test.

Mast cell Mediator cells in the tissues that influence the response of the immune system by releasing vasoactive chemicals (e.g. histamine). Responsible for the inflammatory response and hypersensitivity reactions.

Meiosis A form of cell division, characteristic of eucaryotic cells; it result in haploid progeny cells (male and female gametes).

Messenger RNA The transcript of the DNA from which a polypeptide is synthesized by the ribosome.

Metabolism A general term for all the biochemical processes that occur in a living cell.

Metabolite Breakdown products of the process of metabolism.

Micro-organism A creature too small to be seen with the naked eye (or only just visible); the term includes bacteria, fungi, protozoa, some of the algae and the viruses.

Minimum inhibitory concentration (MIC) The lowest concentration of an antibiotic or other agent that will inhibit the growth of a micro-organism.

Mitochondrion An intracellular organelle that contains the energy-generating systems of eucaryotic cells.

Mitosis Division of a eucaryotic cell into two diploid daughter cells.

Monocyte A white cell of the blood, which develops into the tissue macrophage.

Mutation A change in the sequence of the bases in the DNA strand.

Myalgia Pain in the muscles, a feature of many viral infections.

Mycelium An intertwined mass of filaments (hyphae), typical of the growth of fungi.

Mycoses Infections caused by fungi; can be superficial (e.g. affecting the skin) or deep, invading tissue and causing systemic infection.

Narrow spectrum An antibiotic with activity against only one, or a limited range of, bacteria.

Natural killer cells Large lymphoid cells capable of killing cells with the appropriate receptors on the surface.

Neutrophil A phagocytic white cell of the blood. Accounts for the greatest proportion of white cells circulating in the blood.

Normal flora The community of microbes that colonize a body surface.

Nosocomial Acquired or occurring in a hospital; for example, a nosocomial infection = a hospital-acquired infection.

Nuclease An enzyme that catalyses the breakdown of nucleic acids.

Nucleic acid The organic acids DNA and RNA that carry the genetic code of the cell.

Nucleolus An area in the nucleus of a eucaryotic cell where RNA is synthesized.

Nucleotide The components of DNA or RNA, made up of a sugar, an organic base and a phosphate group.

Nucleus (a) The central part of an atom, made up of protons and neutrons; or (b) the part of the eucaryotic cell that contains the genetic material.

Objective lens The lens of a microscope that forms the primary image of the specimen.

Obligate An obligate organism is restricted to a particular way of life; for example, an obligate parasite cannot live free without a host; an obligate aerobe cannot live without oxygen.

Ocular lens The lens of a microscope that further magnifies the primary image formed by the objective lens.

Opportunistic organism One capable of causing infection when the immune system of the host is impaired.

Organelle A distinct structure within the cytoplasm of a eucaryotic cell that possesses a separate function (e.g. the mitochondria, Golgi complex).

Organic compound Contains carbon.

Osmosis The movement of a solvent (e.g. water) from a less concentrated to a more concentrated solution through a semipermeable membrane.

Oxidation The addition of oxygen to, or the removal of electrons from, a substance.

Pandemic A worldwide outbreak of an infectious disease.

Parasite An organism that lives in or on another creature and obtains food and shelter without benefiting the host. Hence 'parasitism'. *See* commensal, symbiosis.

Parenteral Administered by injection directly into the tissues (e.g. subcutaneously, intramuscularly, intravenously).

Passive immunity Immunity conferred on the host animal by antibodies made in another host.

Pathogen A microbe capable of causing disease.

Pathogenicity The ability of a microbe to invade and cause disease.

Peptide A chain of amino acids.

Peptidoglycan A major structural component of bacterial cell walls, consisting of chains of sugars crosslinked by peptides.

Peptones Short chains of amino acids derived from the breakdown of proteins.

pH The symbol denoting hydrogen ion concentration; the pH ranges between 0 and 14, and its value indicates the relative acidity or alkalinity of a solution.

Phage *See* bacteriophage.

Phagocyte A cell capable of phagocytosis.

Phagocytosis The ingestion of material by a cell either in order to destroy foreign matter or for its own nutrition.

Photosynthesis The use of solar energy by green plants and some bacteria to synthesize carbon compounds from carbon dioxide and water.

Plasma The fluid in which blood cells are suspended. It contains a high concentration of protein and inorganic salts (e.g. sodium, potassium, calcium).

Plasma cell A cell that develops from a B lymphocyte and that manufactures a specific antibody.

Plasmid A small circle of DNA that may be present in the cytoplasm of a microbial cell. Plasmids often carry genes for antibiotic resistance.

Polymer A molecule made up of similar subunits.

Polymorphonuclear leucocyte The blood contains three polymorphonuclear leucocytes: the neutrophil, the eosinophil and the basophil.

Polypeptide A chain of at least four, and usually more, amino acids.

Precipitate The result of a reaction between two soluble substances to form an insoluble material that 'falls' out of solution.

Precipitin reaction A reaction between antigen and antibody resulting in a visible precipitate.

Prevalence The number of cases occurring within a population at one particular time.

Primary response The production of antibody in response to the first contact with the antigen.

Probe A short single-stranded segment of DNA or RNA that is identical in base sequence to a part of a gene, plasmid, ribosome, etc., and which can be used to detect the presence of the gene or plasmid, and hence to identify the microbe of which it is a part.

Procaryotic cell One of two chief types of living cells, in which the nucleus is not delimited from the cytoplasm by a membrane. In general procaryotic cells are smaller and of less complex structure than eucaryotic cells.

Prophylaxis Treatment intended to prevent disease rather than cure it (e.g. prophylactic antibiotic therapy).

Prostaglandin A group of hormones present in a wide variety of tissues and body fluids.

Protein A large molecule, one of the main constituents of living matter; it consists of one or more polypeptide chains.

Protozoa Microscopic single-celled eucaryotic microbes; some are free living, others are important parasites.

Pus An accumulation of fluid as a result of infection; it consists of living and dead microbes, phagocytes and tissue cells, together with the fluid that has accumulated in the tissue because of inflammation.

Reservoir (of infection) The site where a micro-organism normally lives and the permanent source of infection; for example, foxes are a reservoir of rabies in western Europe.

Respiration The generation of energy by the conversion of organic compounds to carbon dioxide and water.

Restriction endonucleases Enzymes that cut DNA strands at specific base combinations.

Reverse transcriptase An enzyme that synthesizes DNA from an RNA template. The human immunodeficiency virus contains a reverse transcriptase.

Ribonucleic acid (RNA) A nucleic acid in which the component nucleotides contain the sugar ribose. The ribonucleic acids of cells are messenger RNA, transfer RNA and ribosomal RNA; in addition the genome of some viruses consists of RNA.

Ribosome The protein-synthesizing 'factory' of the cytoplasm.

Saprophyte An organism that lives on dead organic matter.

Sensitivity The susceptibility of certain organisms to specific agents.

Septicaemia Bacteria present in the bloodstream and accompanied by symptoms and signs of infection with no other recognized cause.

Seroconversion The production of specific antibodies in response to an antigen.

Serotype A strain of a bacterial species that can be differentiated by the antigens present on its surface; these are detected by antibodies (serological methods).

Serum The liquid that separates from clotted blood. Similar composition to plasma, but without substances used in coagulation (e.g. fibrinogen).

Species *See* genus.

Spore A resistant casing that some bacteria use to enclose their cells in adverse environmental conditions. Spores germinate when conditions improve and the cell recommences multiplication.

Sterilization A process that removes or destroys all microorganisms including spores.

Strain A group of bacteria with different properties to other bacteria of the same species. Strains are distinguished in the laboratory by specialist 'typing' techniques.

Subclinical infection An infection that produces no symptoms or signs of disease; said of the early stages or a very mild form of the disease.

Superinfection Acquisition of a more resistant strain of the organism already causing infection, or replacement of normal flora by antibiotic-resistant organisms because of antibiotic use.

Surveillance The systematic observation of the occurrence of disease in a population with analysis and dissemination of the results.

Symbiosis An association between two species in which there is mutual benefit.

Syndrome A set of symptoms and signs that forms a distinctive clinical picture suggesting a particular disease.

Synergy When the effect of two antibiotics (or other drugs) given together is greater than can be accounted for by the effect of each acting alone.

Systemic Involving the whole body.

Teichoic acid A polymer of an alcohol, phosphate and other molecules found in Gram-positive cell walls.

Titre A measure of the concentration of an antibody in serum.

Topical A drug that is applied directly to the affected part (e.g. skin or eye) is applied topically.

Toxin Any poisonous substance produced by a living organism, especially a microbe.

Toxoid A microbial toxin treated (usually with dilute formaldehyde) so that its toxic activity is destroyed, but it is still capable of stimulating the production of antibodies that recognize the microbial toxin.

Trace element A chemical element required for growth, but needed in only very small amounts.

Transcription Copying the sense strand of the DNA into messenger RNA.

Transduction The introduction of new genes into a bacterial cell, by a bacteriophage. The new genes are derived from the bacterium in which the phage previously replicated.

Transfer RNA Small RNA molecules that carry individual amino acids to the ribosome.

Transformation The introduction of new genes into a cell by the uptake of fragments of DNA from solution.

Translation Synthesis of a polypeptide chain from the messenger RNA template.

Transposon A 'jumping gene'; a segment of DNA that can move from one DNA molecule to another or from one site to another in the same DNA molecule.

Tuberculin test A skin test used to detect infection by mycobacteria.

Ultraviolet light Invisible light of wavelength shorter than the light at the violet end of the visible spectrum.

Vaccination The process of inducing immunity by administering a vaccine.

Vaccine A preparation of killed or inactivated microbes, inactivated microbial toxins or microbial antigens used to induce immunity.

Vector An animal, usually an arthropod (insect or tick) that transfers an infectious microbe from one host to another.

Virulence The ability of an organism to cause disease.

Virus A micro-organism capable of reproduction only inside living cells.

Zoonosis An infectious disease of animals that may be transmitted to humans. Brucellosis, rabies and toxoplasmosis are examples.

Index